Medicine in the Beehive State

1940–1990

MEDICINE IN THE

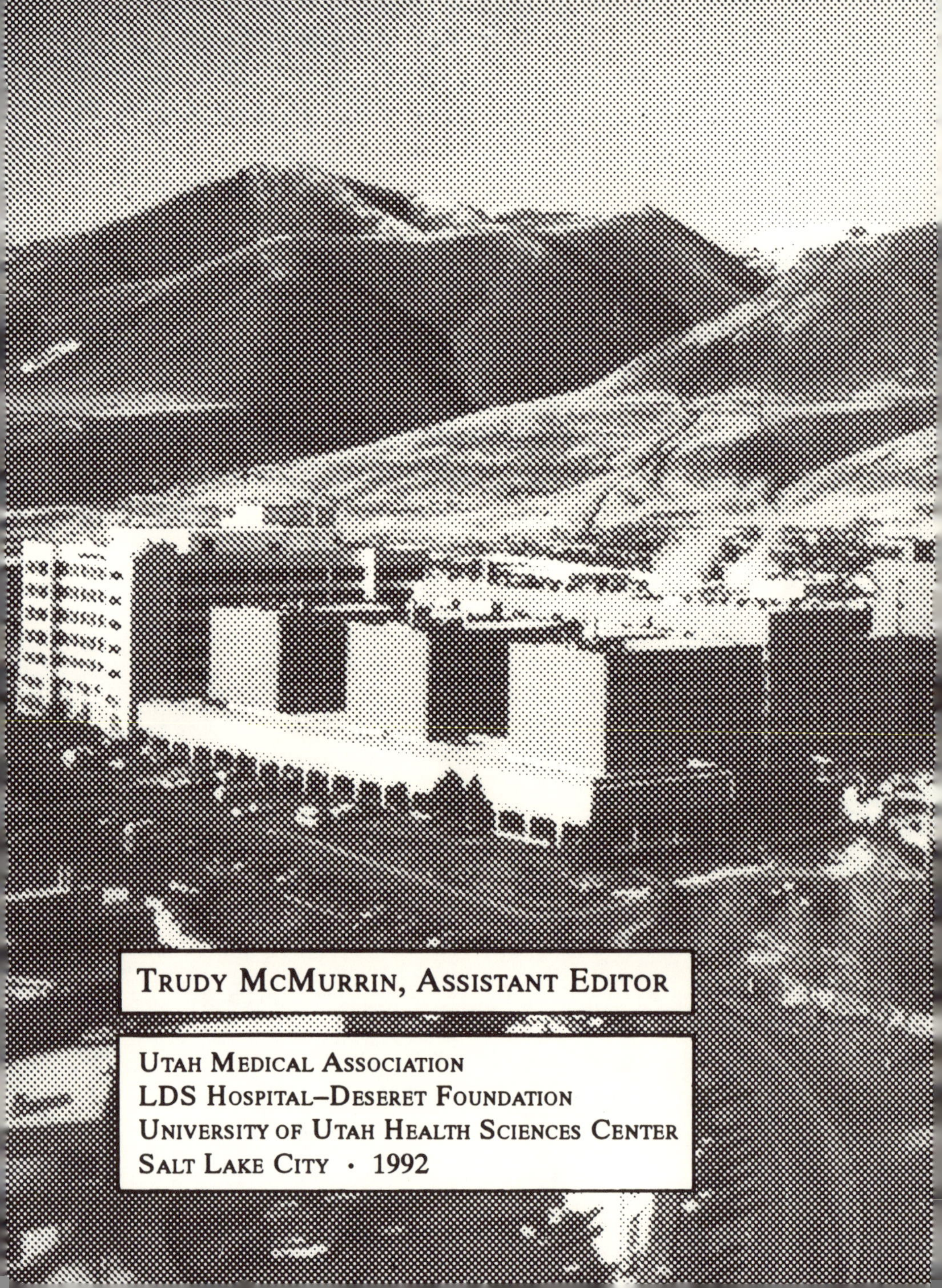

TRUDY MCMURRIN, ASSISTANT EDITOR

UTAH MEDICAL ASSOCIATION
LDS HOSPITAL–DESERET FOUNDATION
UNIVERSITY OF UTAH HEALTH SCIENCES CENTER
SALT LAKE CITY • 1992

BEEHIVE STATE
1940–1990

EDITED BY HENRY P. PLENK

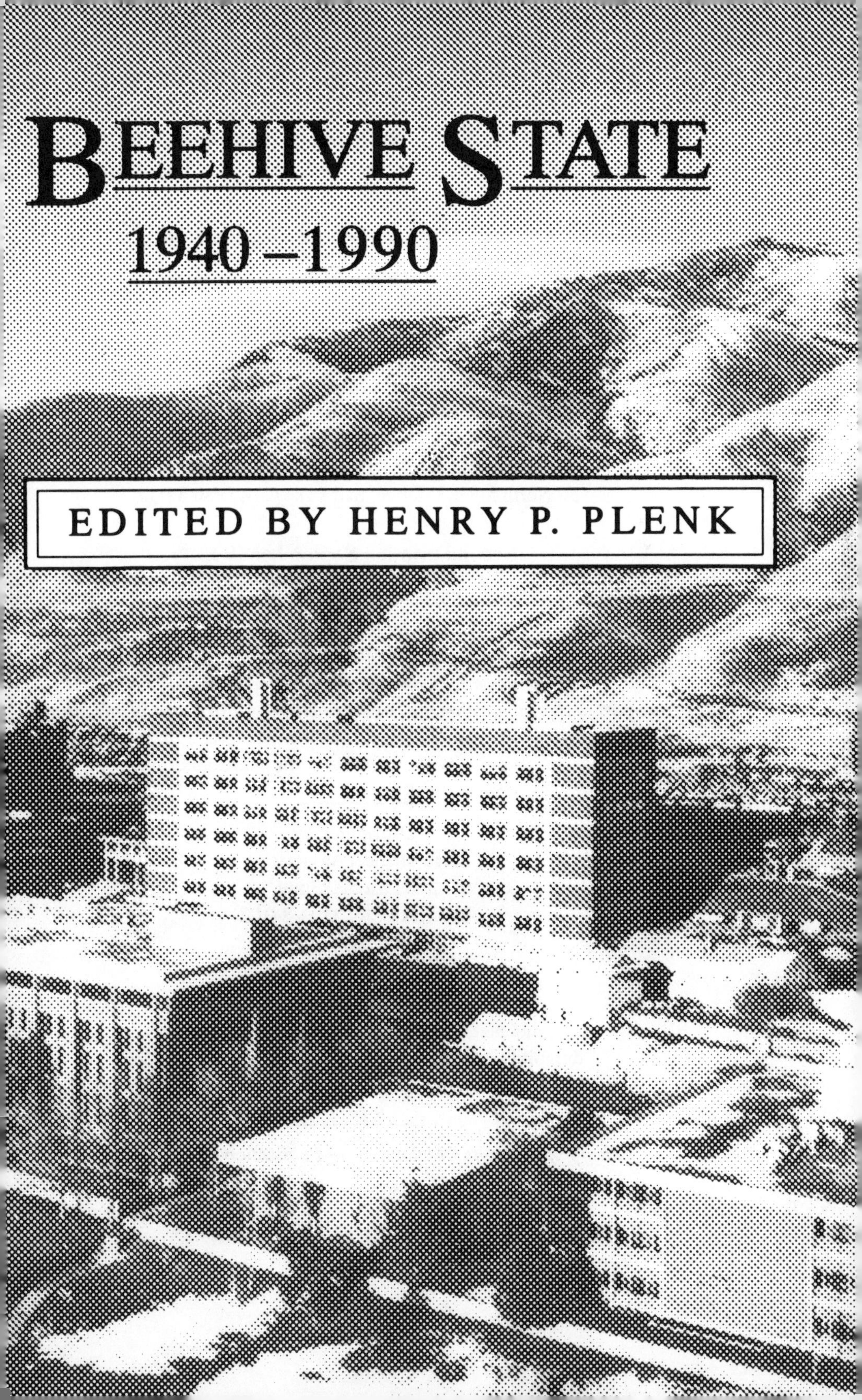

Published by
Utah Medical Association
540 East 500 South, Salt Lake City, Utah 84102
and
LDS Hospital–Deseret Foundation
Eighth Avenue and C Street, Salt Lake City, Utah 84103
and
University of Utah Health Sciences Center
50 North Medical Drive, Salt Lake City, Utah 84112.

Second printing September 1992.

Printed in the United States of America
ISBN 0–87480–396–9

Distributed by
Utah Medical Association
540 East 500 South
Salt Lake City, Utah 84102
(801) 355-7477.

The paper in this book is acid free
and meets the standards for permanence and
durability established by the Committee on Production
Guidelines for Book Longevity of the Council on Library Resources.

Library of Congress Cataloguing-in-Publication Data applied for.

THIS BOOK is dedicated to
Agi Plenk, PhD, a lifelong child advocate,
and to our children,
Bruce and Tim Plenk and Penny Plenk Dalrymple,
who each in their own way have contributed
to making this earth a better place to live.

CONTENTS

— PART THREE —

SURGERY AND SURGICAL SPECIALTIES

— PART SIX —

INDEPENDENT DEPARTMENTS

PROLOGUE

PRIOR TO WORLD WAR II, Salt Lake City and the whole state of Utah were somewhat isolated from the rest of the country. While a few well-trained specialists were available in many fields, the general quality of medicine lagged behind many other metropolitan areas of the United States.

The decision to start a four-year medical school in a relatively poor state with a population base of only 600,000 was certainly heroic. To attract the outstanding nucleus of clinicians and basic scientists in the middle of a war, without adequate financial support, hospital facilities, or equipment, on promises for the future, required salesmanship on Dean A. Cyril Callister's part and faith on the part of the potential faculty rarely found at the start of any institution.

The first time I heard about the new four-year Medical School in Utah was early in the spring of 1947, when Dr. Richard Y. Young, its first full-time dean, came to visit his old friend Earl Crowder, the chief of radiology at Evanston Hospital, Illinois. Before the war, Dick had been attending hematologist at Evanston and part-time assistant to the dean at Northwestern's medical school in Chicago.

Upon completing my residency in radiology at Northwestern, I was interested in an academic career. Dick told me about the new school, which had graduated its first class on September 10, 1944, and aroused my interest in the vacant position for a second man in the Department of Radiology. My wife and I left Evanston April 30, in a snowstorm, and three days later drove into Salt Lake Valley, seeing green grass, lilacs, flowers in bloom, and fresh, glistening snow on the awe-inspiring Wasatch Range.

The sparse facilities at the fifty-year-old Salt Lake General Hospital — with several departments housed in army-type barracks — were anything but impressive, but our warm reception by the entire full-time clinical faculty of about sixteen, average age in the late thirties, made up for the lack of buildings and equipment. Having dinner with Dr. Lou Goodman, head of pharmacology and author of the most widely used text (Goodman and Gilman), and lunch with Dr. Max Wintrobe, author of *the* textbook on hematology, impressed us with the close relationships among the high-quality faculty not found in any other medical school in the country.

The chance to get in on the ground floor of an institution of such high standards created in barely four years, plus the attraction of the community — not to mention skiing in Alta — cast the die for us, and we arrived to stay on June 17, 1947.

Acknowledgments

While president of the Utah Medical Society in 1987, Dr. J. P. Hughes appointed me as chair of a committee with the assigned task of gathering materials and writing the history of medicine in the state. Representatives of most of the existing specialties and subspecialties were invited to submit essays covering their own fields.

The choice was often difficult. In general, the oldest available member of a department or in practice was sought out. If he was unable or unwilling to write, others were approached. A balance between faculty members and practicing physicians was attempted.

Early support from the LDS–Deseret Foundation and a grant from CIBA Geigy Pharmaceutical, matched by the Utah Medical Association, made this effort possible and allowed the selection of Trudy McMurrin, an experienced professional editor, and Helen Eckersley, a very discerning typist. Dr. David Catron, then director of the University of Utah Press, gave much encouragement to the project. The continuous interest and numerous suggestions of Dr. Harold Bauman of the University of Utah Department of History are gratefully acknowledged.

Many of the manuscripts had to be shortened. The original versions, curricula vitae, and bibliographies of the contributors have been deposited in the Special Collections of the Marriott Library, University of Utah. The essayists deserve much credit for their painstaking research. Their effort made this publication possible.

I would also like to thank the number of family members and secretaries of the major players who supplied much valuable information, especially Helene (Mrs. George) Cartwright, Marge (Mrs.

Frank) Gunn, Louise (Mrs. Val) Jager, Laura (Mrs. William) Moretz, Barbara (Mrs. Leo) Samuels, Becky (Mrs. Max) Wintrobe, Dorothy (Mrs. Lowell) Woodbury, and Dr. Kenneth Castleton, who made some of his excellent early essays available to me.

A donation by James L. Sorenson of Sorenson Laboratories helped make the second printing possible.

INTRODUCTION

HENRY P. PLENK, MD, MS

THROUGH THE NINETEENTH CENTURY, medical education in the United States was extremely haphazard and totally unregulated. Most of the medical schools were proprietary and/or sectarian (starting with preconceived ideas about the nature of illness) and had few prerequisites for admission. Their major purpose was to enrich the owners, not to educate. In 1874, 457 such schools existed between the U.S. and Canada, many short-lived and perhaps 50 stillborn.

The state of Utah was not exempt. In a term paper presented at Brigham Young University in 1986, Dee R. Darling stated: "On Saturday afternoon January 31, 1880, at a meeting held [in Salt Lake City] a forty-three year old physician from Pennsylvania legally established Utah's first medical college in Morgan, Utah, forty-two miles northeast of Salt Lake City and about twelve miles up Weber Canyon." The founder, Dr. Frederick S. Kohler, had completed two years of study at Dartmouth and attended the "Ecclectic Medical College of Pennsylvania," graduating in 1860. He continued his formal studies at the Medical College of Ohio, graduating in 1873. In 1882 the Utah "college" honored its only graduating class of six students and closed in 1883.

The American Medical Association, founded in 1847, attempted to raise the level of medical education based on better schools in England, France, and Germany. A permanent Council of Medical Education was formed in 1904 to set American standards that would include one premedical year of science; two years of laboratory science, including anatomy, physiology, pathology, and pharmacology; two years of clinical contact in a dispensary and hospital; and a sixth year for internship.

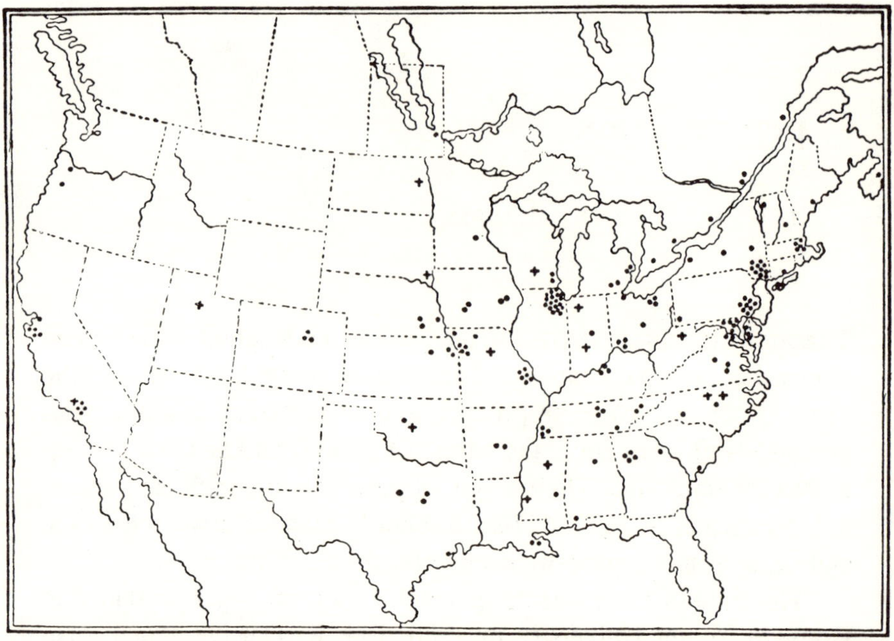

1. Map showing the actual number, location, and distribution of medical schools in the United States in 1908. Dots represent schools; crosses represent "half-schools." Two parts of a divided school in close proximity are represented by one dot.

A rating system for schools was introduced, with three categories: A (acceptable), B (doubtful), and C (unacceptable). In 1907, of 160 U.S. medical schools only 82 were Class A, 46 were B, and 32 C; of these, 29 schools had closed by 1910. By 1929 the number of schools had dropped to 76, but it had increased again gradually to 123 in 1990, corresponding to the increase in both population and specialization.

The Carnegie Foundation for the Advancement of Teaching became interested in the appraisal of the quality of professional education and in 1908 accepted the task of assessing American medical education in the U.S. and Canada. In 1910 Dr. Abraham Flexner issued the Foundation's epoch-making report, which was to revolutionize medicine on the North American continent. Map 1 indicates the location of the medical schools in 1908; map 2 shows suggested numbers and locations of schools as justified by the 1908 population.

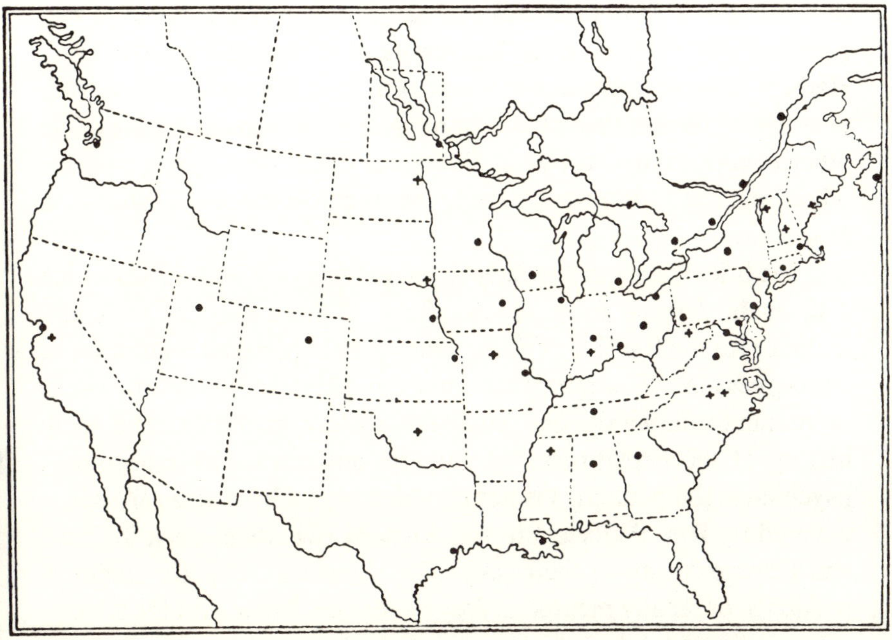

2. Map showing the suggested number, location, and distribution of U.S. medical schools in 1908. Illustrations accompanied the Flexner Report, originally published in 1910.

The "Medical Department" at the University of Utah was started in 1905 as a two-and-a-half-year school operating on a budget of $10,000 per year, with six professors. It is of interest that the program was rated in the report as Class A, with the comment that "more liberal financial support was necessary."

The period from 1940 to 1947, after the start of World War II in Europe, was the beginning of a new era of relationships between the federal government and science. The National Research Defense Council (NRDC) was established by President Roosevelt in 1940 and included the Office of Scientific Research and Development (OSRD), under the direction of Dr. Vannevar Bush. Its mission was to serve as the center for mobilization of scientific personnel and resources, applying the results of scientific research for defense purposes. Expenditures for research jumped from $100 million in 1940 to $1.5

billion in 1945. After the attack on Pearl Harbor on December 7, 1941, pressure was exerted on the University of Utah and Utah Governor Herbert Maw to upgrade the Medical School from a two- to a four-year institution because of the shortage of physicians in the West. No other school existed between Denver and the West Coast, and the whole state of California had only two medical schools, both in San Francisco.

The brief history of the early four-year school (1942–1952) which follows is derived from recollections of the author as a faculty member for the last five of those years, timely personal interviews of colleagues (Drs. Wintrobe, Hashimoto, and Moretz died within weeks or months afterward), and available written materials. The early history of the departments of surgery, obstetrics and gynecology, psychiatry, and pediatrics is not included here. These areas are better covered by Drs. Wallace Brooke, Richard Hebertson, Jack Tedrow, and George Veasy in their respective chapters. As early students, residents, or faculty members, they have been able to provide a much more personal touch concerning the early days as well as discussions of the more recent progress in their respective fields.

The following chapter highlights the very limited number of key people who were responsible for the amazing success of the transition to a full-scale operation and for laying a very solid foundation for the remarkable growth in the stature and reputation achieved by this medical school in a relatively short period of time.

PART ONE

•

EARLY HISTORY OF THE FOUR-YEAR MEDICAL SCHOOL AT THE UNIVERSITY OF UTAH 1942–1952

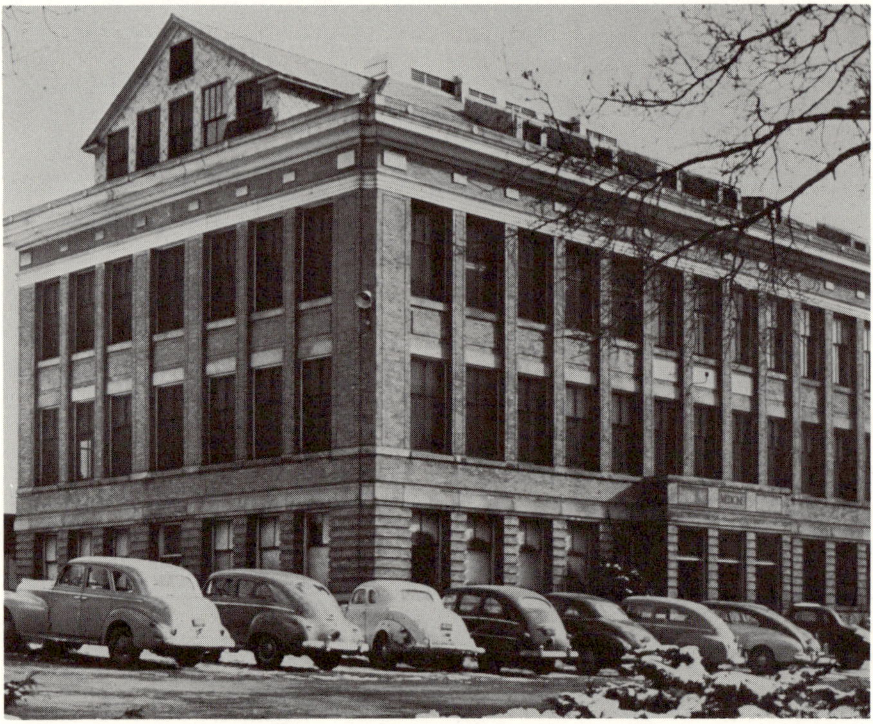

The Basic Science Building, University of Utah College of Medicine, 1920–1965.

PART ONE

Early History of the Four-Year Medical School at the University of Utah, 1942–1952

HENRY P. PLENK, MD, MS

IN THE 1905–06 SCHOOL YEAR, the University of Utah, then fifty-five years old, offered basic medical science courses to qualify students for the first two years of medical school. Fourteen students registered for the program the first year and forty-seven the following year. Not until 1920 was the school housed separately in a red brick building begun by the Army during World War I. In spite of a minimal budget, a minuscule staff, and inadequate laboratories, the school managed to win and maintain a Class A rating, as defined by the Flexner Report. Graduates of the two-year program had to be accepted as transfer students at established four-year schools in the East, Midwest, and South, including Harvard, Jefferson, Northwestern, and Louisville. Stiff competition and scholastic achievement determined which schools accepted the students for their clinical years. The good records of these students assured future admission of graduates of the two-year school.

Dr. Leroy E. Cowles assumed the presidency of the University in 1941, promptly appointing a committee of four members of the Board of Regents, including two physicians, Louis E. Viko and A. Hamer Reiser, to draw up plans for the formation of a four-year medical school. Because of a shortage of physicians during the war and the lack of any four-year schools between Denver and the Pacific Coast and from Canada to Mexico, not only the Army but the American Medical Association encouraged the change. Approval was given by

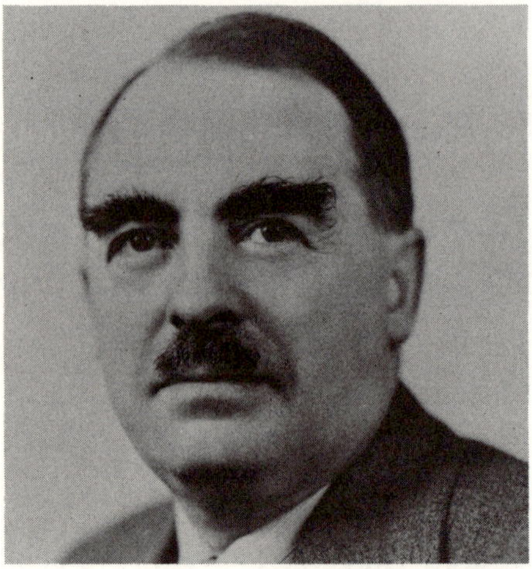

A. Cyril Callister, MD, from 1942 to 1945, the first dean (part-time), responsible for the transition from the two-year to the four-year Medical School.

the Board of Regents on May 18, 1942, and Dr. A. Cyril Callister, a practicing surgeon, was appointed half-time dean, permitting him to continue his practice.

Dr. Callister was short, aggressive, and had a "fighting spirit." He immediately set out to gather a faculty, frequently traveling at his own expense. He desired them to be well known in medical education and to have good teaching abilities and national status for their research — an almost impossible task in the middle of a war with extreme manpower shortages. The dean was ably supported by Dr. Viko; by Alan Gregg, a former medical school classmate of Callister's at Harvard then serving as director of the Rockefeller Foundation for Medical Education; and by former Utahn Dr. Irvine McQuarrie, head of pediatrics at the University of Minnesota.

Even before the arrival of the dean on campus, President Cowles had traveled to San Francisco in September 1942 to recruit Dr. Louis P. Gebhardt from Stanford as associate professor and later chair of the newly formed Department of Bacteriology. Utah was suffering from a severe epidemic of poliomyelitis, and Dr. Gebhardt was involved in the development of a nasally administered polio "vaccine" which held

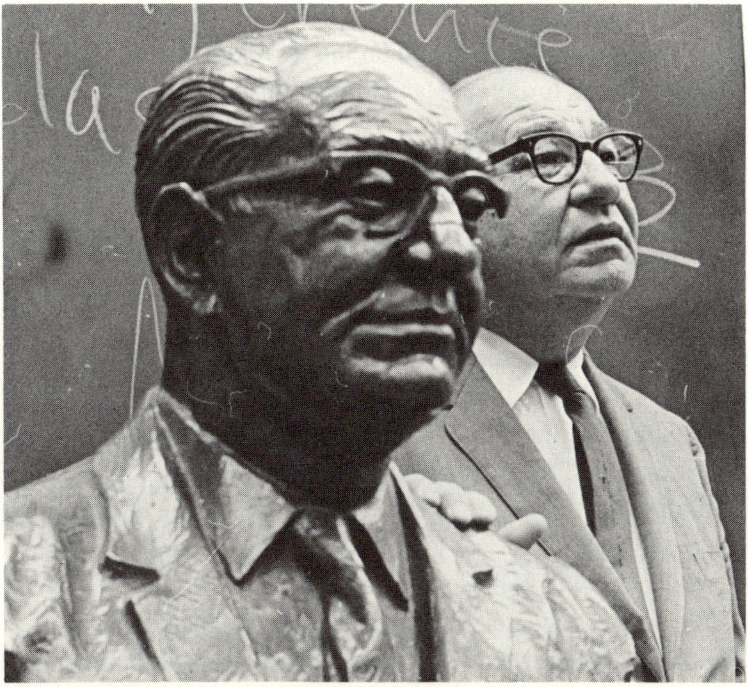

Louis P. Gebhardt, MD, pioneer polio vaccine researcher. The first faculty recruit for the new four-year Medical School in 1942, Gebhardt was chair of the newly created Department of Bacteriology from 1943 to 1971.

promise but which caused patients to lose their sense of smell. Utah was among four laboratories invited in 1948 to cooperate in the development of an effective polio vaccine, which was later successfully produced at the University of Pittsburgh by Dr. Jonas Salk.

Dr. Gebhardt proved to be an excellent mentor. During his tenure, fifty-five students obtained their PhDs in bacteriology. His research centered on western encephalitis as well as poliomyelitis, and he wrote a microbiology textbook. He received many honors and awards and enhanced the reputation of the University of Utah Medical School. Dr. Gebhardt retired in 1974 and died in January 1985 at the age of seventy-nine.

In December 1942, Dr. Philip B. Price was recruited to head the Department of Surgery. Price was born March 7, 1897, in Sinchang,

China, a son of Protestant missionaries. He was schooled by his mother until he was thirteen, when his family returned to the United States for a year's furlough. He graduated from high school at sixteen. After obtaining a BA degree from Davidson College, North Carolina, Price went to medical school at the University of Virginia but graduated from Johns Hopkins in Baltimore, where he had his surgical training at Union Memorial Hospital. He married Octavia Howard, who had just completed her nurse's training, and they went to China as medical missionaries. Dr. Price became associate professor of surgery at Chiloo University in Tsinan, Shantung Province, and was director of the hospital from 1933 to 1938. After China was invaded by the Japanese, the Prices returned to Baltimore in 1938, where Philip progressed to associate in surgery at Johns Hopkins. He assumed the position as professor and head of the Department of Surgery at the University of Utah and surgeon in chief at the Salt Lake General Hospital (SLGH) in February 1943.

Throughout his career Price was deeply interested in research and wrote on such subjects as bladder stones, urinary incontinence, and peptic ulcers. He continued his interest in skin disinfection and the treatment of wounds, burns, shock, and radiation injuries.

Price published approximately 100 papers and contributed a number of chapters to textbooks. He received many honors and distinctions in Utah, the United States, China, and Japan. As a surgeon he was meticulous, gentle, and methodical, but he was thought to be a rather slow operator. He was demanding but extremely fair and was well respected by his colleagues, staff, and students. He was a good tennis player, loved photography, and later in his life took up golf and painting.

Price remained head of surgery until 1955, when he accepted the position as dean of the Medical School. He played a major role in the realization and development of the new University Hospital, which finally opened at the Fort Douglas site in 1965, three years after his retirement. He died in the East on October 27, 1982, of congestive heart failure.

Dr. Fuller B. Bailey was appointed acting head of the Department of Medicine by Dean Callister in late 1942. Bailey organized a

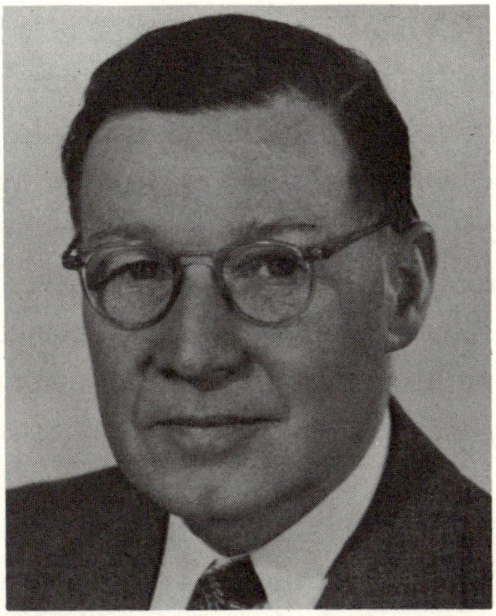

Philip B. Price, MD, the earliest clinician appointed to the four-year Medical School, came from Johns Hopkins to head the Department of Surgery from 1943 to 1955. He was largely responsible for recruiting Dr. M. M. Wintrobe and, as dean of the Medical School from 1955 to 1962, for construction of the new Medical School and hospital building, completed in 1965, three years after his retirement.

teaching program in medicine and attended ward and clinic patients at SLGH with two associates, Drs. Fred W. Clausen and Wayland Macfarlane.

Dr. Bailey had come to Salt Lake City in 1923 from Rush–Presbyterian Hospital in Chicago, with Martin Lindem, a trained surgeon. Bailey was one of the area's first qualified internists. He had spent eight months at the University of Vienna in 1930, where he learned to read electrocardiograms and to use the rigid gastroscope. Bailey developed a busy practice at Holy Cross Hospital and remained an associate clinical professor of medicine from 1943 to 1965.

One of Dr. Price's early accomplishments was to interest Maxwell M. Wintrobe, MD, PhD, his former colleague on the Hopkins faculty, in the position of professor and head of the Department of Medicine. In his first letter to Wintrobe, dated May 21, 1943, after he had spent three months in Utah, Price extolled the great possibilities of organizing a new school "without the restrictions of time-honored conventions and traditions" and stated that the opportunity to develop a program from scratch does not occur frequently. Prejudice prevailed in very low quotas for Jewish as well as female students in many medical schools. It was even more obvious in the selection of department heads, a fact which did not escape Dr. Wintrobe. Price described the old County Hospital in the process of being remodeled and refurbished to hold 250 beds and stressed the need and promise for a larger University Hospital, which he had made one of the conditions of his own coming to Utah. With the commitment of $15,000 for research and a "piggery" to continue his research on anemia, Wintrobe accepted following a personal visit to Utah.

Maxwell Myer Wintrobe was born in Halifax, Nova Scotia, October 27, 1901; he earned his MD degree from the University of Manitoba in 1926 and a PhD from Tulane in New Orleans in 1929. As a fellow in medicine in Manitoba he became interested in pernicious anemia, which stimulated his interest and research in the new field of hematology.

He accepted an instructorship at Tulane in 1927. While studying "Anemia of the South," Dr. Wintrobe devised a flat-bottomed graduated centrifuge tube to determine blood corpuscular *vis-à-vis* plasma volumes; described in 1928, this simple device — named the Wintrobe Tube — was soon used the world over, boosting his reputation. He and Tulane declined to patent the tube or to derive any financial benefits from its manufacture. Medical students sometimes referred to Wintrobe, affectionately, as "the tube."

After three months of bachelorhood, Wintrobe brought his bride, Becky Zanphir, from Winnipeg, settled down to married life, and began to enjoy New Orleans. Charity Hospital provided an extraordinary experience in the volume and variety of tropical and exotic diseases treated. Well run by the Sisters of Charity, the hospital was clean but so crowded that two patients were occasionally put in one bed, head to toe. Once, when he came to examine a patient, Wintrobe discovered that the bedmate was dead.

Max and Becky Wintrobe were warmly received by a most hospitable faculty — a pleasant change from the cold, impersonal attitude at Manitoba. He completed the requirements for his PhD and submitted his dissertation to the journal *Medicine*. The editor-in-chief, Dean Chesney of Johns Hopkins Medical School, was obviously impressed and soon offered him an instructorship in the Department of Medicine.

The Wintrobes left New Orleans in September 1930 to arrive in Baltimore to a chilling reception. The chief's secretary handed them a list of apartments to explore, quickly replacing it with another when she learned that they were Jewish. With the exception of Dean Chesney and a few others, the Wintrobes were not invited into the homes of their faculty colleagues.

Wintrobe taught clinical laboratory medicine to sophomore and junior medical students, held outpatient clinics, and was assigned to the wards. He was successful in bringing history and clinical findings to correlate with laboratory procedures, and what had been a dry exercise became a very popular class. He was the first to observe cryoglobulin in a patient with multiple myeloma and developed a classification of anemia based on various laboratory indices for red blood cell volume and hemoglobin content (MCV, MCH, MCHC). Training good technicians in this field allowed him to develop a full-scale research program in hematology. With the help of an initial grant of $5,000 from the pharmaceutical company Parke Davis, Wintrobe started a project producing pernicious anemia in newborn piglets and studying their various vitamin deficiencies.

After the Japanese attacked Pearl Harbor on December 7, 1941, the decision was made for Dr. Wintrobe to remain in Baltimore to assist in running the department and not to join the Hopkins Army Hospital Unit. In 1942 his textbook *Hematology* was published to considerable acclaim.

It was decided that Wintrobe should team up with Dr. Val Jager, one of the assistant residents, in studies concerning the effects of various poison gases, such as nitrogen mustard. Wintrobe did not realize at the time that this was the first step toward the later development in Utah of chemotherapy as the mainstay of anti-tumor treatment. Wintrobe was promoted to the rank of assistant professor, put in charge of the Clinic for Gastrointestinal, Hematologic and Nutri-

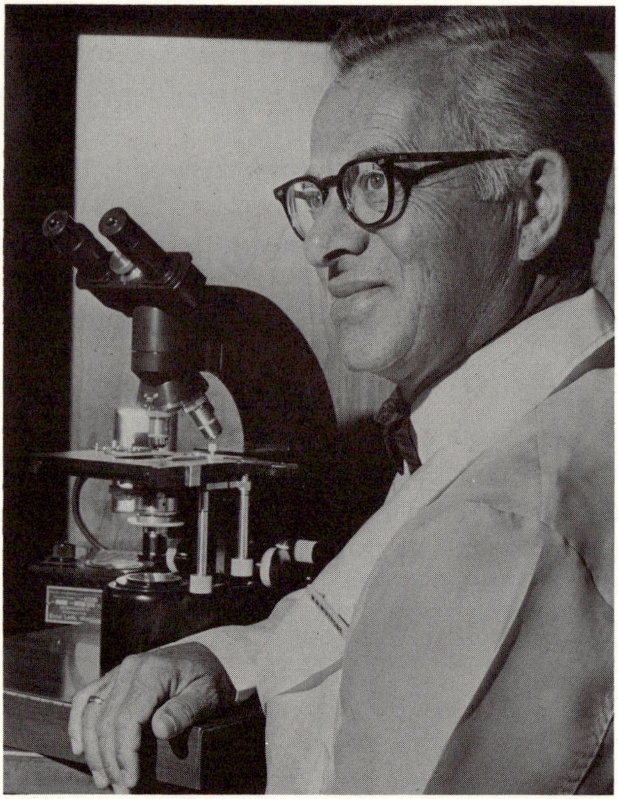

Maxwell M. Wintrobe, MD, PhD, came from Johns Hopkins in 1943 as full professor and chair of the Department of Medicine from 1943 to 1967. World renowned for his research, Wintrobe helped to shape the character of the Medical School and to attract national attention to the fledgling program.

tional Disorders, and made editor of the *Johns Hopkins Medical Journal*, with a salary increase to $5,000 per year.

The letters from Dr. Price and Dean Callister offering the job of professor and head of the Department of Medicine at $8,000 per year were quite a surprise. At Hopkins only the head of the department could be a full professor; associate professorship was Wintrobe's highest attainable goal there.

Following a seventy-two-hour train ride to Salt Lake City, being "wined and dined" at the Roof Garden of the Hotel Utah — the only

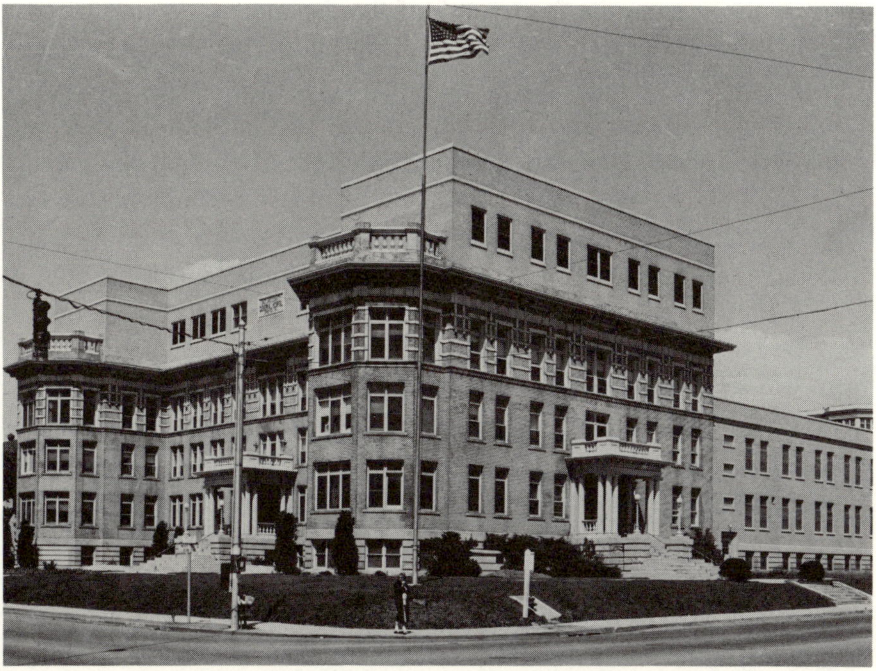

The Salt Lake County General Hospital, at 21st South and State Streets, housed the University of Utah Medical School from 1942 to 1965. Shown is the General Building (housing surgery and operating rooms, radiology, and pathology) and the medicine–infirmary building, about 1950.

good, even elegant restaurant in town — and seeing mountains for the first time, Wintrobe accepted Utah's offer.

Dr. Wintrobe's motor trip west in September 1943, through the desolate eastern part of the state, with restaurants full of flies, reports of the ongoing polio epidemic, and uncomfortable motel quarters in Salt Lake until a house could be found were not good for morale. The antiquated, neglected County Hospital, a political football for the elected commissioners, had hardly a laboratory, no blood bank, and only the most primitive, filthy patient facilities. Wintrobe's first task was to build up a faculty, and his first choice was his labmate from Hopkins, Dr. Val Jager.*

*For photographs of the early members of the Department of Medicine, see "The Quorum" on page 19.

Jager became the "factotum" of the department, having broad knowledge of the entire field of medicine and taking special interest in the study of syphilis (still at that time a very widespread and almost untreatable disease) and neurology. In conjunction with the staff of the Tooele Army Depot southwest of Salt Lake City, Jager continued his work on chemical warfare, which once almost cost him his life in an accidental spill. An enthusiastic teacher, he was loved by his students; he was respected by his colleagues for his forthright opinions, but not always appreciated by those of higher rank and responsibility. Jager remained in Utah as associate professor until 1958, when he left for several medical schools in the East. He ultimately took his Boards in pathology and worked as pathologist at a Veterans Administration hospital in upstate New York after some hearing loss made clinical practice more difficult for him. He retired in 1982 and died on December 5, 1989, at the age of seventy-six.

The next addition to the staff of the Department of Medicine was Dr. Hans H. Hecht, who approached Dr. Wintrobe at a national meeting in the East about the possibility of a position in Utah. Hecht was born on January 23, 1913, in Basel, Switzerland. He received his MD from the University of Berlin in 1936 and came to the United States in 1937. As a nineteen-year-old medical student in Berlin, he had written his first paper on electrocardiography, published in 1935 in the prestigious *Klinische Wochenschrift*. Hecht was an intern and resident in medicine at Wayne County General Hospital in Detroit and a research fellow at the University of Michigan from 1937 to 1944, the last two years under Dr. Frank Wilson. At the University of Utah he advanced from instructor to associate professor of medicine between 1944 and 1955 and was director of the Heart Station at SLGH. He was named L. E. Viko Professor of Cardiology from 1957 to 1964. It is ironic that, as a foreign graduate, he was not permitted a license to practice in Utah. To become eligible, he had to enroll in medical school for the senior year, and he graduated from Utah in 1946.

When Hecht arrived in Salt Lake in 1944, the physical plant at the SLGH was still deplorable. The "Infirmary Building," where the Department of Medicine was housed, had an auditorium where "inmates" worshiped on Sundays. Hecht proposed having the floor rebuilt so that it sloped from back to front, creating a triangular space below the new floor where he could squeeze in an electrocardiography machine, a patient bed, a fluoroscope, darkroom, and desk. In this very limited space he did outstanding research in such diverse fields as pulmonary circulation, cor pulmonale, cardiodynamics, muscle metabolism, and the electrical behavior of the myocardium — as well as various aspects of clinical cardiology, electrocardiography, and pharmacology.

The method of passing a catheter through a vein into the heart was first introduced in this country by Dr. André Cournand at Bellevue Hospital in New York in 1942. Cardiac catheterization is used to measure pressure and oxygen tension in various parts of the heart and pulmonary vessels. Together with angiocardiography (injection of contrast media into veins and, later, arteries, followed by the taking of several x-ray films), cardiac catheterization led in the forties and fifties to the early diagnosis of congenital heart disease. Dr. Hecht was one of the pioneers of the method, beginning in 1945, and by 1951 he had done more than 200 of these studies. The development of early surgical procedures to correct congenital cardiac defects provided a powerful stimulus for more accurate diagnosis.

The first open-heart procedure — a commissurotomy (cutting of stenotic leaflets of the mitral valve resulting from rheumatic heart disease) — was performed by Dr. William Ray Rumel on May 17, 1951, at LDS Hospital on referral by Dr. Hecht.

After the Heart Station had existed for many years in most inadequate quarters, a $60,000 grant from the National Heart Institute provided a new building on the SLGH grounds next to the animal research building. Grants for the facility were also obtained from pharmaceutical houses and the Utah and Idaho Heart Association.

When it became apparent that Dr. George Cartwright would be the most likely chief of medicine upon Dr. Wintrobe's retirement, Dr. Hecht accepted the invitation to become chief of cardiology and professor of medicine and physiology at the University of Chicago Medical School in 1964. In 1968 he was promoted to chair of the entire Department of Medicine. He held many important positions with national and local organizations and scientific journals. He died of a heart attack on August 12, 1971, at age fifty-eight, after a most productive life as an outstanding clinician, teacher, investigator, and basic scientist.

George E. Cartwright was born in Lancaster, Wisconsin, on December 1, 1917. He earned his BS degree at the University of Wisconsin and his MD degree in 1943 at Johns Hopkins, where he first made contact with Dr. Wintrobe. After one year of internship at Hopkins, he came to Utah in January 1944 as a resident in medicine, but was called into the Army in 1945. He rose to the rank of captain MC and spent much of his two years of medical service in China. He returned to Utah in June 1947 as an instructor in medicine and was promoted to assistant professor in 1948, when he also married Helene Cleare, the University's first medical illustrator. He was closely associated with Wintrobe's research in diseases of the blood, nutrition, and the use of nitrogen mustard in lymphomas, initiating the era of chemotherapy. In 1950 Cartwright was put in charge of the hematology section. He achieved national prominence for his important role in the study of the genetic diseases hemochromatosis and Wilson's Disease and for his role in starting the now-outstanding genetics program at Utah. He developed the first broadly based clinical hematology training program and, with Dr. Wintrobe, graduated more than 100 fellows by 1971. After Wintrobe's resignation as chair of the Department of Medicine in 1967, Cartwright assumed the leadership and was responsible for staffing many of the subspecialties in the field. He was an ardent wilderness supporter, liked backpacking and skiing, and served as a member of the Alta Ski Patrol.

Cartwright published a small book on clinical pathology under his own name and played a major role in updating many editions of Wintrobe's textbook on hematology, as well as contributing to Harrison's *Principles of Internal Medicine*, of which Dr. Wintrobe had become the senior editor. Dr. Cartwright gave notice of his impending resignation as department chair effective July 1, 1980, feeling that someone younger should assume leadership and hoping to be able to concentrate on genetic research. He died that April at age sixty-three, however, prior to the arrival of his successor, Dr. William Odell.

John F. Waldo was the first native Utahn to join the clinical department, in 1946. He graduated from medical school and took all his training in medicine and infectious diseases at the University of Rochester. Dr. Waldo's career and accomplishments are described in detail in the chapter on "Infectious Diseases" by Charles B. Smith.

Frank H. Tyler was born in Villisca, Iowa, on January 5, 1916. His family moved to LaGrande, Oregon, when he was six, and he graduated from Willamette College in Salem with an AB in 1938. He received his MD degree in 1942 and stayed for a year's internship in medicine at Johns Hopkins, where Max Wintrobe was on the faculty and George Cartwright was a fourth-year student. In 1943 George W. Thorn, one of the senior staff in medicine at Hopkins, became Hersey Professor of Physic (Medicine) at Harvard and Peter Bent Brigham Hospital. Dr. Tyler joined Thorn as assistant resident in metabolism from 1943 to 1944 to pursue an interest in the field from earlier work he had done with a physical chemist in Oregon. He also worked with Thorn at Hopkins on glucocorticoids and was involved in chemical warfare research with Wintrobe and Jager. After two years in the Navy, Tyler returned to Boston as resident and fellow from 1946 to 1947 to get in on the ground floor of clinical research with ACTH (adrenocorticotrophic hormone). He was recruited for Utah by Dr. Wintrobe in July 1947.

When Army research came to a halt after the armistice, it was decided that the national Public Health Service (USPHS) should develop a system of research grants. Senator Elbert Thomas of Utah sponsored an appropriation of $100,000, and about one hundred institutions applied. Drs. Wintrobe and Fayette Stephens, a geneticist, were already involved in the study of hereditary diseases and applied for $100,000. Senator Thomas was opposed to splitting a relatively limited amount and was instrumental in awarding it all to Dr. Wintrobe and the University of Utah. A phone call from Washington a few weeks later informed Wintrobe that no funds had been provided for administration of grants, and the caller asked that $8,000 be returned.

Wintrobe generously agreed to the refund, since it was the largest grant he had ever received. Dr. Emil Smith, an outstanding biochemist, had already arrived from Los Angeles to work on the project. Wintrobe also needed a "metabolite," and Dr. Tyler was the choice candidate.

Over many years, more than 600 patients with various types of muscular dystrophy were studied with respect to enzymes, proteins, genetic transmission, clinical manifestations, and muscle histology, resulting in numerous publications. The USPHS continued to support the project for thirty-two years, until 1979 — fourteen years after Dr. Wintrobe's retirement. Tyler's laboratory, presently designated "for the study of hereditary and metabolic diseases," has been in the forefront of the field.

The study of steroids, especially adrenal cortical hormones, has been a major interest of various members of the Departments of Pharmacology, Physiology, Anatomy, and Biochemistry, interacting with Dr. Tyler. Drs. George Sayers in pharmacology, Tom Dougherty in anatomy, and Leo Samuels and Don Nelson in biochemistry have been particularly outstanding members of this team (see Chapter 12).

Thus the original "post-war six" (Drs. Wintrobe, Jager, Hecht, Waldo, Cartwright, and Tyler) covered all aspects of internal medicine, handled all the teaching, clinics, and medical wards, and carried on an enormous amount of very productive original research until further expansion of the staff began in the mid-fifties.

During his tenure from 1943 to 1968, Dr. Wintrobe certainly was the guiding spirit of the school. The all-powerful Executive Committee, the ruling body consisting of all department heads, almost never passed any resolution without his consent; and on a few occasions a decision made during his absence was revised the next month. The dean acted as the executive officer of this committee, but deans came and went rather frequently. It is of interest that the first full-time dean, Dr. Richard Young, came from Northwestern University, a school which itself had had few full-time faculty members in the clinical departments. Young, who was appointed in 1946, left after three years to become dean at Northwestern, where he was very successful in

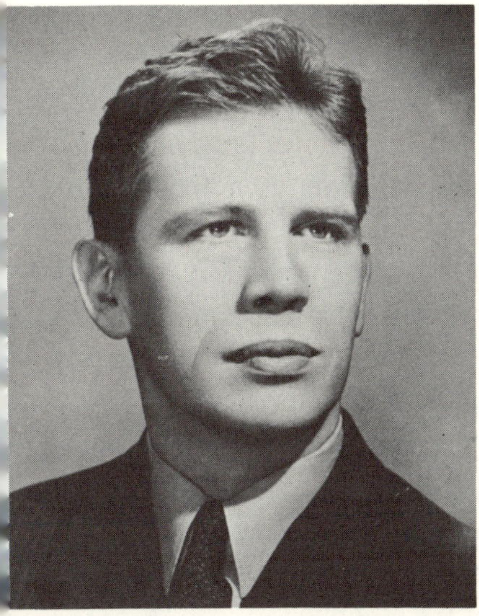 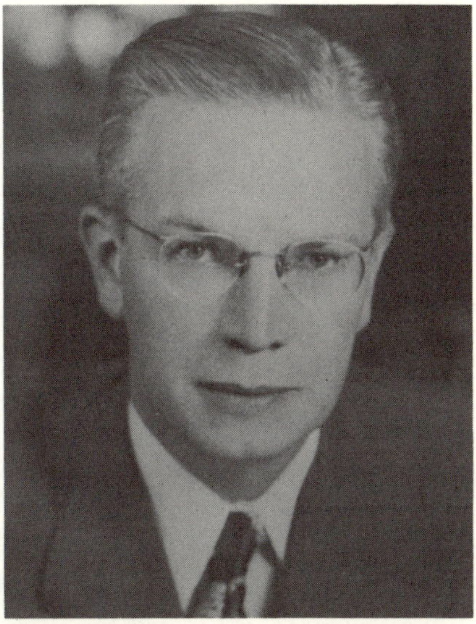

Blair Valdemar (Val) Jager, MD, left, second member of the Department of Medicine, was recruited in 1943. An outstanding clinician and teacher, Dr. Jager concentrated on neurology and syphilology. Richard H. Young, MD, right, was the first full-time dean, from 1946 to 1949, when he returned to Northwestern University as dean of the medical school there.

introducing the full-time faculty system he had experienced in Utah. The interspersed acting deans felt constrained from making any radical changes and often postponed decisions.

Wintrobe was a strict disciplinarian and demanded full commitment from everybody. He would not hire any married house officer and pronounced that you should only have one master: medicine. One chief resident in his last year of training got married secretly for fear he would get kicked out of the program. (This policy was abolished by 1950.)

One of Wintrobe's former interns (also a resident and staff member under him and later a professor at another medical school) described Dr. Wintrobe as a "workaholic," arriving at work about 8 A.M., leaving around 6 P.M., and usually working at home until 11 P.M. each night. He would make "professor's rounds" twice a week at the SLGH and weekly at the VA Hospital. A student or house staff member would present every patient on the wards and was expected to discuss each problem presented.

Dr. Wintrobe was thought to be an outstanding chair of a very good department and seemed to enjoy it. In staff meetings he listened respectfully to others but usually followed his own feelings and beliefs. He was a great critic but would rarely compliment anybody for anything. He was an outstanding organizer, especially of weekly medical rounds — the prime educational experience of the week, which drew not only full-time staff and students but practicing physicians, enough to fill a large auditorium. Four presenters had twenty minutes each to present a subject in depth, with some discussion, all in one and one-half hours. It was the best show in town. If a performance was inadequate, Wintrobe could be scathing in his public criticism. Val Jager was one of the few who would contradict the professor; some of the radiologists were the others.

This story told by a student who later became a professor of psychiatry casts light on Wintrobe's teaching methods. It was the student's first presentation of a patient to the professor. The patient had rheumatic heart disease. The student did a very thorough job of reciting history and physical findings, including a systolic murmur. The student was asked, "So you did not find an aortic diastolic murmur?" "No." The patient was put into various positions, stethoscopes were exchanged, etc. "Now do you hear it?" "No, I don't hear it," until Wintrobe finally said, "You know, I don't hear it either." The student reports that she was held in high regard from then on.

Wintrobe took great personal interest in his staff and students, helping many with personal problems and developing a network with some of the best Eastern institutions to exchange interns, residents, and fellows.

Especially during the early years, very close personal relationships were formed not only with members of the department but among the entire Medical School staff. Becky Wintrobe was a wonderful hostess, and regular parties at the Wintrobe home and picnics including spouses and children were regular features. Wednesday afternoon skiing allowed for relaxation and personal contact in the

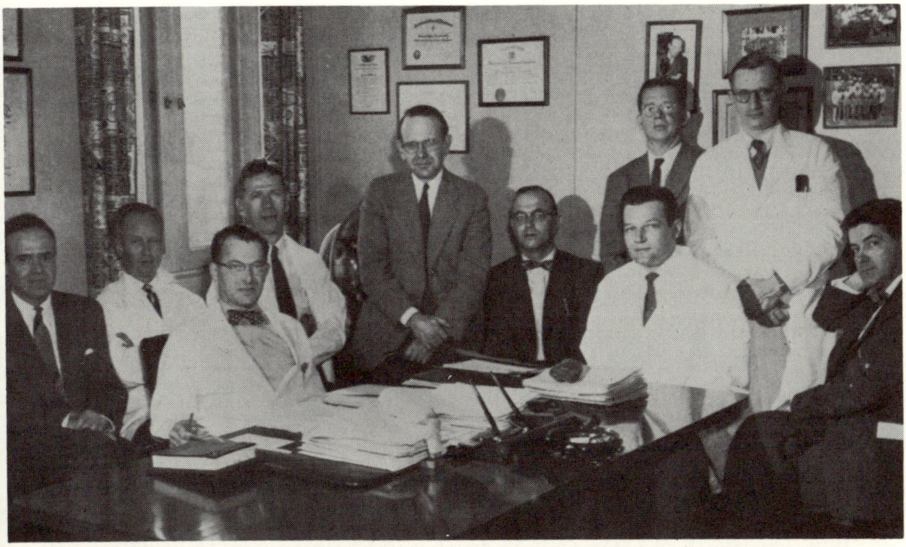

"The Quorum" —the entire staff of the Department of Medicine —photographed and nicknamed by the medical students for their 1956 yearbook. From left to right, Drs. Leonard W. Jarcho, George E. Cartwright, Maxwell M. Wintrobe, B. Val Jager, Frank H. Tyler, Harold Brown, Lyman Fulton, Glen R. Leymaster, and rear, standing, H. William Harris and Hans H. Hecht.

most wonderful surroundings of Alta, but Saturday mornings were used to make up for lost work.

The faculty worked full-time at the SLGH. The clinicians cared for county charity patients and agreed to limit the number of their private patients to direct referrals by practicing physicians. The poor physical facility made admission of private patients quite unattractive unless it was absolutely necessary because of the patient's condition and the unique skills provided mostly by Drs. Wintrobe and Hecht. Thus, time had to be divided between teaching, research, and patient care.

Renewed yearly, the initial epoch-making 1945 grant of $92,000 for the study of hereditary diseases brought in $4,093,689 over the next twenty-three years and was the forerunner of many U.S. government and private grants. Dr. Wintrobe directed this study from 1945 to 1973, and the Cardiovascular Research and Training Institute from

1969 to 1973. He was involved in early studies of pernicious anemia and the discovery that folic acid has the same effect as liver extract. Anemia of infection and nutritional anemia, as well as copper and iron metabolism, were subjected to intense study by Wintrobe and Cartwright in their laboratory.

Dr. Wintrobe's premier textbook on hematology, *Clinical Hematology*, first published in 1942 and now in its eighth edition, has been translated into three languages and is used by medical schools and practicing physicians worldwide.

In addition, Wintrobe was a founding editor of Harrison's *Principles of Internal Medicine*, the most widely used textbook in that specialty, now in its eleventh edition. He was editor-in-chief of the sixth and seventh editions. His *Blood, Pure and Eloquent*, published in 1981, received the American Medical Writers' Association award that year for the best medical book by a physician. His book *Hematology, The Blossoming of a Science: A Story of Inspiration and Effort*, was published in 1985.

For more than twenty-five years, Wintrobe was involved with the World Health Organization, chairing many of its committees and traveling throughout the world to bolster research in the area of nutritional anemias. He also gave many years of service to the National Institutes of Health (NIH) Research Council as a member and chair of its grants committee.

Dr. Wintrobe wrote more than 400 articles for professional journals. His guest lectureships and visiting professorships numbered in the hundreds. He was the recipient of a number of honorary degrees and many other honors, including the Kober Medal of the Association of American Physicians. He served as president of that association, as well as of the Western Association of American Physicians, the American Society of Hematology, and the International Society of Hematology.

Some have asked why Wintrobe was such a dominant factor in the early Medical School. When he came to Utah, Wintrobe had already established his reputation as the pioneer hematologist in the world. He set high standards for himself and demanded the same from others. He was well organized, worked long hours, utilized his time well, and accomplished a great deal. Wintrobe's scientific output was prolific, although it depended largely on the collaboration of his students, fellows, and colleagues. Primarily, he dedicated his life to this Medical School, turning down many attractive offers and preferring to be the "big fish in a little pond." Dr. Louis Goodman in pharmacology played a similar role in the basic sciences, and sometimes competition, if not conflict, existed between the two. Other department chairs — Leo Samuels in biochemistry and Tom Dougherty in anatomy — shared the limelight in the preclinical area.

In spite of the close relationships among the members of the Department of Medicine, inequality of income was an obvious sore spot. Dr. Wintrobe attracted the largest number of private patients, a source of considerable additional revenue, as were his two textbooks on hematology and medicine. These resources were not shared in proportion to the contribution of other members in patient care and in scientific input to the textbooks. Inadequate credit for authorship of papers may have aroused some resentment. Yet the general atmosphere of cooperation in a well-organized, productive department caused few faculty desertions, especially in the early years.

Department of Medicine at the Veterans Administration Hospital

A unique contract between the University of Utah and the Veterans Administration, worked out in 1946, placed Salt Lake's 12th Avenue institution under the control of the Medical School Dean's Committee, allowing the school to make all professional appointments. In view of the state's meager financial support, the agreement was of tremendous importance in adding numerous salaries, equipment, and laboratory space for additional University faculty.

Dr. Jack Nunemaker was appointed the first chief of medicine at the VA under the new agreement. Having trained at the University of Michigan with Dr. Richard Freyberg, his special interest was arthritis.

Dr. Harold Brown, a Harvard Medical School graduate with excellent training (an internship, residency, and chief residency in medicine at Boston City Hospital), arrived in 1947 as half-time chief resident and half-time instructor in pharmacology. He became assistant chief of medicine at the VA Hospital in 1948. National Institutes of Health (NIH) grant support allowed him to do research in endocrinology, particularly in steroid metabolism. He became the proud owner of the first flame photometer in Utah and developed an interest in potassium and magnesium metabolism. In cooperation with Dr. Hans Hecht, he used the earliest kidney dialysis machines on patients as well as dogs.

An active residency program at the VA produced more internists who went into practice in Utah than did the SLGH program, which concentrated on future academicians. An internship which was integrated with the University program was added a few years later.

When Nunemaker assumed a position at the central VA office in Washington in 1952, Brown became chief of medicine. His term was interrupted by a two-year stint as visiting professor of medicine at a medical school in Bangkok, Thailand, from 1957 to 1959. During this period, Dr. Jerry Perkoff acted as chief.

A four-bed metabolic ward was set up at the VA Hospital early in Brown's tenure, providing an excellent opportunity for very productive scientific studies.

In September 1961, Dr. Brown accepted a position as chief of staff of the VA Hospital and professor of medicine at Baylor College of Medicine in Houston, Texas. He later became the first director of the Baylor General Research Center at Methodist Hospital and left the VA in July 1962.

Department of Public Health and Preventive Medicine

The major functions of the Department of Public Health and Preventive Medicine were teaching and responsibility for student health. Some of the later faculty members participated in the activities of the Department of Medicine and took their turn in rounding on medicine wards.

One of the few native Utahns of the early four-year Medical School faculty, a carryover from the two-year school, was Dr. H. Leo

Marshall, professor of Physical Welfare and University physician from 1920 to 1944, and professor and head of Public Health and Preventive Medicine from 1944 to 1950.

Marshall was born on September 10, 1884, in a one-room log cabin with a dirt floor, later used as a chicken coop. As a child, he worked on his family's fifteen-acre farm, tending the animals, picking fruit, and harvesting vegetables. His sister Annie was a school teacher in Tooele and taught young Leo in her class. There was no high school in Tooele; in fact, there were few in the state outside of Salt Lake City and Ogden. However, the preparatory section of the University of Utah, which then constituted a major portion of the school, served as a high school for students who came from a considerable distance. Marshall spent three years in the preparatory division, four years in the college, and graduated with a BA degree in history in 1908. While still a student, he was appointed an instructor in physical education. After graduation, he taught physical education at the LDS High School for one year. He then completed the two-year course at the University of Utah Medical School before entering Columbia University Medical School, where he was granted his MD degree in 1914. He rejoined the University of Utah faculty, but with the outbreak of World War I, he joined the U.S. Navy as a lieutenant and served as a medical officer in the North Atlantic.

The twenty-four-year period Marshall served as professor of Physical Welfare and University physician was interrupted only by his attendance at the University of Michigan, where he received an MS degree in public health in 1930. From 1942 until his retirement in 1950, he served as professor of Public Health and Preventive Medicine and director of the Student Health Service. During this period, he also served on many committees and commissions.

Upon Dr. Callister's resignation as part-time dean in 1945, Dr. Marshall was appointed acting dean for one and a half years until the arrival of the first permanent full-time dean, Dr. Richard Young, in 1946. During his tenure, Marshall played a major role in obtaining a part of Fort Douglas for construction of a new VA Hospital and one-third of the remaining land as a gift to the University.

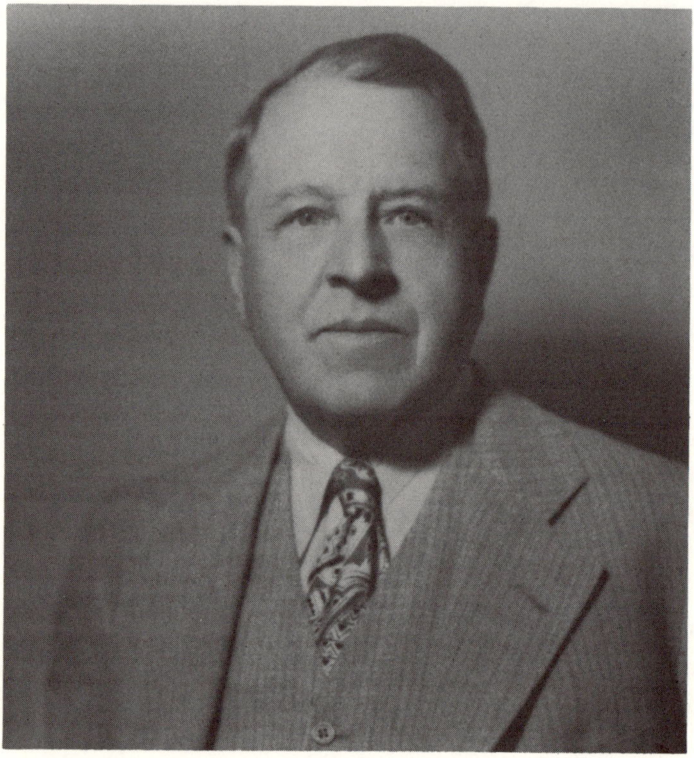

H. Leo Marshall, professor of Public Health and Preventive Medicine from 1944 to 1950, and acting dean in 1945–46 and 1949–50, was one of the few native Utahns on the Medical School faculty in the early years.

On many occasions, Marshall was influential in obtaining financial support for the University, and in 1954 he became very much involved in the planning and financing of the new University Hospital, which was finally completed in 1965.

When Dean Young resigned in July 1949, Dr. Marshall was called upon again to serve as acting dean until Dr. John Z. Bowers was appointed to the position in November 1950. At that time Marshall resigned his University position and left for the Pacific to become medical director of the Trust Territory of the Pacific Islands.

Dr. Glen Leymaster succeeded Dr. Marshall as head of the Department of Public Health and Preventive Medicine from 1950 to 1961.

After a long period of reorganization and redefinition, Dr. John R. Ward was put in charge from 1965 to 1970, when it became the Department of Family and Community Medicine under Dr. C. Hilmon Castle.

Pathology: Written with Assistance from Ernst J. Eichwald

As a specialty, pathology plays a dual role as a preclinical department by teaching the sophomore course and as a clinical department in charge of anatomical and clinical pathology and of the hospital's laboratory.

John H. (Jack) Carlquist, a Salt Lake native, received his MD at Cornell University in 1935, completed a residency in pathology at St. John's Hospital in New York City, and returned to Salt Lake City in 1939. He affiliated with Dr. Lyman Daines, who was both pathologist at LDS Hospital and dean of the two-year Medical School, where he also taught pathology. Carlquist was appointed instructor of pathology in 1941 and welcomed with open arms because Daines had suffered a heart attack which led to his death that December (see Chapter 40).

Dr. Orin Ogilvie, the only other pathologist in Utah, covered Holy Cross, St. Mark's, and Salt Lake General hospitals, maintained a private laboratory (Wasatch Laboratory), and also taught at the Medical School, which he had done since 1927. He was appointed chair of the department in 1943, but resigned in 1944 as a result of friction that developed after the transition to the four-year school. This left Carlquist the only faculty member in pathology. Dr. Louis P. Gebhardt, a bacteriologist, arrived in 1942 and became professor and chair of the newly created Department of Bacteriology in 1943. Finally, in the summer of 1944, Dr. Francis (Frank) D. Gunn, an associate professor of pathology at Northwestern, was recruited to head the Department of Pathology at the Medical School and arrived in the early spring of 1945, providing considerable relief for Carlquist. A few months later Gunn developed active pulmonary tuberculosis, and Carlquist was by himself again until Gunn was able to resume some of his duties toward the end of the year.

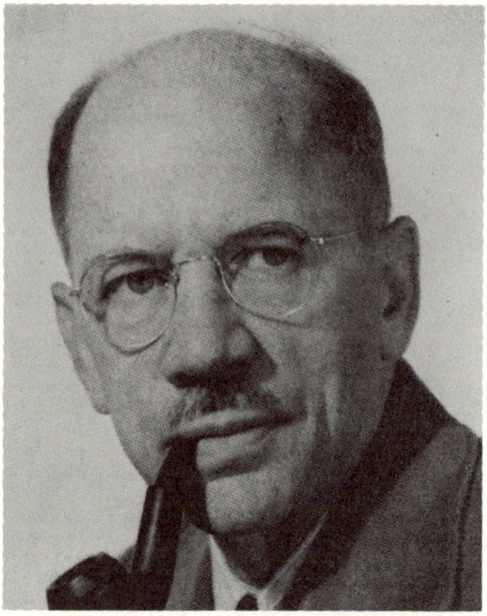

Francis D. Gunn, MD, PhD, arrived from Northwestern in 1945 as professor and chair of Pathology until 1953; he left the University in 1954 and served on the LDS Hospital staff until 1966.

Dr. Gunn was born in 1900 and received an AB degree from Cornell in 1921, where he also attended the first two years of medical school. He married his classmate Jo Dickmann. The couple disliked New York, and Frank was accepted at Northwestern University in Chicago, graduating in 1924. Jo had to complete her medical training at the University of Illinois, since Northwestern did not admit women at the time. Frank interned at Buffalo City Hospital in 1924–25 and became a National Research Council Fellow in Pathology under Dr. Benjamin Roman at Buffalo General Hospital from 1925 to 1927. He took specialty boards, joined the Northwestern faculty as an associate, and earned a PhD there in 1930. Gunn was an assistant professor of pathology from 1931 to 1939 and associate professor from 1939 to 1944.

When Gunn arrived in 1945, he, like the other new faculty, found the physical plant at SLGH abominable. The department consisted of one office, one room for storing museum specimens, and a lecture room. He pleaded for and organized a more up-to-date service facility

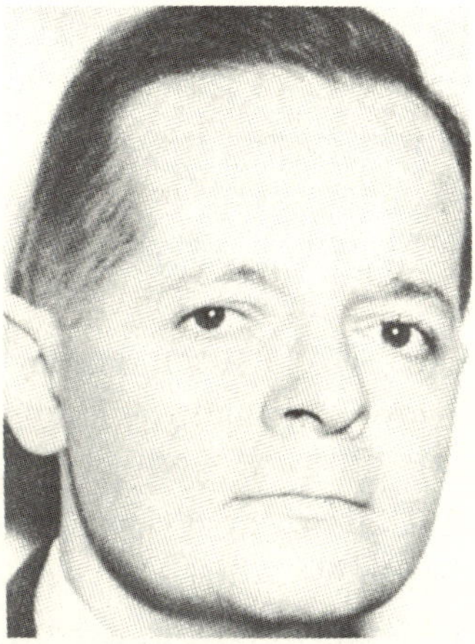

John Z. Bowers, MD, came to the Medical School from the Atomic Energy Commission. He served as dean from 1950 to 1955, when he went to the University of Wisconsin.

on the top floor of the hospital. He also established a residency program, and among his first graduates were Cyril D. Fullmer, later department head at Holy Cross; Richard Call, later head at Utah Valley and founder of the Utah Medical Examiners Program; Harlan Spjut, later professor at Washington University in St. Louis and co-author of Ackerman and del Regato's first textbook on cancer; and Roscoe Anderson, who left the faculty over a dispute with Dean Bowers and went to the University of Washington in Seattle. Gunn's first staff person was Dr. John Sheehy, who, during a stint in the Army, would meet Ernst Eichwald and help tie his future to Utah as well.

Gunn was a nationally known academician in tuberculous infections, his major field of endeavor. He was a man of very serious mind and unquestionable integrity, and he could be intimidating to newcomers and young faculty members. He was free of pretense, but also free of charisma. His departmental emphasis was on the autopsy service, which in consequence reached the highest standards. He was not well, suffering from diabetes in addition to tuberculosis. Gunn stepped down as head of the department in 1953 and left the University in 1954 to continue as a staff pathologist at LDS Hospital until he retired in 1965. He then transferred to Holy Cross Hospital and pursued research in cytogenetics with Sister Ann Josephine.

Ernst J. Eichwald was born in Hannover, Germany, in 1913. He started medical school in Frankfurt, Germany, in 1932 and transferred to Freiburg in 1933. After graduating from Freiburg in 1938, he entered the German Army but was able to get a year's leave "to do postgraduate work in the U.S.," never intending to return. He obtained an internship in Covington, Kentucky, which he completed virtually without supervision. He tells a fairly typical Eichwald tale: Having never before attended a delivery on his own, he was awakened at 3:00 A.M. to be informed that an out-of-town physician had a complicated delivery and was at a loss as to how to handle it. The fetus was in a transverse position with one arm hanging out of the vagina. Eichwald remembered his German theoretical learning (an approach totally lacking in practical training) of seventeen steps to be undertaken: the arm was pushed back into the uterus, the fetus was turned around, and a normal baby was delivered. His reputation was made!

After a second internship in Dayton, Ohio, which paid $50 a month, Eichwald became a resident in pathology in the same city at $75 a month. His chief turned out to be a near-terminal alcoholic who relied on Eichwald to do all the work, again without teaching or supervision. There he became acquainted with an attractive x-ray technician who became his wife for twenty-four years. Through another physician he heard about a residency in pathology with Dr. Sidney Farber at Children's Hospital in Boston at *no* salary. His well-known chief was a disappointment, but he learned much pediatric pathology from Farber's chief resident, C. K. Mostofi (of later urology fame), and gynecologic pathology at Boston Lying-in Hospital from Arthur Hertig, who was later chair at Harvard. In the U.S. Army, from 1944 to 1946, he was made chief of laboratory services of a "paper" general hospital in New Guinea which never saw any patients. Two weeks after the bombing of Hiroshima and Nagasaki, he was sent to Osaka, Japan, to test the water supply, yet another task he had never done before. Upon his discharge and return to Dayton, he found an eight-month-old daughter and a letter from Farber offering him a position as assistant pathologist at Boston Children's Hospital for $2,000 per year — a 2,000% raise.

Eichwald became involved in a joint study with Harry S. N. Greene at Yale doing anterior chamber transplants of human tumors into the eyes of guinea pigs. This experiment was essentially a failure except for one fibrosarcoma of a child at Children's Hospital which started to grow for a few days. Publication of a description of this one incident resulted in an invitation to the important Gordon Conference at Colgate University and established Eichwald's reputation as a tumor transplant "expert."

On the suggestion of his Army colleague John Sheehy, Eichwald was recruited by Dean Richard Young in November 1947 and arrived in Utah in 1948. He obtained the use of an old wooden building, former stables at Fort Douglas, where he installed his mouse colony from Boston. He taught Dr. Plenk the technique of anterior chamber transplants and started a fruitful cooperative project with the radiology department, having found an excellent model for testing the effects of various drugs, such as ACTH and cortisone, on tumor growth and metastases.

Like Dr. Hecht before him, Eichwald registered for the senior year at the University of Utah to receive an American MD degree in 1953 in order to obtain a license to practice in Utah. By that time he had the rank of associate professor.

Eichwald continued to study the problem of tissue rejection in the early fifties, when serious tissue transplantation was just on the horizon. In 1952 he proposed a symposium to be called by a new NIH study section to discuss various aspects of tissue transplantation and rejection. The gathering was attended by geneticists, immunologists, surgeons, and plastic surgeons, several of whom, including George Snell and Peter Medawar, became Nobel Prize winners. At a CIBA-sponsored transplantation meeting in London in 1953, it was decided to publish a journal. Eichwald was appointed editor of the *Transplantation Bulletin*, later renamed *Transplantation*, a position he was to hold for thirty-eight years.

Eichwald left the department in 1953 because of a disagreeable relationship with Dean Bowers. He entered private practice in pathology at the Montana Deaconess Hospital in Great Falls, with the understanding that he would have time, space, and funds to carry on his research. It was there that he discovered "H-Y," initially called the Eichwald–Silmser Effect: skin grafts from male donors to female recipient mice are regularly rejected, but not in any other sex combination. The study served to center attention on the Y chromosome. Detection that the identical gene was present in males of all vertebrate species (including fish) gave rise to a speculative wave that H-Y was *the* signal for sex differentiation, and life as we know it was inconceivable without H-Y. This research bandwagon came to a fairly early halt, however: "Wrong gene, wrong chromosome."

Eichwald was appointed chair of a transplantation committee of the National Academy of Sciences, a position he held for twelve years. He also was one of the speakers at a seminar in Forest Hills, Illinois, attended by Dr. Keith Reemtsma, who was just taking over as chief of surgery at Utah. Reemtsma was bringing Dr. Willem J. Kolff from Cleveland to head a department of artificial organ research, and he wanted "Eich" to come to Salt Lake City for a combined appointment as professor in surgery and pathology. Eichwald returned on Christmas Eve 1967. Organ transplantation became a high priority at Utah, leading eventually to the development of the artificial heart and its application in animals and humans.

Dr. Oscar Rambo became chief of pathology at the VA Hospital in 1950. He stood out among devoted lecturers and beloved teachers, and his departure for the University of California at San Francisco in 1955 was a serious loss to the medical community.

Dr. Richard H. Follis from Johns Hopkins was appointed head of the University's pathology department in 1954. Follis was a brilliant, charismatic investigator and pathologist, and a vigorous new wind seemed to sweep the halls of the well-designed, albeit limited space assigned to the department on the top floor of the SLGH. Follis managed to recruit two excellent younger men to his liking, Drs. Richard Jones and Terry Cochrane. His stay was limited because of personal circumstances, however, and disagreements with those in

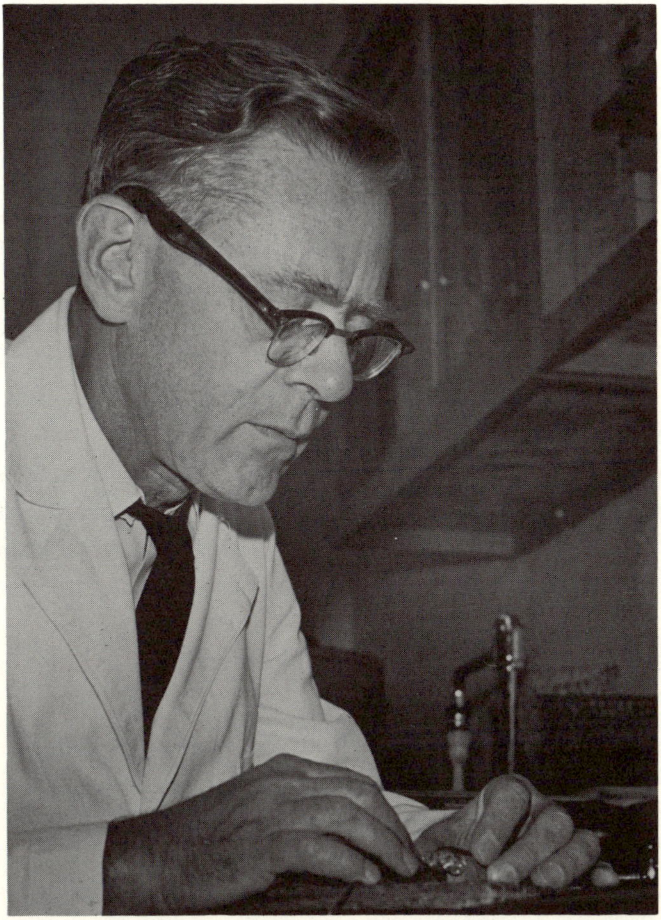

Ernst J. Eichwald, MD, came to the Department of Pathology in 1948 from Boston Children's Hospital and served as chair from 1968 to 1979. A pioneer in tissue transplantation and editor of the journal Transplantation *for thirty-eight years, Eichwald has had a varied and accomplished career.*

power. He "just didn't fit." Follis left in 1955, and his mysterious, untimely death in Amsterdam a few years later was never explained satisfactorily.

After Follis's departure, William H. Carnes from Stanford was appointed chair in 1956. In some aspects he resembled Frank Gunn: serious, impeccably honest, considerably prestigious; and, like Gunn,

Carnes considered the autopsy service the highest priority. He also undertook and assisted with cutting-edge research in the area of murine (viral) leukemia, in association with Henry Kaplan of Stanford, and in atherogenesis, with biochemists in the field of mucopolysaccharides and elastin precursors.

Carnes attracted and trained some outstanding young doctors, for example, Pat Cancilla, now chair at UCLA; Wally Coulson, author of an important book on surgical pathology; and Elizabeth Hammond, well known in the fields of ultrastructure, immunopathology, and human heart transplants — now at LDS Hospital. It was during Carnes's stewardship that Eichwald was re-recruited. Within a year of Eichwald's return, Carnes himself had resigned because of his dissatisfaction with the dean's office, and Eichwald was asked to take over, becoming chair in 1968, a position he held for twelve years.

Eichwald had some difficulties with one of Carnes's basic concepts, namely, that all academic pathologists should qualify in service, teaching, *and* research. Eichwald believed instead that excellent service and excellent research were incompatible — except in cases of "clinical" research. To demand research from service people would detract from patient care and yield mediocre results, and vice versa. He also aimed to raise the priority of surgical pathology and the clinical labs at the expense of the autopsy service, except to the extent that the latter affected patient care. This change of emphasis after so many years remained a sore and unresolved issue in the department until very recently.

Inspired by more recent recruits in the late sixties, including Drs. Charles DeWitt, David Steinmuller, James Swanson, and James Prahl (who came to a most untimely end while mountaineering in 1990), the Division of Experimental Pathology (renamed Division of Cell Biology and Immunology) was established in 1969 and has increased continuously in quantity and quality of research being conducted. At present the division accommodates a fairly large number of independently funded investigators of national and international renown. Their activities include research in the fields of ultraviolet biology, receptor kinetics, and complement genetics, among others. As in Dr.

Carnes's time, all the researchers have PhDs, and MD pathologists are rare within this division.

Three MD pathologists should be cited here for their service and teaching contributions. Robert McDivit (1981–86) was the first surgical pathologist of world renown to increase the department's visibility. His presence, together with that of Dr. James Weston, at that time State Medical Examiner, served to revive the sorely lagging residency training program. McDivit's successor, Tom Colby (1986–89), was also a superb role model for applicants and trainees, and the number and quality of residents has been exceptionally high ever since. The tendency to separate service pathologists from full-time investigators has also pervaded the service field, which clearly has been broken up by super-specialization. Within anatomic pathology, for example, cytopathologists do cytopathology; others limit themselves to dermato-, neuro-, or hematopathology. Specialization offers advantages, however, and within the latter two areas, Drs. Jeannette Townsend and Carl Kjeldsberg have raised the department's performance to widely recognized heights.

The search for a new chair upon Eichwald's retirement was a tedious and drawn-out process, despite the presence of two well-qualified in-house candidates. The final choice in 1979 was Reginald Mason from Tampa, Florida, who had published extensively on platelet function. A few years later, after several days of absence, Dr. Mason was found in his apartment, having terminated his own life.

Dr. John Matsen, who is not a "card-carrying" pathologist, took over in 1981. In view of impending restrictive federal legislation pertaining to the outside income allowed radiologists and pathologists, a better choice could not have been made. He organized an off-campus clinical laboratory, the Associated Regional University Pathologists (ARUP), from which the department and the Medical School could derive financial support. The ARUP has certainly strengthened not only the area of clinical pathology, but has also allowed the recruitment of new investigators of national and international distinction to enhance the experimental division. Dr. Eichwald is still active in research and teaching in 1991.

Radiology

Before 1946, radiologic services were largely in the hands of Dr. M. Lowry Allen, who covered the SLGH on a part-time basis, keeping his major emphasis on his private practice in the Judge Building downtown. Dr. James P. Kerby, the first Board-certified radiologist in Utah, provided what teaching was offered in the two-year program and during the first few years of the four-year Medical School. Kerby was the radiologist for the St. Mark's, Holy Cross and VA hospitals and concentrated his activities in his own office at 343 South Main Street.

From 1944 to 1946, Henry H. Lerner, Maj. MC, a Boston-trained, Board-certified radiologist, was stationed at the Army Hospital in Kearns, Utah, as head of the radiology department. He inaugurated conferences and seminars for Air Force and Army personnel at the bases scattered around the Intermountain area and also participated in medical rounds at the SLGH. Dr. Lerner had made an impression on the faculty during his Army career and expressed an interest in staying in the area. No search committee had been created to find a radiologist for the position of department chair. Lerner was offered the position after his discharge in March 1946 and assumed his new duties that May. According to Dr. Wintrobe, "Lerner brought good radiology to Utah, previously unavailable, and was able to apply radiology to the diagnostic and therapeutic aspects of medicine. He was a stimulating teacher and contributed to some very good debates on various cases at medical rounds."

With a large number of physicians being discharged from military service at this time, residencies were very much in demand. Dr. Lerner started two residents in the 1946–47 academic year and three more on July 1, 1947. Lerner could be quite critical and was known for making provocative statements, such as "radical mastectomy never cured anybody," which certainly aroused heated protests among the surgeons. The radiologists' participation in clinical conferences gave the department considerable stature among attending and house staff. The residents in radiology made rounds with the clinical house staff,

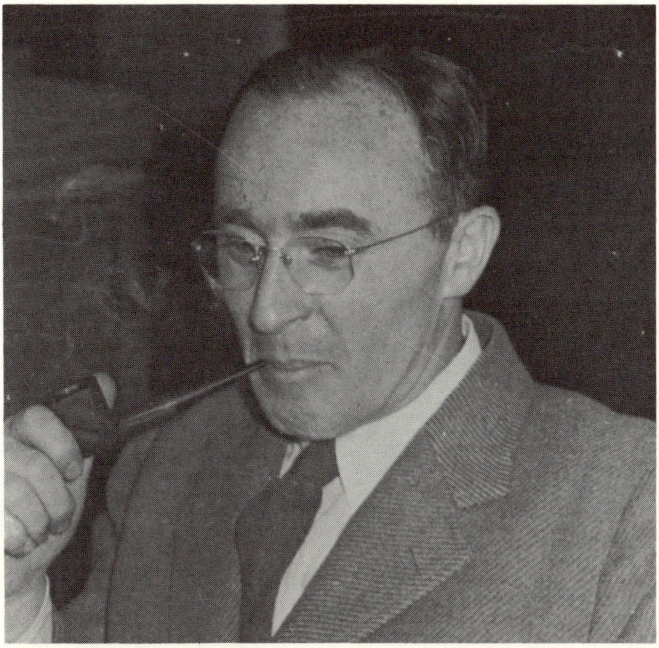

Henry H. Lerner, MD, was stationed in Utah with the Army during World War II and stayed to become the Medical School's first full-time chief of radiology, from 1946 to 1948. He is now Distinguished Professor of Radiology at the University of Miami School of Medicine.

and good interplay existed within the department as well as with the staff of other clinical areas.

Lerner established a small experimental laboratory and conducted studies on mice, comparing chemotherapy and radiation in the treatment of lymphomas and leukemia. This endeavor was never adequately funded. He co-authored and published several papers, mostly clinical case reports, with residents and medical students.

Dr. Wintrobe recalled that Dr. Kerby considered himself the kingpin of education in radiology. When not he but Henry Lerner was named chair of the department, Dr. Kerby became the nucleus of a group of physicians who were very critical of the new full-time faculty at the Medical School. Their complaints led to a meeting of the Board of Regents and the president of the University with a number of practicing physicians in the community, and the faculty's strong stand against outside interference was accepted by the Regents. However, Dr. Lerner was not permitted to join the local society of radiologists and through their efforts was blackballed nationally.

In June 1947, Dr. Henry Plenk arrived as second man in the department, with the rank of assistant professor. Born in Vienna, Austria, in 1917, he graduated from Real-Gymnasium in 1935 and completed the first half of the six-year medical school curriculum at the University of Vienna. Austria had become a fascist state in 1934. Faced with continuing political uncertainty, as well as the threat of induction into the German Army following Hitler's invasion of Austria in March 1938, he and his fellow student Agi Mero decided to marry and leave for the United States in August of that year. After moving to Chicago, Henry was accepted as a special student in the sophomore year, to make up for some lacking credits, and he graduated from Northwestern University Medical School in 1941. As a medical student he also did graduate work in physiology and pathology leading to an MS degree in 1946. During Plenk's internship at Evanston Hospital (a Northwestern affiliate), Dr. Earl Crowder, head of radiology, inspired him to go into radiology. After fifteen months of combined residency in radiology and pathology, Plenk entered the Army Medical Corps in April 1944 and was assigned to the Army School of Roentgenology at the University of Tennessee for a three-month course. He spent almost two years as a radiologist in evacuation, station and general hospitals, mostly in the European Theatre. He returned for his last year of residency at Evanston Hospital in 1946–47.

Dr. Richard Young, former attending hematologist at Evanston and assistant to the dean at Northwestern Medical School, had become the first full-time dean of the new four-year Medical School at the University of Utah in 1946. On a visit to Evanston in the spring of 1947, he recruited Dr. Plenk for the Department of Radiology. Plenk's first assignment was to organize an x-ray department at the VA Hospital, which had recently formed its close affiliation with the Medical School. This required a complete reorganization as well as hiring a new technical staff, improving radiographic techniques, establishing filing systems, etc. Clinical conferences were initiated. A joint medical, surgical, and radiology conference on Saturday mornings attracted the heads of both medicine and surgery, Drs. Wintrobe and Price, which had not been accomplished before.

Plenk's afternoons were spent at the SLGH, with the primary task of reviewing x-ray films with residents and supervising the limited therapy that was performed. A considerable load of teaching medical students and technologists filled up what time remained.

While taking his specialty boards in Chicago in June 1948, Plenk received a phone call from Dean Young informing him that Dr. Lerner had resigned his position and was returning to Boston. Dr. Plenk was appointed acting chair. After several months of exploration by a search committee and several visits of potential candidates, the attempt to find a well-known radiologist was abandoned. Plenk was promoted to associate professor and given full responsibility for developing the department, and his salary was raised to that of a full professor and department chair — $8,000. The difficulties of running a department, especially for someone only a year out of residency, seemed quite overwhelming. The annual budget provided by the University was $30,000 to cover all staff salaries, a secretary, and a chief technologist. While the department was remodeled between 1946 and 1948, no space was added. The whole area for radiology consisted of two radiographic and fluoroscopic rooms, a darkroom, a therapy room, and minimal office and x-ray reading space. The departmental operating budget for the year, provided by the county, was exhausted after six months, and getting enough funds to purchase film and other necessary supplies required a combination of diplomacy and table pounding. Under threats of closing the department, money was usually forthcoming before the last film was used.

The major task at hand was to organize a good teaching program for medical students as well as for the residents, nine of whom started their training in radiology between 1946 and 1952. Students were taught in front of view boxes in groups of about sixteen. Organ systems were reviewed from a teaching file through class participation.

All students attended sessions for an hour a week on diagnostic problems throughout their junior year and for one quarter on therapy problems during their senior year.

A weekly tumor conference was instituted with the help of Dr. Edwin Lawrence, a thoracic surgeon who was the first cancer coordinator, followed after a year by Dr. Ernst Eichwald, then the second man in the Department of Pathology. These conferences were well attended by the surgical and gynecological staff and to a lesser extent by the medical staff and students. Several other clinical conferences were held with various subspecialties. With the new tools available for assistance in making more accurate diagnoses — such as cardiac catheterization and early angiographic techniques — the cardiology conference was of great importance in arriving at joint diagnoses, especially of congenital heart disease, between Dr. Hecht's group in medicine, Dr. Robert Alway's group in pediatrics, and the radiology staff.

Research laboratory space on the County hospital grounds was unobtainable. Through the courtesy of Dr. Eichwald, who had established an experimental laboratory in the stables of the old Fort Douglas, a room with running water was made available. An amount of $6,000 per year was adequate to support a technologist and purchase lab supplies. Over the years, research grants were obtained from the James Picker Foundation and the American Cancer Society to carry on Plenk's work of transplanting tumors into the anterior chambers of the eyes of mice to determine the effects of radiation and various drugs on growth and metastases. A number of published papers resulted from this investigation.

Several practicing radiologists, including Drs. Ralph Meyer at Holy Cross and Lou Matthei at St. Benedict's Hospital in Ogden, helped greatly with the teaching load. Dr. Irwin Winter spent a couple of hours a day supervising residents for a minimum stipend while waiting for his own office to be ready for occupancy. In 1950 Dr. Marshall Landa completed his residency and remained for a year as an instructor. During the same period Dr. John Karr, who finished his training plus an extra year in therapy at the University of Rochester,

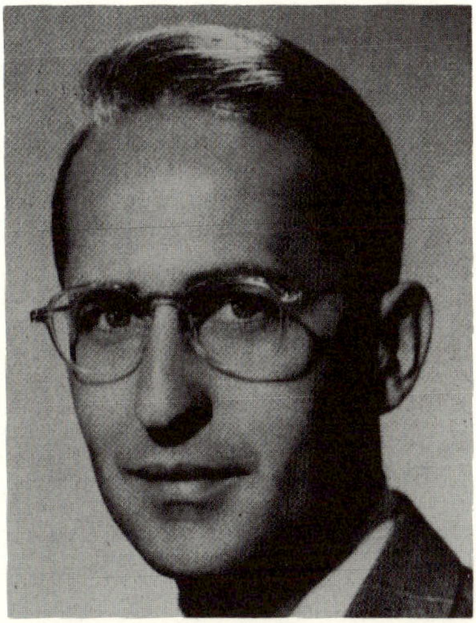

Henry P. Plenk, MD, MS (in pathology), came from Northwestern in 1947 and chaired the Department of Radiology from 1948 to 1952. Plenk left the University in 1952 and became the pioneer radiation oncologist at St. Mark's from 1960 to 1969 and at LDS Hospital from 1969 to 1986.

joined the faculty to take over therapy. Unfortunately, both men left after only a year. Dr. Ru Kan Lin, graduate of a Chinese medical school with a residency at Peter Bent Brigham Hospital in Boston and a year of therapy with Dr. Juan del Regato in Colorado Springs, took their place and stayed until 1954, when he left the state because as a foreign graduate he could not be licensed. All of the radiologists in the area participated in a regular film-reading session, bringing many interesting problems from their own practices, and in a resident seminar which took place the same evening. The staff also took an active part in monthly clinical pathological conferences and outstanding weekly medical rounds.

Dr. Plenk was involved in a study of a family with polyposis and peculiar benign subcutaneous soft tissue tumors. In the course of examining a male patient who had polyps and a carcinoma of the large bowel, the unusual appearance of his face was noted. X-rays revealed striking bilateral osteomas which also affected numerous other bones of his body. A review of the skeletons of all the patients with polyposis revealed that this was a constant accompaniment of the polyps and of the soft tissue tumors and led to the discovery of a new triad, Plenk–Gardner Syndrome.

Other research leading to publication or presentation included an evaluation of x-ray therapy for tendinitis of the shoulder, at that time the treatment of choice. In a randomized study, no benefit of x-rays was discovered. The ability to differentiate by x-ray between benign and malignant gastric ulcers was demonstrated on the basis of a citywide correlative study. The value of barium enema in the reduction of intussusception (the infolding of a part of the bowel into another) in childhood was confirmed, and with Dr. Chester Powell, a neurosurgeon at Holy Cross Hospital, the findings of 328 cases of cerebral angiography were reported.

Toward the end of 1951, Dr. Kerby could no longer perform his duties at St. Mark's because of the progressive spreading of radiation-induced cancer that started in his hands. A search committee approached Dr. Plenk about the position early in 1952. The lack of adequate state funding, making it impossible to attract qualified staff, and the extremely limited, outdated physical plant and equipment at the SLGH — with no prospect of a new University Hospital — convinced Dr. Plenk to accept the offer from St. Mark's to build a new department consisting of two floors, with a diagnostic department on one and nuclear medicine and therapy facilities on the other, including the first supervoltage unit in the Intermountain area. He assumed his new duties on March 1, 1952, covering both St. Mark's and the SLGH until July and the arrival of his successor at the Medical School, Dr. William Christensen.

Basic Sciences

PHARMACOLOGY AND PHYSIOLOGY. Dr. Louis S. Goodman was appointed the first chair of the University's combined Department of Pharmacology and Physiology and arrived in December of 1944. A native of Portland, Oregon, he received a BA degree from Reed College in 1928 and was appointed an assistant in psychology at that institution. In 1932 he received both MA and MD degrees from the

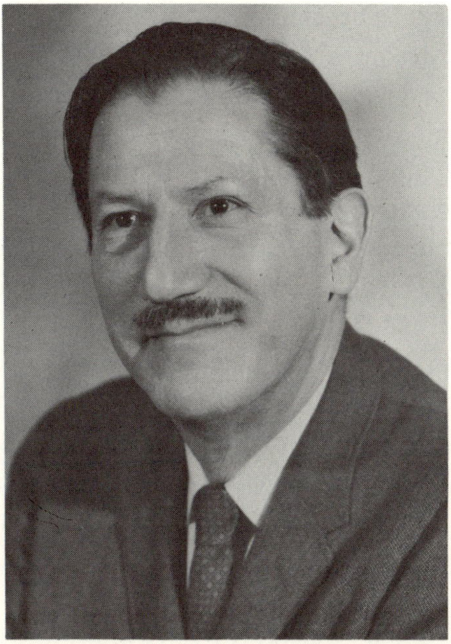

Louis S. Goodman, MD, came to Utah in 1944 from Yale and Vermont as first chair of the Department of Pharmacology and Physiology until 1945 and of the new Department of Pharmacology until 1971. His very productive research involved neuro- and psychopharmacology, epilepsy, adrenergic blocking agents, and early experiments with nitrogen mustard, among others. His greatest claim to fame was The Pharmacologic Basis of Therapeutics, the *textbook used the world over.*

University of Oregon School of Medicine. He was a house officer at Johns Hopkins in 1932–33 and in 1934 became a National Research Council Fellow in Pharmacology at Yale. He was appointed an instructor in pharmacology in 1935 and assistant professor in 1937. In 1943 he became professor and chair of pharmacology and physiology at the University of Vermont College of Medicine.

At Yale Goodman had become involved in the study of anticonvulsive drugs, and in 1942, with Drs. Alfred Gilman and Thomas F. Dougherty, was the first to use nitrogen mustard as an experimental anticancer drug in the treatment of lymphomas.

In Utah, with his associate Dr. Mark Nickerson, Goodman discovered the first alpha adrenergic blocking agent. With Dr. Lincoln

Clark in psychiatry he became involved in psychopharmacology, and his department became widely known for research in neuropharmacology. Goodman developed a new anti-epileptic drug, which is used mainly in Europe, and obtained a large grant to work on the physiology and pharmacology of convulsive disorders.

One of Goodman's greatest honors was the selection of five of his associates and trainees in seven years for the prestigious Abel Award for research: Drs. George Sayers, Herb Borison, Dixon Woodbury, Mark Nickerson, and Don W. Esplin.

Dr. Goodman was a masterful teacher himself, who carried a large teaching load and attended many of the lectures given by his staff. By rotating the assigned topics every year, he made sure that lectures were always up to date and of superb quality. He encouraged student participation in research projects and established summer research fellowships. His textbook *The Pharmacologic Basis of Therapeutics* emphasized the clinical aspects of pharmacology. First published by Goodman and Gilman in 1941, it was soon used widely all over the world, selling more than 1.5 million copies. By 1987 eight editions had been published.

Dr. Dixon Woodbury, born in 1921, obtained his PhD in physiological chemical biology from the University of California in Berkeley and started to work with Dr. Goodman in pharmacology. Woodbury became an important contributor to the textbook and was interested in anticonvulsive drugs as well as in various joint projects with the Departments of Biochemistry and Anatomy. With Dr. Frank Tyler he organized the first course in endocrinology. He stated that the cross-fertilization of ideas from members of various departments fostered a very stimulating and productive atmosphere for creative research. While somewhat overshadowed by the other outstanding faculty in the early years, Woodbury gradually gained increased recognition, especially after receiving the Abel Award, and he became Dr. Goodman's successor as department chair upon the latter's resignation in 1971. Dr. Woodbury in turn resigned as chair in 1980, continuing to work on his own funded projects. He moved into the Department of Physiology in the University of Utah Research Park when the pharmacology departments of the Medical School and the School of Pharmacy were combined.

With the recruitment of Horace Davenport, PhD, as professor in physiology, a separate department of physiology was created in 1945. Davenport is described by one of his colleagues as a towering six-foot-eight perfectionist, somewhat inflexible, and not easy to get along with, but a good teacher. His major research activity dealt with gastric secretions. Davenport was never able to build a strong department and left for greener pastures as head of the Department of Physiology at the University of Michigan in 1956.

One remarkable member of the physiology staff was Dr. Lowell Woodbury, Dixon's older brother, whose broad interests in electricity, physics, radiobiology, and epilepsy made him an important collaborator with many investigators in various departments. He developed an electric shock machine and, with Dr. Hecht, was the first to produce intracellular recordings of electrical potentials in muscles,

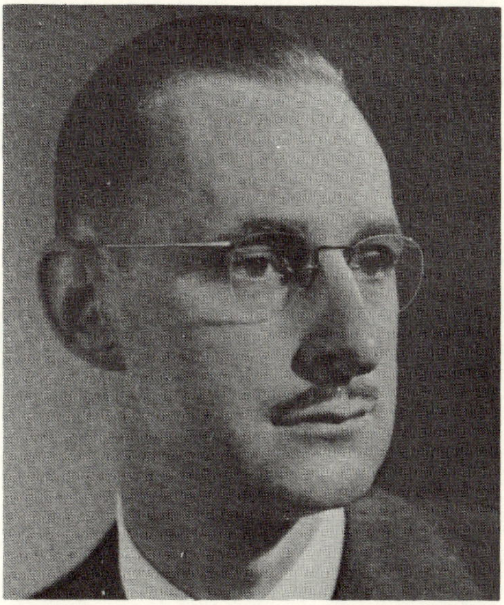

Horace W. Davenport, PhD, a Rhodes Scholar, came to Utah from Harvard in 1945 to head the newly created Department of Physiology, split off from Pharmacology. He left in 1956 for a similar position at the University of Michigan.

especially frogs' heart fibers. Woodbury was the first statistician in the Medical School and helped with the statistical analysis of data for many papers. He taught statistics to medical and postgraduate students and radiobiology to the radiology residents. With his brother Dixon he became involved in the study of convulsive disorders and maintained a lifelong interest in epilepsy. Before his death he had prepared a large manuscript for a textbook on epilepsy.

Because of a conflict with his department chair, Woodbury resigned from the Medical School in June 1952 to work for the Atomic Bomb Casualty Commission in Japan, investigating the long-term effects of the two atomic explosions. In 1958 he returned to the University of Utah to work with anatomy's radiobiology laboratory as radiologic health officer, only to embark on a new international career with the World Health Organization (WHO) a year later. For the next seventeen years he set up medical records systems and initiated the gathering of health statistics in many Asian countries, including South Korea, Thailand, and Malaysia, and was also assigned to WHO headquarters in Geneva, Switzerland. After his retirement in 1975, he returned to the radiobiology lab of the University for several years, then moved to Toquerville, Utah, to continue with statistical consultation, his work on epilepsy, and a federal grant to identify varieties of desert cactus.

Lowell Woodbury and his wife Dorothy, among the very few "locals" on the early Medical School faculty, played an important role in making newcomers feel welcome in the community. They introduced them to many interesting members of the University faculty outside the Medical School, as well as to their love for the desert and home canning of the area's abundant fresh fruit.

ANATOMY. The 1944 yearbook of the first graduating class of the four-year school (kindly donated by Dr. Fuller B. Bailey) lists the following members of the department: Clay B. Freudenberger, AB, MA, PhD, MD, associate dean, professor and head; Chester A. Swinyard, BS, MS, PhD, associate professor; Edward I. Hashimoto, BA, MA, MD, associate professor; and Edward D. LeCompte, AB,

MD, instructor. Dr. Freudenberger died during a leave of absence; Dr. Swinyard became chair of the department, but left in 1949 to pursue his own medical education and specialty training in physical medicine and rehabilitation. This left only Dr. Hashimoto, who taught gross anatomy, and Dr. Thomas F. Dougherty, PhD, who had arrived in 1947, teaching histology. Dr. Dougherty succeeded Swinyard as chair of the department.

Dr. Edward I. Hashimoto was born February 24, 1911, in his family home at 315 So. 12th East in Salt Lake City. He was brought into the world by Dr. W. R. Tyndale, who arrived by horse and buggy

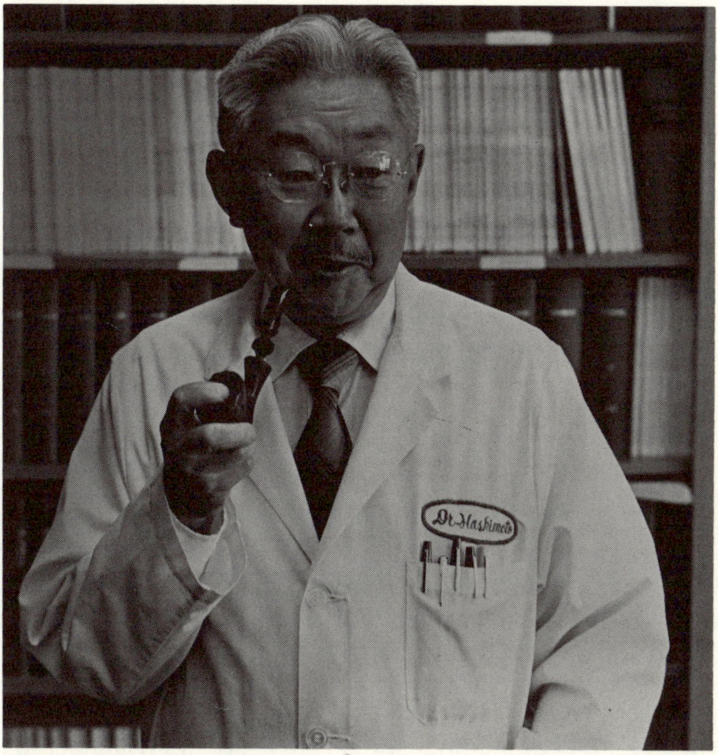

Edward I. Hashimoto, MD, became a teaching fellow in anatomy in 1935 and the Medical School's longest tenured professor until his death in 1987. The popular and productive Hashimoto also carried on a busy practice as a physician and surgeon from 1933 onward.

in a severe snowstorm and was unable to leave the house for two days because of the weather. Hashimoto graduated with an AB degree from the University of Utah in 1930 and after two years of medical school transferred to Harvard in 1932. After one year of internship he was slated to be one of the early residents in pediatric surgery in Boston, but, as an only son, he was obliged to return home when his father became ill. At age twenty-two he started a practice in the family home, where he maintained his office, until his death on August 23, 1987, in the same bedroom in which he was born.

In 1935 Hashimoto became a teaching fellow in the anatomy department for $90 per month to supplement the meager income from his Depression-era practice. After apprenticing with trained surgeons for eight years, he had become a competent surgeon in his own right.

As an anatomy teacher Hashimoto was most appreciated by his students for his animated, often humorous approach to making a dry subject stimulating. He was known for his masterful anatomical drawings, made with both hands, as well as frequent "off-color" jokes. In 1972 he was honored with the Outstanding Professor Award, accompanied by $500 which he used to establish an emergency loan fund for students. He led a full, productive life and was held in high esteem by his many patients as well as by his students.

The following information on Thomas F. Dougherty is taken, with few omissions, from an excellent essay by Dr. Kenneth B. Castleton and reproduced here by permission:

> Tom Dougherty was one of the brilliant young department heads recruited to the new University of Utah School of Medicine in 1947. He was born March 27, 1915, in the little town of Forman, North Dakota, the son of an Irish farmer. He attended the local schools and then entered the University of Minnesota where he received a BS degree in 1936, an MA in 1937, and a PhD in 1942. He was a research fellow at the University of Oklahoma School of Medicine (1937–39), then returned to the University of Minnesota as a teaching assistant (1939–42). From 1942 to 1944, he was an International Cancer Research Foundation Fellow and research assistant at Yale University School of Medicine. At the

same institution, he was an instructor during 1944–45, then a research assistant during 1945–47. He came to the University of Utah in 1947 as professor of anatomy, and in 1949 was appointed chairman of the department, a post that he held until his death. On May 1, 1955, he was also appointed director of the Radiobiology Laboratory at Utah.

Dr. Dougherty is perhaps best known and remembered for his research. His interests were very broad and included the fields of cancer chemotherapy, radiation biology, steroid chemistry, and experimental endocrinology. While at Yale he became involved with Dr. Louis Goodman and Dr. Alfred Gilman in research on nitrogen mustard as a chemotherapeutic agent. They were the first to use it in the treatment of lymphosarcoma. Indeed, August 27, 1942, marked the first use anywhere of a chemotherapeutic agent in the treatment of malignancy.

Dr. Dougherty was a pioneer in demonstrating the anti–inflammatory effects of cortisone and became a world authority on inflammation, steroids, the nature of malignancy, leucocytes, and chronic radiation intoxication. He also demonstrated the anti–inflammatory properties of heparin and studied the role of the adrenal cortex in the production of antibodies and in the regulation of lymphocytes. He laid the groundwork for many synthetic analogs which have greater anti-inflammatory effects than the original compound.

Under his direction, the Radiobiology Laboratory achieved international renown and is a major component of the U.S. Atomic Energy Commission's biological program. He wrote the handbook on permissible isotope doses distributed by the National Council on Radiation Protection.

According to some, he always felt that others who later became involved in chemotherapy never gave him the credit that he deserved for his early work in the field. He experimented with adrenal cortex as a crude extract, including its local use in an ointment. He was interested in the rejection phenomenon of transplanted organs and in the role of cortisone preparations in an effort to prevent rejection. Bleeding following administration of aspirin was another of his interests, and he discovered that it was related to the production of heparin, serotonin, and histamine. These are found in mast cells where the granules are dissolved by aspirin, releasing heparin, which causes the bleeding. He also found that aspirin prolonged coagulation time.

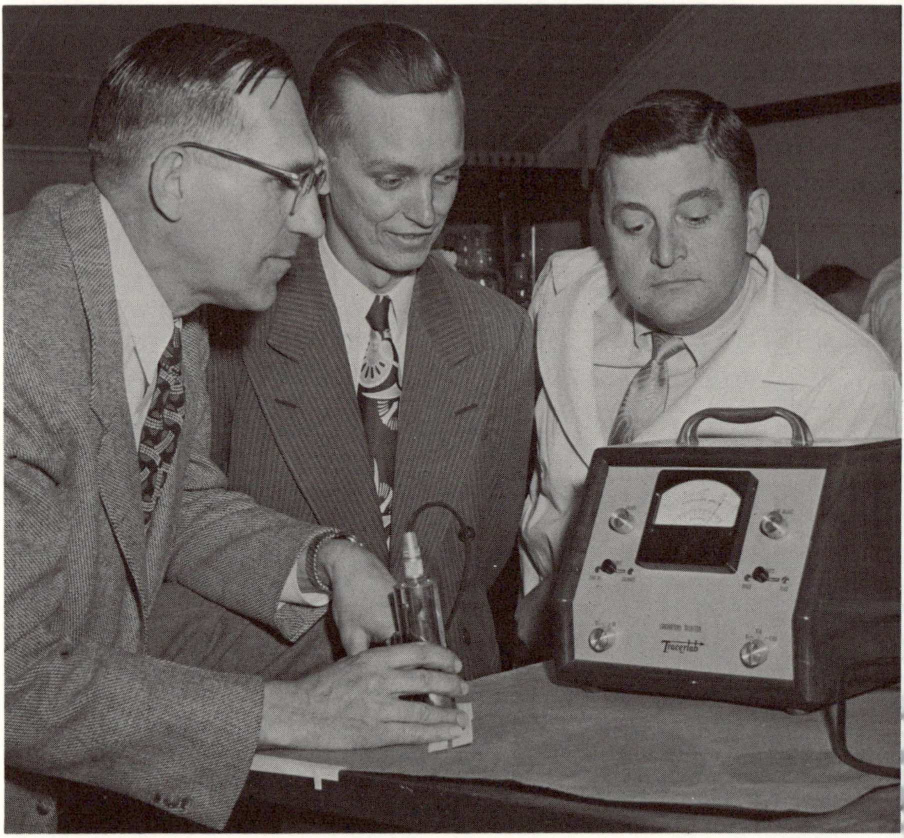

Drs. Leo T. Samuels, Don H. Nelson, and Thomas F. Dougherty, left to right, about 1950, collaborating on a project in adrenal corticosteroid hormone chemistry.

He was a good teacher and the students liked him for his keen mind. He taught histology, a rather dull subject, but he made it interesting. He was very patient with students. He was especially good with graduate students, who loved him. He had some conflicts, however, with other members of the faculty in other departments. One of his long-time associates tells this story about him. His lectures were often accompanied by slides. However, he had a tendency to wander from his subject, and it was up to the projector operator to bring him back to his subject by showing the next slide. On one occasion he wandered more than usual. He was talking about the skin and his own research on the action of steroids on skin. This went on for some time. Finally, the operator slipped in a slide of a nude woman. Dr. Dougherty was facing the class and did not see it. The projectionist then went to the next slide before Dr. Dougherty saw it. The class was much amused and applauded vigorously. He thought they were applauding his lecture.

He was a good administrator and attracted a superb staff which he stimulated and coordinated. During his years at the University of Utah, he served on numerous committees, including those on pre-clinical promotion, examinations, cancer teaching, curriculum, leukemia research, electronic, and isotopes, and he was chairman of most of them. He was also on the powerful Executive Committee and was chairman of it at one period.

He liked the outdoors and took long hikes. He played a fairly good game of tennis and did some skiing. He loved to sing and had a fine voice. He told one of his associates that he had always wanted to be an opera singer. He was liked by his staff and respected by them. One of his former associates said that he was like a second father to him. He liked to tell stories. He drank, sometimes too much. He said, shortly before his death, probably tongue in cheek, that he wanted to be embalmed with grain alcohol. He had a good sense of humor.

He received many honors and was a member of numerous scientific societies. He was a member of the American Association for Cancer Research; American Association of Anatomists; Society for the Study of Internal Secretions; American Society for the Study of Arteriosclerosis; Western Clinical Society; New York Academy of Science; American Physiological Society; and served as president of the International Reticuloendothelial Society. He was a member of the faculty of the Army Medical Research Institute and a Special Consultant to the Surgeon–General of the U.S. Army. Other societies in which he held membership include Sigma Xi; Society of Experimental Biology; the Histochemical Society; Gamma Alpha; and he was a Fellow of the International Society of Hematology and a Fellow of the International Cancer Research Foundation and others.

He had many health problems. He had severe diabetes. He had surgery for a carcinoma of the colon in 1968. He died about seven years later in 1975 following surgery for a fractured hip. At autopsy no evidence of recurrence of cancer was found.

He married his wife Jean while both were at the University of

Minnesota. She is said to have been a brilliant student, graduating first with an AB degree and later receiving an MD degree. She then received postgraduate training in hematology. She had a faculty appointment at Utah, but not in her husband's department because of the rule against nepotism. She did, however, work with him on many of his projects. They had no children of their own but adopted two, a boy and a girl.

BIOCHEMISTRY. This essay on Dr. Leo T. Samuels was kindly supplied by Dr. Ken Castleton and is reproduced with his permission and a few omissions and minor changes:

> Dr. Leo Samuels was chairman of the Department of Biochemistry in the University of Utah School of Medicine from 1944 to 1964.
>
> He received his early education in Indianapolis and graduated from the Arsenal Technical High School in 1916. His father had suffered a stroke in 1913, so Leo and his mother were forced to support themselves. While in high school, he had become interested in chemistry, but the school did not have a chemistry laboratory. While working in an automobile accessory plant, he took chemistry courses at night at the YMCA. These included general chemistry, qualitative analysis, and organic chemistry. He then obtained a job as a laboratory assistant in the local food research laboratory of the U.S. Department of Agriculture. This was probably the beginning of his interest in biochemistry.
>
> With the outbreak of World War I, he joined the ROTC and attended Butler College, where he studied qualitative analysis. When the war ended in November 1918, he was discharged from the ROTC and got a job as a laboratory assistant in the research laboratories of the Van Camp Packing Company, which made soups and other canned goods.
>
> Dr. Samuels' father died in 1920, when Leo was twenty-one years old. Leo and his mother sold their equity in their little house and moved to Berrien Springs, Michigan, where he entered Emmanuel Missionary College. There he got a job as a laboratory assistant in general chemistry. The college owned a farm of 365 acres and was eager to establish a plant to can the crops. College authorities assigned him the task of establishing and equipping a canning plant. He was so successful that by the time he graduated from the college three years later, the plant was shipping ten to

twelve carloads of canned goods each season. He actually never took a course in chemistry in college, although the college gave him credit for the three courses he had taken at the YMCA night school. The school also assigned him the task of teaching a course in physiological chemistry to home economics and premedical students. This continued for several years. He also taught a course in agricultural chemistry and received credit for it on his record. He was, in effect, a self-made chemist.

After teaching and operating a canning plant for three years, he decided that he wanted to go to graduate school. He went to the University of Chicago to see Dr. Fred C. Koch, head of biochemistry. Because of insufficient credits, Dr. Koch accepted him for one quarter on a trial basis and told Samuels that if he did well, he would try to get a fellowship for him. He brought his mother down from Michigan. He continued on his fellowship until his graduation in 1930 with a PhD degree, completing his work in a little over two years.

Dr. Samuels' first job was with the W. K. Kellogg Cancer Research Foundation in Los Angeles in October 1930. In January of 1931 he was appointed a research biochemist at the White Memorial Hospital in Los Angeles, affiliated with Loma Linda Medical College. His salary at this time was $1,600 per year. By this time, he was very interested in endocrinology, probably influenced by the fact that Dr. Koch at the University of Chicago was a leader in the isolation of the male hormone. Dr. Samuels' first publication dealt with the effect of nutrition on the male hormonal system.

While he was in Los Angeles, Dr. Samuels gathered several people interested in endocrinology and cancer, and together they developed a small group which met monthly. This stimulated his interest in the subject and influenced his own development in this field.

The group included Mrs. Walter Wanger, wife of the movie producer, who kept a colony of mice for cancer research; Dr. Bennett Allen, head of zoology at the University of California at Los Angeles; Dr. Clinton Thienes, head of pharmacology at the University of Southern California; Dr. Harry Deuel, also at USC; and Dr. Samuel Hershfeld, who was the physician for a number of movie personalities.

Dr. Samuels became interested in the possibility of determining the presence and amount of estrogen in blood. He enlisted the help of Dr. Hershfeld, who drew weekly blood samples through two menstrual periods of Claudette Colbert, Joan Bennett, and Mrs. Wanger. All of these women were having menstrual problems and were willing to pay $100 per sample to support the research. Dr. Samuels attempted to develop a bio-assay for the hormones in blood, but it wasn't until several years later that he discovered a chemical method.

Dr. Thienes offered Dr. Samuels an appointment in the Department of Pharmacology at USC. From that position (1937), he went to the University of Minnesota in the Department of Physiological Chemistry on invitation of Dr. Maurice Visscher. There he continued his work on the role of the pituitary and also did some work on the influence of hormones on tumor growth and also on the metabolic factors such as the role of fat, carbohydrates, and protein. While in Minneapolis, he began the first work on chemical methods of measuring steroid hormones. He also carried out the first work on demonstrating enzymic metabolism of steroid hormones by tissues. It was not until after he had come to Utah that he developed methods for extracting other steroids in tissue extracts as well as estrogens. At the University of Utah, Dr. Don Nelson, with Dr. Samuels, developed the Nelson–Samuels laboratory method for estimation of adrenal corticosteroids in blood.

In 1953 Dr. Samuels married Barbara Katherine Petri, also a native of Indiana. They had known each other for a long time and their families had been friends. Barbara had BA and MA degrees from UCLA and was working on a PhD in Western history at the same institution. For many years — up to his retirement and beyond — she worked in his laboratory and was of enormous help to him. A more loyal, supportive, and devoted wife would be difficult to find. They had no children.

Dr. Samuels' decision to come to Utah is an interesting story in itself. While in Chicago to investigate an offer from another university, he was told about a position at Utah and was able to meet Dr. L. E. Viko, chair of the search committee. He already knew that Drs. John Anderson in pediatrics, Emil Holmstrom in obstetrics, and Robert Hoyt in bacteriology had left the University of Minnesota to go to Utah. He decided to accept the offer to join the faculty — a very fortunate "accident" for Utah.

After his arrival, Dr. Samuels concentrated on research predominantly in the field of steroid hormones. In the early years here, he received some financial support from the Works Project

Administration, the American Medical Association, and the Donner Foundation. Later he got support from the Army Quartermaster Corps and the Office of Naval Research. When the extramural programs of the National Institutes of Health (NIH) were initiated, the school obtained a grant for the Laboratory of Hereditary and Metabolic Diseases. The American Cancer Society and the National Foundation also gave support. He was appointed to the Advisory Committee of the National Foundation and retained that appointment until 1968.

When he first came to Utah, the tiny Department of Biochemistry consisted of Dr. Harold Goldthorpe and Mr. John Kohnhorst, a laboratory assistant. It is said that Mr. Kohnhorst, who had only a bachelor's degree in pharmacy, was given a faculty appointment when the AAMC threatened to deny accreditation because the only full-time faculty member was not engaged in any ongoing original research. It is said that Dr. Goldthorpe started some research, but President Thomas found him working at night and ordered him out of the building because it was too expensive to burn the lights.

The general student laboratory was in the attic of the old medical building. Dr. Samuels was successful in some remodeling that improved the situation somewhat, and he also obtained permission for two additional faculty members, Dr. Sherman Dickman, who recently retired from the faculty, and Dr. Garth Hansen, who later became head of the Department of Biochemistry at the University of California at Los Angeles.

Gradually the number of graduate and postdoctoral students increased and they came from all parts of the world. Everyone on the staff participated in the teaching program because Dr. Samuels believed that anyone teaching benefited by it, as much as the students.

Many of Dr. Samuels' trainees entered academic careers, and eighteen of them became heads of departments or full professors. Dr. Samuels believed that student contact with good researchers was essential. He also knew that institutions with the greatest reputations are the ones with the best research. A good research program, he felt, should accompany a good teaching program, and a good teacher will interest students regardless of the curriculum.

After the four-year school was established, it was not long before the need for a new physical plant became apparent. One of the important decisions that was made early was to place the new facility on the University campus, although many people thought the new center should be developed at the Salt Lake General Hospital grounds to save expense.

In 1950 the National Cancer Institute awarded the Medical Center funds to build the Cancer Research Building at the recently acquired Fort Douglas site. One floor was assigned to biochemistry and the other two to anatomy and physiology. Later funds were obtained from the state and a public fund drive, as well as from numerous federal sources, to build the new Medical Center. About this time, Dr. Samuels was asked to serve on the advisory committee of the Eleanor Roosevelt Cancer Research Foundation, which had been established by James Roosevelt to honor his mother. One day Dr. Samuels got a telephone call from James Roosevelt asking if the Medical Center could use $350,000 for building facilities that might be considered as representative of the Eleanor Roosevelt Foundation. This was, of course, accepted with great enthusiasm, not only because it was a sizable sum of money, but also because it could be used as matching funds for an equal amount of federal funds. This money was used to construct the E wing of the Medical Center.

Dr. Samuels retired as chairman of the Department of Biochemistry in 1964, one year before the usual retirement time. He did this because he felt that the new department head should have the opportunity to assign space in the new building according to his own preferences, and plans for the department would take place under the new head. This was typical of Dr. Samuels' fairness and generosity. He remained on the faculty as professor of biochemistry and continued his research program. Later he stopped accepting graduate students but continued to have postdoctoral fellows.

In the summer of 1954 he was invited to Germany for a series of conferences in Marburg, Tübingen, Heidelberg, and Berlin as a member of the Unitarian Service Committee medical team in endocrinology. In 1958 he spent a year at Cambridge University in England, where he was associated with Dr. Thaddeus R. R. Mann in the Unit for Reproductive Biology and Biochemistry.

Over the years he became good friends with many of the great biochemists of the world, including Drs. Gregory Pincus, Herbert Evans, Roger Guilleman, Adolf Beutenandt, and Percy Julian.

During the time he was department chairman, the federal government established two steroid training institutes. One was at Worcester, Massachusetts, under Dr. Gregory Pincus and the other was at Utah under Dr. Samuels. Because he was so involved in his other work, he appointed Kris Eik-Nes to direct the center. Scholars from all over the world trained at the center.

Dr. Samuels became associated with Dr. Heinz Goetze in 1964, when the latter, as head of the Springer Verlag Publishing Company in Heidelberg, Germany, asked him to serve as a member of the editorial board of a projected series of monographs in endocrinology. Dr. Samuels was an active member of this board until the time of his death.

Dr. Samuels was a foremost leader in the field of endocrinology and steroid chemistry. He trained more than 100 scientists from all over the world and was a wonderful role model for all. He provided unselfish leadership and devotion to the school and to science. He was a "gentleman of the old school."

Dr. Samuels died March 30, 1978, beloved by all. He is survived by his wife Barbara, who continues to find many ways to be of service to people and to the community.

Postscript

The initial appointments for the new four-year school of Dippel and McLennan in obstetrics and gynecology (see Chapter 30), Price in surgery, John A. Anderson in pediatrics (Chapter 31), and Wintrobe in medicine in the clinical areas and Gebhardt (bacteriology), Samuels (chemistry), and Goodman (pharmacology) in the basic sciences were extremely fortuitous. Together with very few additional recruits, a few holdouts from the two-year school, and some help from practicing physicians, they initiated an excellent program of education for fifty medical students on an accelerated wartime schedule of admission every nine months, and they laid the groundwork for some outstanding research programs.

The yearbook of the first graduating class in 1944 lists thirteen faculty members in the basic sciences: anatomy (four), bacteriology (two), biochemistry (two), pathology (two, both part-time), and pharmacology and physiology (three). In the clinical areas: medicine

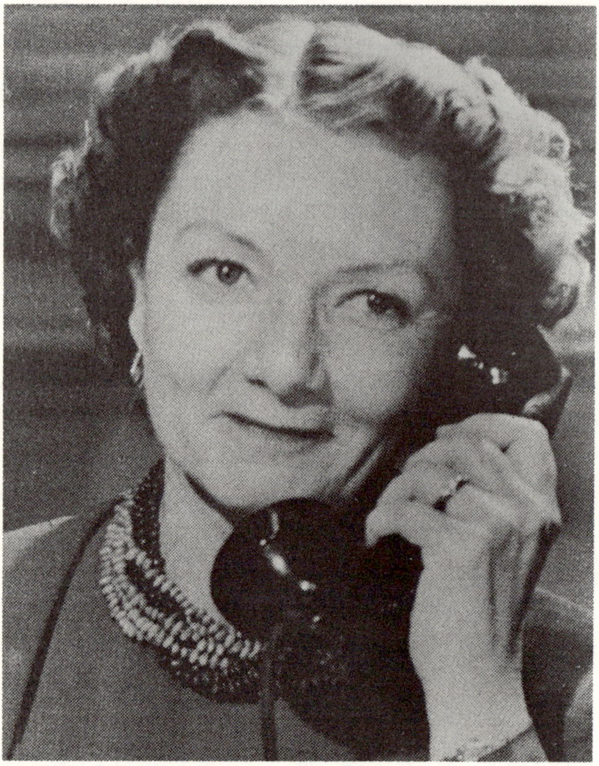

Florence Strong, the original secretary from the beginning of the four-year Medical School, became the "Dean of Students" as well as the indispensable administrative assistant to six deans over a twenty-five-year period. She was described in the yearbook Medicine Man 1952 *as "friend to everyone, mother to all medical students."*

(three), surgery (three), Ob-Gyn (two), pediatrics (three), public health and preventive medicine (one), for a total of twelve.

Even after the 1946–47 recruiting spree that followed the release of much talent from the military, the total full-time faculty of the clinical departments had increased only to twenty by 1949. The dean's office consisted of the dean himself, Florence Strong, a former secretary who acted as the dean of students, and a secretary. By 1954 the total faculty had increased to eighty-one.

With the availability of abundant grant money from Washington and the formation of many divisions of various subspecialties in medicine and surgery in the sixties and seventies, the faculty mushroomed almost beyond belief and now exceeds 800 full-time and 300 clinical members. The opening of the University Hospital and Basic Science Building at Fort Douglas in 1965 and the new hospital in 1981 accelerated this process.

While the original faculty had to be recruited from out of state, some of the best graduates from the new four-year school began to take some or all of their training elsewhere. They have returned to provide great talent not only for the staff of the Medical School, but also for the private hospitals and the community at large.

The relatively plush facility of the 1965 Medical School and University Hospital had become overcrowded by 1974, and plans were developed for expansion of the hospital from 200 to 450 beds and dedication of the existing building to research and teaching. These plans came to fruition in 1981. The Medical School budget allotment from the State of Utah for early and more recent years provides an interesting comparison:

1943	107,000
1946	141,000
1947	387,000
1948	442,000
. . . .	. . . .
1981	8,400,000
1989	11,600,000.

In addition to Price, Wintrobe, and Anderson (pediatrics) in the clinical areas, and Samuels, Goodman, and later Davenport and Dougherty in the preclinical sciences, a number of unsung heroes of the early four-year school deserve special mention: Val Jager and Hans Hecht as the first wartime recruits in medicine — Jager as a master clinician and teacher, and Hecht as a pioneer clinical and research cardiologist who took over as chair of the cardiology section at the University of Chicago in 1965 with a larger staff than Utah's entire Department of Medicine.

Ernst Eichwald, who came as the second man in pathology, developed a national and international reputation as an expert on tissue transplantation in spite of the fact that he left the University in 1953 for private practice in Montana. He was re-recruited in 1967 to help with the transplant program and later became chair of the pathology department.

Lowell Woodbury, who introduced statistics, radiobiology, and electrophysiology to heart research and later helped to improve medicine throughout the Pacific working for the World Health Organization, returned to work in radiobiology and epilepsy.

Homer Warner, who helped to develop cardiac catheterization at the Salt Lake General and LDS hospitals, is largely responsible for introducing computers in medicine, an undertaking which has resulted in a knowledge revolution.

Mark Skolnick, a PhD candidate in population genetics who was attracted to Utah by the resource of the genealogical library of the LDS Church, helped to computerize this resource. He developed the database for mushrooming genetic studies which resulted in numerous landmark discoveries in the field and which has contributed greatly to making Utah a prime institution for genetic studies in the world.

Hilmon Castle, who developed the outreach program of the IRMP (Intermountain Regional Medical Program), provided early postgraduate programs which increased the prestige of the Medical School as well as the referral base of the entire Medical School faculty. His leadership in the Department of Family and Community Medicine is responsible for the training of 245 family physicians in twenty years, of whom 50% are now practicing in medically underserved areas. This group has also swelled the number of primary care physicians in the large communities to replace the dwindling numbers of general internists.

A special tribute is also due the early University faculty wives. Octavia Price, Becky Wintrobe, and Peggy Holmstrom in particular made newcomers feel at home and fostered close relationships with house staff and medical students. Helene Cleare (Mrs. George) Cartwright, the University's first medical artist, raised the quality and put her own stamp on illustrations for all the research papers emanating from the institution.

All in all, a small band of dedicated, enthusiastic, and innovative people deserve an enormous amount of credit and the gratitude of the state, the region, and the medical profession for creating a world-class clinical and research center from the most humble beginnings.

PART TWO

•

PRACTICE OF MEDICINE AND MEDICAL SUBSPECIALTIES

CHAPTER ONE

Family Practice: The "New" Specialty

JOSEPH M. HEATH, MD

BY THE 1960S THE FAMILY DOCTOR, idealized by novelists, placed on a pedestal by television series, and revered by the public, was on the list of endangered species. The old country doctor was considered as anachronistic as the horse and buggy or the Model T he drove to make house calls. A rush for specialization, and the attitude in medical schools further fostered this trend. The term "LMD," local medical doctor, used by medical educators, suggested a bumbling incompetent who couldn't be expected to make the diagnosis. This negativism, plus the virtual explosion of medical knowledge, dissuaded students from considering general practice.

The total effect of these attitudes is shown dramatically by statistics. The numbers in general practice showed a precipitous decline between 1931 and 1970. In 1931, GPs totaled 112,116 of the 150,425 physicians in this country (74%). By 1970, they totaled only 50,816 of the 310,845 (16%), an attrition rate that raised serious questions as to how the medical profession would fill the key position occupied for so long by the general practitioner.

The same factors affecting medicine were operative in Utah in the 1950s. On the surface, everything seemed to be in balance. Good family doctors, loved by their patients, practiced in the major cities, with many dedicated "country doctors" in isolated rural communities. To be sure, even then many areas of the state were underserved, but this was nothing compared to the crisis that would come as the "old guard," overworked, with little help in sight, were dying "with their boots on."

The "Old Days"

The history of family practice in Utah would not be complete without a few examples of those great old general practitioners. Dr. Stanford Rees, a retired physician from Gunnison, writes about his father, one of three doctors in Nephi. In the period around 1915, he made house calls from Mona to Levan and surrounding areas with "a good team of horses, bridled, harnessed, and hooked onto a solid buggy. . . . Rain or shine, snow or mud did not stop him." Stan went with him on a few deliveries that kept his father up all night. Anesthesia in those days included a water glass with a piece of cotton in it soaked in chloroform, which the expectant mother held up to her nose and mouth. Stan relates, "I don't remember any real trouble any of the women had." A patient came to his father with a vial of medicine, arsphenamine in powder form. His father soaked a piece of cotton with 'rub alcohol' and lit it. With the good flame he dissolved the yellow powder, made a sterile solution, and gave it intravenously for syphilis. Stan also remembers the old quarantine signs in big red letters for scarlet fever and other diseases.

Dr. Frank Daughters started the Olympus Clinic in Holladay in the late 1940s, taking over the practice of Dr. Root. He and his partner, Dr. Ronald King, epitomized the model of hard-working physicians. They delivered a dozen or so babies a month, did their share of surgery, took care of the fractures off the ski slopes, saw the coronaries and strokes, and were the trusted counselors in times of crisis. After a long day in the office, they still had twenty or thirty phone calls to make and then the house calls (probably ten or more) on the way home. A typical day would end around 11:00 P.M.

One story from their experience concerns an elderly patient who had decided she needed a checkup. It was about 1960, in the "pre-Medicare" era. Dr. Daughters did a complete exam, CBC, U/A, BUN, FBS, EKG, and a chest x-ray. After all was done, the patient told Lucille, the nurse, that she wanted to pay the bill. Lucille went to

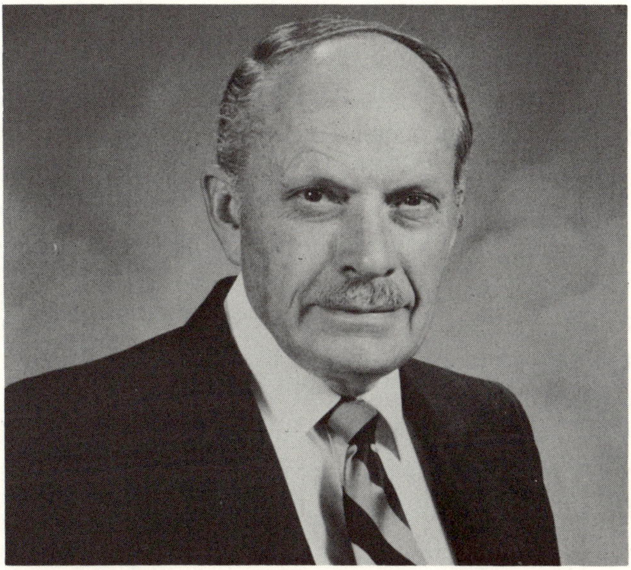

Joseph M. Heath.

Frank to get the amount. He said, "Oh, she doesn't have much, just charge her $5.00." When the patient was told the amount, she retorted, "Every time I come here you charge me more. You're just after my money."

Dr. Eldred Wright started practice in 1937 in Midvale, then moved to Kamas about two years later. During his seven years in that rural setting he had many challenging experiences. These were the days when penicillin was becoming available for the doctors in the trenches. He saw a gravely ill two-year-old with meningitis. In the old days, these patients had died, but Dr. Wright decided to try penicillin intrathecally. For nineteen days he went to the home, did a spinal tap, and introduced about 100,000 units of penicillin. This patient, Jodi Hoyt, now nearly fifty years old, survived without sequelae (complications).

There are lessons to be learned from these early family doctors. Dr. Wright returned to the Midvale area and was practicing with Dr. Hosmer. An eight-year-old patient with severe leg pain and high fever presented. They suspected osteomyelitis, but without today's modern technology they had to depend on clinical acumen alone. Treatment had not been standardized, and with penicillin as their only nonsurgical option, they decided on a thirty-day regimen of injected penicillin. Dr. Hosmer knew the father. "The kid's father's no good. He'll never pay, but I don't want this boy to be crippled. Go ahead with the treatment." The patient recovered without complication, and, as predicted, the doctors went without compensation.

Medicine had more "heart" in those days. Dr. Wright had a case of endometrial carcinoma needing a hysterectomy — a widow with no money. He went to the administrator at St. Mark's, who said, "We'll take care of her. If you don't charge, we won't." It was not unusual to excuse a bill or accept a chicken for payment. In the thirties the total charge for a delivery and ten days in the old Cottonwood Maternity Home was $56.00; $25.00 for the doctor and $31.00 for the hospital. Office calls were $2.00, often less for older people.

Today's practitioners, burdened by "the system," can remember the advice given by Dr. John Z. Bowers, dean of the University Medical School, "Illegitimum non carborundum" (Don't let the bastards get you down). Dr. Graham, practicing in the Midvale area, knew how to handle those exasperating, completely frustrating moments. One night after his sleep had been interrupted umpteen times by phone calls, not all of which were really emergencies, he just reached over the side of the bed and jerked the telephone cord out of the wall! It worked. There were no further phone calls. Another time, he was fed up with the constant haranguing from the medical records department at the hospital, so he took his large stack of charts out of the hospital and threw them in the Jordan River. A stroke of freedom for the beleaguered doctor!

Dr. Tom Robinson is a living example of the old-style general practitioner. He started practice in Sugarhouse in 1932 in an office over the old Granite Mart at 1086 East 21st South, rented for $35.00 a month. Now, fifty-seven years later, the "Iron Man" of Utah medicine still sees patients four afternoons a week. He was really a generalist, doing operations such as hysterectomies, thyroidectomies, and gall bladders, deliveries and C-sections, medicine, pediatrics, orthopedics, psychiatry, and the rest. He related his experience with polio, which took its toll in the early years of his practice. He had his own theory that the extent of paralysis was related to edema around the anterior horn cells. He restricted fluids and gave a hypertonic 50% sucrose solution. Many polio patients, including his own daughter, made remarkable recoveries.

Many physicians from the ranks of the general practitioners have made significant contributions to the advancement of medicine in Utah. Dr. Stan Rees followed his father's example and became a general practitioner in Gunnison in 1932. Before he opened the Gunnison Valley Hospital in 1940, he routinely traveled to Salina, twenty miles away. He remembers a case of gangrene of the hand and forearm in a seventy-year-old diabetic. Dr. Rees took him to Salina in his Chevy coupe, and on the way the old man sang "I'm Heading for the Last Roundup." It wasn't his last roundup, however, because after the amputation of his arm he recovered and lived for several more years.

Practicing in a remote area of rural Utah, Rees and another physician, Dr. J. A. Hagan, had to care for all who lived there or traveled on Highway 25. Frequent serious accidents required emergency care. They had a small hospital but no ambulance in the early days, and certainly no air lift or other way of transporting severely injured patients. Dr. Rees rigged up his car to transport those injured on the highway. Later they acquired an ambulance and a very modern hospital which the community is trying to keep open and financially solvent.

Dr. Rees was a state senator for twelve years. During one of his terms of office, legislation to establish the University of Utah Medical Center was being considered. Rees was very active in pushing the enactment of the bill, realizing the importance of that institution for the future progress of medicine in Utah.

Similar accounts of experiences and contributions of the doctors in many cities and towns of Utah could be related, the unsung heroes at the "front." These were the model family doctors. They earned the complete faith and confidence of their patients.

Changes in the Wind

The only training available for general practitioners was in the form of a one-year general practice residency after medical school and internship. This training was invaluable, but it did not change the trend toward specialization.

In 1946 a group of twenty met as the GP section of the AMA national convention, held in San Francisco that year. Utah's own Tom Robinson was one of that small group. He said that during a "bull session" they decided that general practitioners should organize nationally. A Dr. Paul Davis from Akron, Ohio, was selected as chairman by 150 family doctors. In Atlantic City in 1947, the American Academy of General Practice (AAGP) was formed with Paul Davis as the first president. Utah was represented in that vanguard group by Drs. Tom Robinson and Ulrich Bryner. Dr. Bryner, now nearing ninety years of age, played a leadership role in the early history of the AAGP, becoming the national president in 1953.

The Academy became the first medical association to require continuing postgraduate education. Each member is required to complete 150 hours of accredited study every three years, and this requirement has done much to inspire the respect of the rest of the profession. Many specialty groups have since followed this example.

Utah was not far behind the national move to organization. On June 14, 1948, during an AMA meeting in Cincinnati, the charter of the Utah chapter of AAGP was accepted. The first president of the Utah chapter was Tom Robinson, with Galen O. Belden as vice–president, E. M. Jeppson as secretary, and J. J. Weight as treasurer.

Too Little, Too Late

The goal of the AAGP was to save the cause of general practice and reverse the rapid decline in its ranks. The GPs had no intention of revolutionizing their approach to medicine. Their confidence was based on close relationships with their patients and the complete acceptance they felt. They worked to sell this concept by expanding preceptor programs, with medical students spending time in the general practitioners' office; they pushed for general practice departments in medical schools and organized students.

With all the noble efforts of the national AAGP and the dedicated officers of the Utah chapter, the years from 1947 to 1969 saw the percentage of family doctors drop from 50% to 16%. Patients may still have preferred the family doctor, but the medical students, whose support was needed, were picking the specialties. General practice seemed headed for a dinosaur-type demise.

The Visionaries

While the rank and file of AAGP worked for preservation of their style of practice, there were those who could see the need for change. Dr. Thomas E. Rardin, chairman of the Section of General Practice of the AMA in 1962, gave the following concept in an address before the Section:

> By common agreement . . . comprehensive medical care for individuals and their families on a continuous basis is desirable and essential. . . . [An] individual doctor of medicine specifically trained to render service over broad areas of medical knowledge, securing, integrating, and coordinating other highly specialized skills and knowledge according to the needs of his patients, should guide individuals and family units.

Dr. Rardin was urging formulation of a specialty in family medicine. Two years later, following a conference entitled "The Family and the Doctor," co-sponsored by the Family Health Care Program and Harvard Medical School in January 1964, Dr. E. Maurice Backette stated:

> Family medicine . . . must be of quite a new kind, a kind which springs from and meets changing medical needs. In democratic societies, it should also go some way toward meeting changing demand. This is just another way of saying the obvious: That the kind of medicine we have should always keep up with or — better still — be one jump ahead of the changes which are going on in the society it serves. This, it has *palpably not done and is not doing.*

The conference summary proposed a new kind of training: "The family doctor should be trained in the medical school and in post-graduate courses to be patient-oriented or family-oriented, not disease-oriented . . . . He needs to become a specialist in family medicine and to concentrate his training and efforts on family-centered medicine."

The year 1966 was a landmark year in medical education circles. Three significant reports were published: (1) "The Graduate Education of Physicians" commissioned by the AMA (Millis Commission Report); (2) "Health Is a Community Affair" (Folsom Report); and (3) "Meeting the Challenge of Family Practice," report of the Ad Hoc Committee on Education for Family Practice of the AMA Council on Medical Education (Willard Report). All of these urged the formulation of a specialty in family practice and the preparation of plans to educate this new style of family doctor.

1969 — The Year of Decision

The idea of general practice becoming a specialty was not without controversy or detractors on both sides of the issue. Many medical educators saw this movement as an attempt to stem the tide toward greater specialization. They doubted that this was possible or even desirable. They questioned whether the public really wanted the family physician or would use a general physician if they had access to specialists. Many of the "old guard" general practitioners resisted the idea of change. Their concept of being generalists had worked well for them, and becoming a "specialist" was diametrically opposite their long-held philosophy.

However, nothing could stop this idea whose time had come. On February 8, 1969, by action of the Liaison Committee of the Advisory Board of Medical Specialties and the Council on Medical Education of the AMA, family practice was recognized and approved as a specialty. Thus the twentieth primary specialty came into existence!

For two years the AAGP Core-Examination Committee had made an extensive study of the type of examination necessary to evaluate the specialty of family practice. The Board moved quickly forward, and the first examination was held February 28 and March 1, 1970. Thirty-six major centers throughout the U.S. were designated as testing sites. Stringent requirements had to be met to qualify for taking the exam, which included 150 hours of continuing medical education (CME) in the preceding three years. The new specialty insisted on two unique provisions: no "grandfather clause" for the older practitioner and periodic recertification.

The hopes of those pioneers who forged the new specialty are evident in the seal of the American Board of Family Practice. The mythological Phoenix is depicted rising out of its nest of fire and represents Family Practice arising from its general practice heritage.

Help from Unexpected Places

It was one thing to have the turnaround nationally, but the problems needing solutions in Utah had to be addressed at home. Six months after family practice became a specialty, and with training programs starting to crop up around the country, Governor Calvin L. Rampton set up a blue ribbon committee to study medical care needs in Utah in August 1969. This committee was composed of the dean of the University of Utah Medical School, Frank Ebaugh, other university educators, and doctors, one of whom was a family doctor. After three months they made three main recommendations: (1) Form a new department of Community and Family Medicine; (2) do community-related medical research; and (3) train family physicians and physician assistants. The Governor acted upon these recommendations, and the budget in January 1970 included an item of $91,000 to perform the operation of grafting family practice onto the University. The dream of general practitioners for years was actually happening!

Obstacles had to be overcome. The Board of Regents had made a strict policy of no new departments. The Department of Medicine under Dr. George Cartwright had always been opposed to the concept of general practice. The main problem of no new departments was solved by proposing the expansion of the existing Department of

Preventive Medicine, then headed by Dr. John R. Ward. Dr. Cartwright did a turnaround with the prospect that the new department would take over the outpatient clinics, relieving his department of this onerous duty. The department came into existence under the name of Community and Family Medicine in July 1970. John Ward elected not to remain as head, and many others were considered before Dean Ebaugh asked Dr. C. Hilmon Castle, then head of the Intermountain Regional Medical Program, to be the new chair.

Dr. Castle, a cardiologist, had been at the University since the early fifties and was known by many in the practicing community as their mentor in medical school. Well-respected because of his position as an educator, and especially in his ability to organize and procure grants for research projects, Castle was a good choice. Not everyone agreed, however, as many of the family doctors felt that one of their own should have been in that position. Dr. Castle took the helm of a ship in largely uncharted waters, with many storms ahead in an ocean full of sharks called the University of Utah.

The family physicians of Utah had found an unexpected friend in Hilmon Castle. One of his first actions was to change the department's name to Family and Community Medicine, putting the challenge of training family physicians first. He moved swiftly to get into the business of training residents. The program was initiated in July 1971, starting with six residents in both the McKay-Dee and St. Benedict hospitals in Ogden. He recruited Dr. Bill Daines, an internist, and later Dr. George Snell, an experienced general physician from Kaysville, to bring the touch of practice to the programs. In 1972 the residents from St. Benedict's were transferred to Holy Cross Hospital in Salt Lake City, and a training program with ties to the University of Utah, long the dream of Utah's family doctors, had finally come into existence. Dr. John Guyman, a well-respected name in Family Practice education circles, came to Utah in that same year. The programs in Salt Lake and Ogden grew rapidly, with a total of thirty-six residents by July 1974.

Dr. Castle recruited able educators such as Drs. David Feigal, John Tudor, David Sundwall, Jerry Gardner, and many practicing family physicians. An effective group was formed early in the 1970s, the Family Practice Advisory Committee, composed of practicing physicians from all parts of the state; it became the liaison between "town and gown." As a member of this committee for more than fifteen years, Dr. Joseph M. Heath saw Castle in action and can attest to his fierce loyalty to the department. He fought "the good fight" to establish family practice as a respected member of the University community.

Doctors in Transition

With the exciting developments occurring both nationally and in Utah, the practicing general practitioners faced the challenges of changing with the times. If they wanted to be counted in the new specialty, they had to prepare to take the rigorous two-day exam and then keep up their CME requirements. They needed their state organization, the Utah Association of Family Physicians, all the more. The UAFP became very active in promoting educational opportunities and became a political force as well, lobbying for legislation that supported the residency financially. Dr. Jack Johnson, Tremonton, was a particularly effective lobbyist. One important area of UAFP involvement was contact with medical students. In the early 1970s the Family Practice Club was formed with financial backing from Marion Laboratories. Members met with students socially and in educational pursuits to encourage them toward the new specialty.

Many capable presidents of UAFP, along with their boards of directors, guided the transition of the more than 200 general practitioners who were finding their way in the new specialty. A typical example of the doctor in transition is Dr. Maurice Baker, who started his practice in the Taylorsville area in 1960. He graduated from the University of Utah Medical School in 1958, following which he had a two-year rotating general practice internship at St. Mark's Hospital, one of a very few such programs in existence. His practice covers broad areas of medicine, including some major surgery and a very active OB practice (more than 4,000 deliveries at the time of this writing). He took his family practice Boards in 1970, the first time offered, which gave him specialist status, a message to his patients that he was a competent as well as a caring family doctor. He is the author of two patient-education books entitled *Doctor, What Do I Do?* and *The Doctor's Advice Without the Price.*

Dr. David Symond has practiced in the remote area of Milford since the mid-1950s. His training after medical school was a rotating internship and a one-year general practice residency. When he started in this old railroad town, it had a very inadequate hospital housed in a large old home. He rallied the community to build a first-rate thirty-two-bed hospital with modern operating and delivery rooms, an emergency room, and an area equipped to treat myocardial infarctions. Many lives have been saved because of the immediate availability of emergency services. Dr. Symond tells of a case of extreme shock following abdominal trauma. He diagnosed a ruptured spleen, but this was not a problem he had seen in training. Time did not permit transfer, so he "read the book" and performed the splenectomy cookbook style. The patient recovered without complication. Recently a seventy-year-old man had repeated cardiac arrests. He was resuscitated more than fifty times by doctors and the hospital staff. During one of the episodes he looked up with resignation. "Doc, you might as well let me go." They didn't, and now he is doing well with a permanent pacer.

Dr. Symond also took his Boards with doctors from throughout the state. When his son joined him in his practice after finishing his residency at the University, Dave was free to make his contribution to the cause of family practice. He went full time to the "U" as associate chair of family practice services. For two years he saw to it that other departments at the University Hospital gave admitting privileges to family practice faculty and other family physicians. He was able to accomplish this in departments such as medicine, surgery, orthopedics, and even obstetrics. He also pushed for the Family Practice Center, a separate model clinic for the training of residents, which is now a reality, located in the old Red Cross building close to the campus.

"The New Breed"

The family practice residency program at the University of Utah has lived up to its expectations. Since its inception in 1971, Salt Lake and Ogden have produced 236 graduates, approximately fifteen each year. This is a group of well-trained family specialists on a par with other primary specialists. They have been well received by the public as heirs apparent of the "Marcus Welbys" of the past. The "U" graduates have made their way into many areas in Utah where urgent need of physicians existed. Ninety have stayed to practice in Utah, fifty-nine located in rural areas. To cite a few examples: Konrad Kotrady in remote Emery County, Kim Bateman and Bruce Burnham in Ephraim, David Flinders in Spanish Fork, Brent Black in Delta, and Brent Jackson in Fillmore. Relief needed in those underserved areas was starting to come.

Dr. Kim Bateman is a remarkable example of what this new breed has accomplished. He graduated from the University of Utah Medical School in 1974 and took his three-year family practice residency at McKay-Dee in Ogden. He went directly to a place where he was really needed: Ephraim, in central rural Utah. New, well-trained doctors provided the impetus to build a modern twenty-bed hospital. Dr. Bateman, as the new man on the block, was asked to represent that part of the state on the Board of Trustees of the Utah Medical Association. He states, "That opportunity has changed my life." He took that assignment seriously, and because of his abilities and contributions, attained the office of president of the UMA in 1983–84. He has remained on the Board of Trustees and is also on the important Committee of Rural Health for the state.

No Finis

There is no end to this story. At this juncture, the life of the family doctor has been preserved. What appeared to be an almost certain demise was rescued by the likes of Ulrich Bryner, Tom Robinson, Stanford Rees, L. D. Nelson, Bob Kelly, Hilmon Castle, George Snell, Dave Symond, Kim Bateman, and scores of others who have believed in the family practice cause.

A recent article, "Is Marcus Welby Dead?," suggests that the very entity which struggled for survival a short twenty years ago is again in jeopardy. Now the behemoths are Medicare, malpractice, and "red ink" in rural hospitals. There is strength in many places. The residency program is under the very capable leadership of Dr. Marian Bishop, producing an excellent crop of residents each year. The UAFP, with Dr. Roslyn Taylor at the helm, is a strong advocate for the practicing physician. For the first time in several years, Utah has one of its own, Dr. John Tudor, in a national position on the Board of Directors of the AAFP. Most important, the individual family physician is still beloved by patients who prefer a doctor who treats people rather than diseases. Let us all be optimists that the Phoenix will continue to soar, with the family doctor's future secure.

CHAPTER TWO

Recollections of a Coal Camp Doctor

J. ELDON DORMAN, MD

I ARRIVED IN CONSUMERS, UTAH, on January 3, 1937. I was a native of Colorado but had gone to medical school and served my internship in California. In July 1936, I went to Spanish Fork, Utah, to work for a doctor who was ill. He had recovered, and since we did not get along very well, I was pleased when, about midnight on January 2, I got a phone call from Terry McGowan, then superintendent of the Blue Blaze Coal Company at Consumers. He offered me a job as the doctor for the coal camps of Consumers, Sweets, and National and asked that I report to work "for sure" at noon on the following day.

I did not quite make it by noon. As a flat-land driver I failed to negotiate the snow-packed curve just west of old Tucker and clobbered my car when it ended up in the creek. So I entered Carbon County riding in the back of a flatbed coal truck, clutching my medical bag and rubbing my contusions.

I found patients waiting for me. I saw several sick people and handled some injuries. Before midnight I delivered a baby boy. I received the surprise of my life when the father pressed a twenty-dollar bill in my hand shortly after I severed the umbilical cord. Never in my previous practice had I been paid so promptly. I had learned to settle many of my bills by barter — a sack of spuds, a box of apples,

Reprinted, with adaptations, from Philip F. Notarianni, ed., *Carbon County, Eastern Utah's Industrial Island* (Salt Lake City: Utah State Historical Society, 1981), with kind permission of the publisher.

or perhaps some eggs, butter, or chickens. That crisp new bill in my otherwise empty pocket made me think I had come to the right place, and indeed I had. I spent three of the most pleasant and enjoyable years of my life in the coal camps of Carbon County. I was called Doctor, Doc, or Mr. Doc (a title of special respect); most frequently, however, I was "Little Mr. Doc," since I tipped the scales in those days at less than 130 pounds.

The Medical Association and the Company Doctor

Consumers, Sweets, and National were the three coal mines in the Gordon Creek area located about twenty miles west and a little north of Price, Utah. In the early 1930s these three camps formed a Medical Association that was not dominated by the coal company, as were most of the others in Carbon County.

A committee made up equally of company and union personnel administered the association. The company representatives were the superintendents of each mine. The presidents of each union represented the miners. In 1937 this committee consisted of Terry McGowan and Charles Semken from Consumers, Lloyd Quinn and Ted Gentry from Sweets, plus Harry Elkins and Joe Matich from National. I attended the meetings but had no vote, and I never had any problems with this group.

The association charged $1.50 per month for a man with a family and $1.00 per month for a single man. Money was collected by the check-off system; it was automatically taken out of the miners' wages by the company and deposited to the association, which then paid the doctor, nurse, medical bills, office expenses, and hospital rent. All medicines were covered, as were office calls and house calls for any type of illness. Coverage did not extend to some surgical items; deliveries were $35 extra, tonsillectomies, $15, appendectomies, $125, and simple fractures, $15. Treatment for venereal diseases was also excluded. All the Gordon Creek companies either carried industrial insurance or were self-insured.

My salary was $300 per month. Consumers provided living quarters and an office. A small five-bed hospital equipped with x-ray,

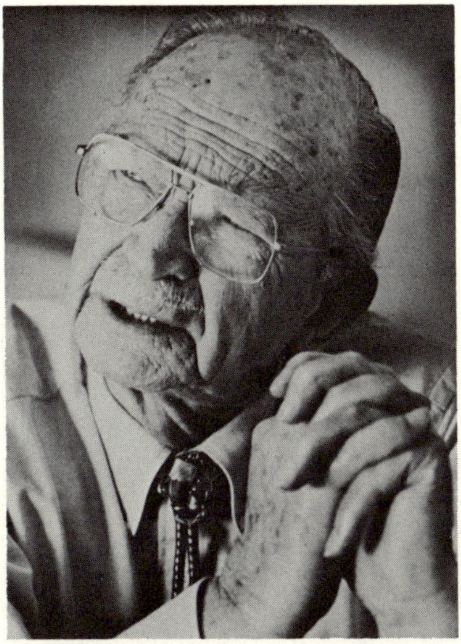

J. Eldon Dorman. Deseret News *photo.*

microscope, and other clinical laboratory facilities, besides a well-stocked drug room, were all operated by the doctor. Daily office hours were held, plus house calls to all three camps and visits to the Price hospital, where the most seriously injured patients were taken. During the winter the roads were often closed by snow.

The coal camp doctor helped to contribute to the morale of the miner and his family, often making the difference in the success or failure of a mining operation. The men insisted on having someone at the portal when they were hurt. This was why I got my job, although I did not know it until after I arrived in Consumers. The previous doctor had left during the Christmas vacation without telling anyone his destination and was gone for a week. A serious accident occurred at the mine, and the doctor was fired upon his return.

As the winter progressed, the demand for coal increased. My office was flooded with men waiting to be examined so they could go to work. The age limit was forty-five years. Strange as it may seem, I "never" had a patient who was over forty-five years of age. They would actually hide their canes and crutches outside my office. The physical examination was just a rough screening test. There were no pre-employment x-rays of chest or back, and anything that fooled the doctor was "legal." But welfare was not yet a way of life. All a coal miner asked for was a chance to work — to dig the coal to pay off his debts, feed and clothe his family, and perhaps send his son to school. He never missed a shift. Often he fought in line to get an extra shift or doubled back to work overtime without extra pay.

I hold a personal respect for the old-time Austrian, Italian, Greek, or Welsh coal miners. I still recall their nicknames — Flat Nose Mike, Fat Mary, Tony Bolony, and Mexican Joe. Each camp had several men known as Big John. The nicknames were always appropriate. A man called Buffalo came into my office one day. His incredible size prompted me to ask him the size of his pants. "Well, Mr. Doc," he replied, "these are fifty-six, but they're getting a bit snug."

I had a mine telephone in my office and one at home. If an accident happened, I was frequently requested to meet the more seriously injured at the portal. It was quite an uphill walk, so I started driving my car. No road existed, but I could drive almost to the mine entrance. The entrance stood in view of the entire town, however, and every woman in camp recognized my car. Soon each was standing on her front or back porch, wringing her hands on her apron and wondering if her husband or son was hurt or killed. I only drove up there twice. The ever-present fear of death in mine accidents, explosions, or afterdamp already haunted the families enough.

The practice of medicine was quite different in those times. No sulfa drugs or antibiotics were available. At Consumers we had a new portable oxygen tent which was extremely useful for treating pneumonia.

Of the various types of cough medicines, syrup of wild cherry was the most popular. It cost $2 per gallon, and I used to buy it in ten-gallon lots. One day I was over helping Dr. Ira Cummings in Standardville, and I mentioned the popularity of this syrup. He set me straight in a hurry. "You're stupid," he said. "Do you realize that a good portion of that syrup goes on these people's pancakes?" His statement was literally true. I watched for it and saw it happen. So, I thought I would

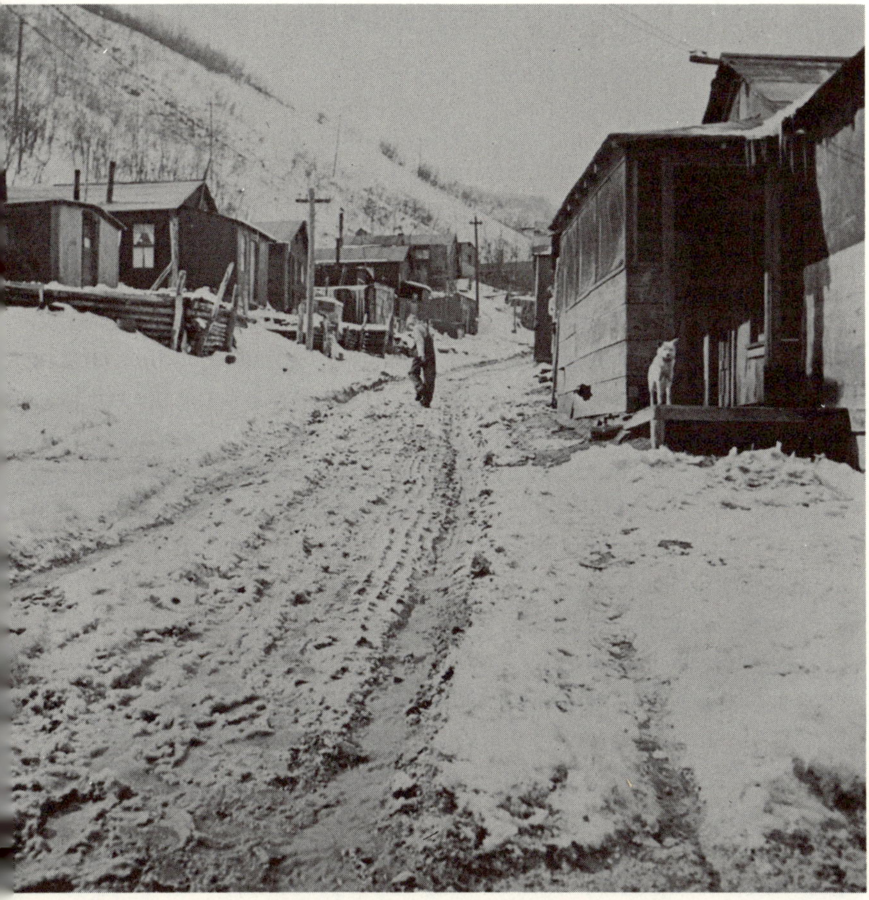

Main Street, Consumers, Carbon County Utah, in 1936. D. Lange.

stop this practice. I bought syrup of white pine tar, which had essentially the same ingredients but tasted terrible. The patients put up a fuss when I tried to switch. Elixir cheracol was another cough medicine used for pancakes. Elixir terpin hydrate with codeine (TH&C) cost $8 a gallon then. It contained 40% alcohol, which is equal to 80-proof vodka, and almost two grains of codeine. TH&C was a popular medicine. It cured a lot of things besides a cough.

The five kinds of aspirin came in different colors. The white and the green worked best for me. The pink and the orange did not seem very popular. Dr. Orson Spencer found it best to use the variegated color.

Mail-Order Nurse

When I first went to Consumers I was unable to find a nurse to assist me. I finally phoned California and by offering $125 per month was able to hire a registered nurse away from her $85-a-month job.

Over the years I continued to have nursing problems. One Catholic RN quit when I asked her to set up a tray for a male sterilization operation. It was simple: she said, "If you are going to do that kind of surgery, I quit." She walked out the door, literally leaving me with my patient's pants down.

In those days there were various correspondence schools offering nurses' training. At least one woman in camp took such a course. She was a young married woman, and I used her a lot both in the hospital under the supervision of the RN and to help me out with home deliveries. She was pleasant, willing, and hard-working.

I was glad to have her with me when I experienced a problem home delivery. The patient was in her early thirties. She had one child, a boy, about eleven years old. Eight previous, more or less full-term pregnancies had ended in stillbirths. She had come to me in about her fourth month of pregnancy. I had found her Wassermann to be a 4+, had treated her with mapharsen, and had hopes of getting a live baby. But when I next saw her, there was a new problem.

My nurse and I found that the baby was well on its way with the head partially exposed, but the patient's labor pains had stopped. I was afraid that the baby might start to breathe and choke to death in the birth canal. So I handed my nurse a 10-cc vial of pituitrin and a 2-cc syringe and said: "give her 2 minims right away." I thought I would have a few minutes for this drug to act, so I rushed into opening the sterile O.B. bundle and getting out sterile sheets, my sterile gown, gloves, and other necessary items. Somehow I chanced to look up just as the nurse injected the medication into the patient's arm. I stood spellbound with my mouth open but unable to say a word as I saw 2 cc instead of 2 minims, or sixteen times the amount I had asked for, being injected. I did not get my gloves or gown on but caught the baby in my open arms against my chest as it shot out of the birth canal like a shot from a cannon. It was alive and apparently healthy.

The baby's cord Wassermann was negative, but the people moved away, so I had no real follow-up. I do not think I even scolded my nurse. It was my fault for not checking whether or not she knew hypodermic dosages. I continued to use her when she was needed and appreciated her help.

Measles and Mumps and "One Night with Venus . . ."

The acute infectious diseases were a great menace in the coal camps. If one child showed up with the measles after a weekend visit to friends or relatives in Castle Valley, the disease spread like a plague to all the children of the three camps. Otitis media, a middle ear infection, was an almost certain complication of the measles in those days. I carried a myringotomy knife in my medical bag and opened many bulging eardrums as I made house calls. The adults did not escape the childhood diseases. I vividly remember an epidemic of mumps that swept the area like wildfire and resulted in the tragic illness of two young men that certainly changed their lifestyle.

Active immunization clinics were held each year for diphtheria, whooping cough, tetanus, typhoid, paratyphoid, and smallpox. In general, the response to these clinics was good.

The venereal diseases also posed a problem in the coal camps. The per capita rate of VD, however, was probably no greater in the coal camps than in Salt Lake City.

The biggest problem, of course, was that we did not have the proper medicines to handle these diseases. Gonorrhea often had to be treated for a year or more to effect a cure. Lues, or syphilis, was more serious. It was treated by various arsenicals such as "606" or mapharsen. Injections of mercury were often used in the chronic stages, which led to the well-worn medical cliche of the 1930s, "One night with Venus and the rest of your life with Mercury."

Each new case of venereal disease afforded considerable interest to the camp doctor. By simple observation and deduction he was able to trace its progress and to discover, often with surprise and amazement, who was doing what and to whom. Any coal mine doctor could have been a blackmail expert. For me, however, keeping the medical and social secrets of the camp was part of the fun.

Pool-Table Surgery

I never dared to leave camp on Saturday nights. These towns really cooked on weekends. Parties, fights, brawls — you name it, they did it with enthusiasm.

I was new in the Gordon Creek area when I received a midnight call on Saturday night to rush to the beer parlor at Sweets. This beer joint was something special. Its floor was covered with several inches of sawdust hiding the blood and gore of previous Saturday nights. I found an older man sitting in a chair against the wall with his head hanging down against his blood-covered chest. When I spoke to him he raised his head and revealed a cut on his throat from ear to ear that gaped open an inch or more. To my amazement I discovered that it was a superficial cut through the skin that exposed but did not damage the major blood vessels of the neck. I also noted that my patient was drunk.

I was disgusted, since I had already patched up several bloody noses and left quite a mess back at my office. There would be a problem transporting a drunk and bleeding patient to the office, probably in my car, to sew him up. Since there was a pool table in the saloon, I decided to work there. I took out a couple of small sterile towels and the necessary instruments and proceeded to sew the man up. This, despite the helpful and sometimes critical audience, did not take too long. The thump of the jukebox never died, and the drinking, smoking, and revelry only paused momentarily while my stitches were inspected.

As I did my barroom surgery I heard most of the story. I was surprised and chagrined to learn that my patient was the assistant mine foreman. He loved to drink and he loved to play poker. He had been doing plenty of both while the jukebox was pounding out polka after polka. Due to the chronic shortage of females in the Sweets beer joint, many of the Austrian men were dancing with each other. One Austrian fellow kept asking the mine foreman to dance with him, making quite a nuisance of himself. Finally, the foreman, more interested in poker and booze, cursed and told the fellow in no uncertain terms to leave him alone. The Austrian left but soon returned with an open clasp knife, stood behind the foreman's chair, and proceeded to cut his throat from left to right.

I had finished my throat repair job and was patching up the hand of Osby Martin, who had grasped the open blade of the assailant's knife as he wrestled it away from him, when somebody suggested, "Maybe you had better go see Sam" — the knife wielder. Then I found out the rest of the story.

When business was good, the right-hand end of the bar held an open case of warm beer. When he removed a cold beer from the cooler, the bartender could replace it with a warm one from the top of the bar. In the excitement of the knife episode, the bar patrons had proceeded to break thirteen full bottles of beer over Sam's head without knocking him out.

I found Sam at the bunkhouse, squatting in a galvanized tub of water and holding a bloody washcloth to his bleeding, lacerated scalp. I asked him how he felt. He looked up and said, "I feel pretty good, but I do got a leetle bit headache"! I spent the next few hours picking glass out of his bald head. I got back to my bed in Consumers just in time to hear the celebrants at the boarding house next door greet the dawn with loud, discordant verses of "It's Only a Shanty in Old Shanty Town."

Osby Martin

Osby Martin was a bachelor who lived in the Sweets mine bunkhouse. It was said that he had killed a man and served time in the Colorado penitentiary, and that he had been an exhibition shooter for the Winchester Repeating Arms Company.

Everyone in Sweets was scared of Osby. On occasion he would take his .30-.30 Winchester 94 rifle, stand in the main street in front of his bunkhouse, toss ordinary glass marbles in the air, and break them one by one. Many heated arguments in Sweets came to an end when Osby threatened to get his "Turty-Turty."

Osby had quite a racket going. The main line in the mine at Sweets used electric motors for haulage, but horses were still used for dispensing and gathering the coal cars to and from the various working entries. Osby Martin was one of the drivers who dispensed the cars. The miners at Sweets were paid fifty-five cents per ton for loading coal, but without coal cars they could not load the coal. If Osby failed to get his proper "cut" on payday, the miners failed to get the cars they needed. Eventually the situation became tense and a union meeting was called. The problem, however, was resolved outside the meeting. The Sweets union hall was reached by a narrow footbridge five or six feet above the small drainage creek that ran through the bottom of the canyon and was fed by the kitchen sinks, dishpans, and slop jars of the cabins lining its banks. Under several inches of slimy gray dishwater was about a foot of malodorous primeval ooze that not even a trilobite could live in.

The problems of the union hall boiled over onto the footbridge. A little five-foot-six-inch, 135-pound miner named Elmer Brinley confronted the brawny Osby. He landed a haymaker on Osby's chin that staggered him back against the flimsy railing. Osby sailed through the air, landing flat on his back in the ooze and slime.

Then the miners sent for me. I never understood why they never called the sheriff, the mine superintendent, or the mine foreman in these situations. Perhaps they thought my services were about to be needed and that I should be handy.

When I drove into Sweets at early dusk I found an armed camp. A man standing behind the corner of his house holding a six-shooter waved me up the road. The closer I came the more belligerent the situation looked, with a shotgun here, a deer rifle there, and an automatic pistol or two in the hands of determined coal miners. I was flagged to a stop by a couple of armed men shielded by a building. They told me that Osby was in his room. I was the logical one to go in and talk to him, they explained, since he might have been hurt in his fall from the bridge. So I pounded on his door. There was no answer, so I pounded again and said, "It's Doc." The door was unlocked and opened. Osby set the .30-.30 by the doorjamb. He had just finished taking a bath in a galvanized washtub. I hastened to sympathize with, and even magnify, his leg and chest injuries. I convinced him to go with me to the hospital at Consumers for x-rays and other first-aid treatment. We did not see a soul as we drove through and out of Sweets with the .30-.30 upright between Osby's legs.

I x-rayed him and bound up his wounds. When he complained of pain, I gave him some "pain" pills well laced with sleeping pills. It was now dark outside. I let him get a little drowsy, and he forgot about his .30-.30, which I had put out of sight. I delivered him back to his room and tucked him in. After a couple of days I took his gun back to him. I was told that this episode finished Osby's days of extortion at Sweets, and Elmer B. was the camp hero.

Father Ruel's Request

In 1937 the Catholic priest at Price was Father William A. Ruel and his assistant was Father Jerome Stoffel, just out of the seminary. They came to Consumers to see a patient for whom I had given up all hope. When the young six-months-pregnant woman had become seriously ill with pneumonia, the community was snowbound. I had her carried to the small mine hospital, where I put her in the new oxygen tent. Without penicillin or other antibiotics, my only hope for her was oxygen, but she had gone steadily downhill. The roads were cleared, but it seemed unwise to move her to the Price hospital, which had nothing more to offer than oxygen.

Quite early one cold, snowy morning, Fathers Ruel and Stoffel appeared and administered the last rites. But about this time another complication came up: she had gone into rather active premature labor. I explained the situation to Father Ruel and his quiet, somewhat shy, young assistant. It looked as if the mother was sure to die; she might, while breathing her last, give birth to an infant who might live but a short time.

I became busy with my other tasks of the day, pausing frequently to check my patient. At dusk I answered a somewhat demanding knock. It was Father Ruel, who needed to talk with me about a matter of great importance. He indicated that he, too, was a busy man, and many duties required his presence back in Price. He and his assistant had spent the entire day in the camps waiting for the baby to be born in order to baptize him, but they must leave at once. Therefore, he wanted me to baptize the new baby if he was born alive. Since I had been raised under a rigid Protestant family and educational regime, my face must have indicated some question. Father Ruel hastened to assure me that this procedure was ethical and honorable. He had me memorize the words that would save a tiny soul from Purgatory. I was further concerned when I thought I discerned a hint of skepticism in the eye of Father Stoffel, as if he, as surely I did, doubted my ability to say the proper words at the proper time and in the proper sequence. Perhaps someone up above was skeptical as well. In any event, within a few hours the premature labor pains stopped, and the patient went on to a rapid recovery from her pneumonia and eventually a normal full-term delivery.

Dental Practice

I was routed out of my bed early one Sunday morning by an older Austrian fellow still somewhat inebriated from a Saturday night party. He held his lower right jaw in both hands and swung his head back and forth and up and down as he moaned and groaned with a toothache. He could not stand still, but paced my office floor in agony, swinging his head in rhythm with his steps. I offered him pills or even a shot of morphine for his pain, but he had brought his own painkiller and proceeded to gulp at frequent intervals from a bottle of Old Crow.

He demanded in no uncertain terms that I pull the offending tooth. I explained that I was not a dentist and that he should visit one in Price or Helper. He objected strongly and pointed out several dental forceps in the glass-enclosed instrument case in the corner. He also informed me that a previous doctor had pulled a tooth for him with no problem. I argued against playing dentist while he took turns pleading and berating my ability. Finally, I reluctantly selected a formidable forceps as he pointed out the offending second molar with his forefinger. I thought his selection was questionable, since several other teeth looked worse. He insisted, however, so I applied the forceps and started to pull, twist, and yank. I gradually backed the patient and chair against the wall, put my knee on his chest, and, eventually, ended up with the tusk. The patient spat out a mouthful of blood in my wastebasket, took another slug of booze, and thanked me profusely as he backed out the door.

When I saw the patient on the street the next day, he ignored me completely. The following day the same thing happened. I wondered if he had been too intoxicated to remember what had happened. I could no longer endure his ungratefulness, so I asked him if he did not appreciate what I had done. He let forth a tirade of blasphemy, shook his fist under my nose, and said he had gone to see Dr. Joe Dalpiaz in Helper because I had pulled the wrong tooth!

Dr. Claude McDermid

Recent medical school graduates often came to Carbon County to work for mine companies, staying just long enough to accumulate enough money to return to the East and open up a practice. Utah historian Helen Papanikolas says that one of these young doctors, Claude McDermid, arrived in Sunnyside in 1911 to assist Dr. Andrew Dowd. After the financial deprivations of his schooling, he intended to stay only long enough to afford to buy another blue serge suit. He stayed.

After a year in Sunnyside, he became the Castle Gate company doctor and won the miners' respect. Florence Reynolds recalls waiting in his office when a new manager stormed in, bent on economizing. It was a cold day in winter, and the manager warned Dr. McDermid that he was going to turn off the electricity in the miners' company houses.

"You are not," said the young doctor.

"I am," the manager answered. "They don't need it and don't deserve it."

Whereupon Dr. McDermid rose to his full six-foot-six, hit the manager with his fist, and sent him sprawling.

Dr. McDermid practiced in Carbon County for twenty-eight years and was the Castle Gate company doctor at the time of the tragic 1924 explosion that took 172 lives. He and his three sons were left with rheumatic hearts from a bacterial epidemic, and he died soon after leaving Carbon County.

I did not have the physique or the ability to be as aggressive as Dr. McDermid, but this story illustrates how many of the early doctors were willing to jeopardize their jobs with the companies that hired them in defense of the coal miners and their families.

Immigrant Sons

Helen Papanikolas points out that "insults to the miners' dignity were commonplace." But the browbeaten first-generation immigrant could attain instant status and respect if he educated his son to be a doctor. One reason this was true, I believe, was that the camp doctor was one of the most respected people in the community.

A large number of Carbon County immigrants' sons became medical doctors and dentists. Often two sons in one family entered the respected professions. Second-generation Italian-American Charles Ruggeri, Jr., became an ophthalmologist, while his brother James practiced dentistry. A. R. and John Demman were another pair of Italian immigrant sons who practiced medicine. Drs. Nick and Mike Orfanakis were sons of a Greek immigrant. The Austrian Gorishek brothers, William and Frank, opened their practices in Carbon County. Today a number of second- and third-generation sons continue to contribute to the professions.

Then and Now

Two hundred miners died in the explosion at the Pleasant Valley Coal Company mine at Winter Quarters (Scofield) in 1900; another 172 men died at Castle Gate in 1924, not to mention dozens of smaller life-taking disasters and countless amputated arms and legs, shattered bones, and broken backs. Life was cheap. Workmen's Compensation did not exist. After the Winter Quarters catastrophe, families received

$500 for the loss of each life. The amputation of an arm or leg sometimes brought $300 to $500, *if* the company paid. It has been said that in the early days of coal mining the life of a miner approximated the value of a prize mine mule. These conditions no longer exist, but they are still part of the coal miners' heritage and must not be forgotten.

Today we are living in boom times, but not too long ago Carbon County was the Appalachia of Utah, the unwanted child. But without its coal, Utah's industries and power plants would grind to an abrupt halt.

Carbon County is also Utah's melting pot. At one time its immigrants outnumbered the "native" Americans. Thirty-two nationalities are recorded as having lived in Helper during the early part of this century. Due to its polyglot population — refined and tempered in the melting process — Carbon County supports a broader, more tolerant and cosmopolitan lifestyle that sets it apart from the rest of Utah. The Greeks, the Austrians, the Italians, the Welsh, the Finns, the Japanese, the Chicanos, and the Native Americans have all left their imprint on its rough, often cruel, yet proud heritage.

I am glad and proud that I had a chance to participate in the formation of this heritage. I am glad and proud that I live and work in Carbon County.

CHAPTER THREE

The Practice of Internal Medicine

A. HAMER REISER, JR., MD

MANY OF THE EARLIEST MEDICAL PRACTITIONERS in Utah Territory were followers of the Botanical or Thomsonian system of medicine, an herbalistic folk medicine which some offered part-time in addition to their work as farmers, shopkeepers, horse breeders, and cattlemen. Their philosophy was "puke 'em, sweat 'em, and purge 'em." The Thomson diploma cost $20.00 and conferred the title of "Doctor" upon the holder, entitling him also to use and sell the medicines secured by Samuel Thomson.

After the Civil War the unskilled practiced throughout the Territory. Later, as doctors began arriving who had graduated from recognized medical schools, their practices were of a general nature, caring for any medical problem which arose. It was not until near the turn of the century that doctors appeared in Utah who had special postgraduate training in and limited their practices to internal medicine.

Dr. Albert Leonard Castleman was the leading internist of St. Mark's Hospital during his time, the first thoroughly trained internist to be appointed to the staff. He graduated from McGill University in 1888, came to Utah and settled in Bingham Canyon in 1892, then moved to Mercur from 1895 to 1903. When the Utah Copper Mine at Bingham Canyon was opened, Mr. Daniel Jackling (president of Utah Copper Company) asked Dr. Castleman to be in charge of the medical department, a position he assumed after a year of postgraduate train-

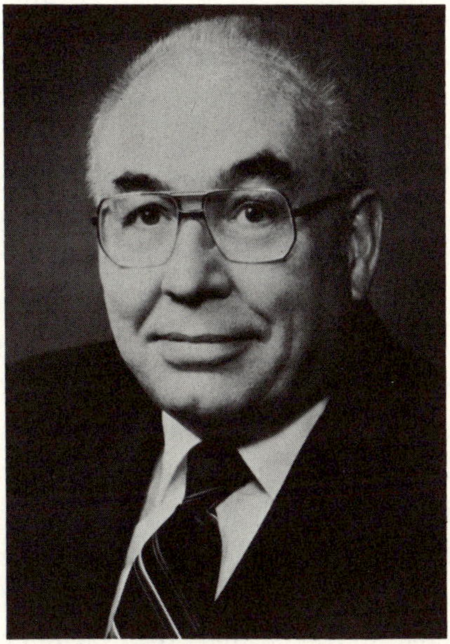

A. Hamer Reiser, Jr.

ing at Johns Hopkins (1903–04). He remained at Bingham until 1907, when he moved his office to Salt Lake City.

Dr. Castleman was a man of omnivorous interests. An accomplished pianist, he enjoyed listening to good music and was an avid reader of good books. He traveled extensively, observed keenly, enjoyed the companionship of good friends, and was known for his charming smile and kindly ways. He enjoyed playing poker, although the stakes were never high. Dr. Castleman retired in 1929 because of poor health and moved to Santa Monica, California, where he died in 1941.

Dr. Clarence Snow was born in St. George, Utah, in 1874. He graduated from Harvard College in 1897 with a degree in electrical engineering and was invited by the General Electric Company to work as a research assistant to Charles Steinmetz. After two years he returned to Utah and became professor of mathematics and physics at the Utah State Agricultural College in Logan. After four years at USAC he went on a mission for the LDS Church in 1902. In 1904 he entered the medical school at the University of Michigan, graduating in 1908. Internships were not required at the time, so he began his practice in Salt Lake City that year and became a member of the Salt Lake Clinic when it was organized in 1915. He had special training in pathology in medical school, so he was in charge of pathology as well as an associate in internal medicine at LDS Hospital.

Dr. Snow was especially interested in problems of clinical diagnosis and was helpful as a consultant. Always concerned with education, he served on the Board of Regents of the University of Utah for thirteen years. Dr. Snow was the first doctor in Utah to own an electrocardiograph machine, the first physician in Utah to use the newly developed Salvarsan in the treatment of syphilis, and the state's pioneer blood transfusionist long before any pre-transfusion testing for incompatibilities was available. A master conversationalist, he was the first doctor on the staff of Dr. W. H. Groves' Latter-day Saints' Hospital who could be classified as an internist. His wide knowledge of internal medicine and keen diagnostic acumen earned him the sobriquet "the doctors' doctor" until his death in 1938.

The first Fellows of the American College of Physicians (ACP) in the Utah region were Drs. G. Gill Richards and William Rich, who were elected in 1920, five years after the College was incorporated. The first College membership directory (1928) lists four more Utah Fellows: Maurice Critchlow, T. C. Gibson, Leon Shackell, and Frank Steele.

At the eleventh annual ACP meeting in 1927, Drs. Richards and L. L. Daines presented a paper, "Recent Observations on Pernicious Anemia." They summarized fifty cases hospitalized at Dr. W. H. Groves' Latter-day Saints' Hospital from 1915 through 1925 and concluded that, "the results of treatment, i.e., diet and dilute hydrochloric acid, were entirely discouraging; benefits from transfusions were often striking, but only temporary; splenectomy possibly prolonged remission . . . . There were only three survivals." The paper was the first by Utah physicians to be published in the *Annals of Internal Medicine*.

In the early 1940s Drs. Richards, Fuller B. Bailey, William R. Tyndale, and Louis E. Viko were the only physicians in Salt Lake City with formal training in internal medicine. Dr. Viko later limited his practice to cardiology.

Dr. Tyndale was born in Iowa in 1873, a small, wiry man with a quick, spry step. An excellent clinician and diagnostician, he was the first thoroughly trained internist to serve on the Holy Cross Hospital staff. He graduated from Rush Medical College in Chicago and served an internship at Presbyterian Hospital, after which he spent eighteen months in Berlin and Vienna, the Meccas of medicine at the time, studying pathology and diagnosis. He came to Salt Lake City in 1904 and soon developed a reputation as a skilled diagnostician. He practiced alone at first, later joining a group which eventually became the Intermountain Clinic.

Dr. Ralph T. Richards wrote of him, "Dr. Tyndale had the fine attributes of a real physician. He was a man of character. He knew his business. He was extremely careful in all the details that go into making a diagnosis. He maintained his interest in his patients at all times, no matter how rough the going. Above all, he had sympathy, not of the emotional type that is so enervating to the giver, but of the intellectual and constructive kind which makes the patient's welfare the guiding motive for all his treatment" (page 72 of *Medicine, Hospitals & Doctors*, University of Utah Press, 1953). Dr. Tyndale served as president of the Utah State Medical Association, 1936–37. He retired in 1945 and moved to California; he died in 1948.

Dr. G. Gill Richards was born in Mendon, Utah, in 1883 and graduated from the New York University School of Medicine in 1906. He practiced with his father as a family doctor for four years. In 1910 he went to Vienna to study for a year, later returning to Vienna and Berlin for two more years. In 1915 he was one of the founders of the Salt Lake Clinic. He became a member of the American College of Physicians in 1920, serving as governor from the Utah Region from 1927 to 1934 and as regent from 1934 to 1937. He developed a national reputation as a fine internist and served as second vice president of the American College of Physicians, 1937–38. In 1932 he was chairman of the Section on Internal Medicine of the American Medical Association. A founder of the American Board of Internal

Medicine in 1936, he was a member of the committee of examiners for ten years.

Dr. Richards was a master clinician. He made diagnoses by carefully obtaining detailed case histories and by using his senses in physical examination. A great bedside teacher, he loved to gather a group of medical students or house staff around a bed, where he would ask one to examine the heart disease patient and describe what murmurs one could expect to hear. The unsuspecting youngster would reach immediately for his stethoscope and place it on the patient's chest. Dr. Richards would say, "Let me hold your stethoscope," and after pocketing it would say, "Now go ahead with your examination." The poor student would be completely disarmed and unable to proceed.

Dr. Richards would then explain how the clinician looks at the patient's lips and skin color, looks at the neck veins, and looks for a capillary pulse by gently compressing the patient's fingernail. He carried a glass slide in his pocket which he pressed against the mucosa of the patient's lip to demonstrate a capillary pulse. He demonstrated how to feel the precordium and to differentiate between wide, heaving precordial thrusts and more circumscribed, forceful thrusts. He showed how to feel for precordial thrills. He demonstrated how to feel in the suprasternal notch to detect dilated, pulsatile aortas. Syphilitic aortic aneurysms were not uncommon at that time. He would percuss or feel for an enlarged liver. He would look for edema of the feet or legs or sacral area. He showed how to palpate radial and brachial arteries and pulses to estimate blood pressure and the degree of hardening of arteries. He showed how to feel femoral and dorsalis pedis pulses. Then, after discussing what murmurs were likely to be heard, he would allow the students to place their stethoscopes on the patient's chest: The murmurs heard were usually exactly as he had predicted.

Dr. Richards' warm personality inspired confidence in his patients, many of whom said they felt better as soon as he came into the room. He literally followed his patients who needed surgery right into the operating room. He would poke his head through the door and ask the surgeon what he had found. If necessary, he would put on a cap and mask to go to the surgeon's side for a better look. He was keenly interested in correlating the clinical history and findings with the surgical or pathological findings. Dr. Richards, the ideal physician, died in Boston in 1950 while attending the annual convention of the American College of Physicians.

Dr. Louis E. Viko, born in Park City, Utah, in 1896, attended the University of Utah and graduated from Harvard Medical School in 1920, helping to pay his tuition by working as an instructor in the anatomy laboratory. He returned to Salt Lake City and practiced with his father for a few months. In 1921 he returned to Massachusetts General Hospital, where he worked for a year under the tutelage of Dr. Paul Dudley White. In 1929 he went to London for a year to study with Sir Thomas Lewis and later studied in Vienna. He was appointed Salt Lake City Health Commissioner in 1932 and served until 1936. For several years he was a member of the Board of Regents of the University of Utah and was instrumental in effecting the change of the Medical School from a two-year to a four-year school. A member of the Intermountain Clinic, he also served on the staffs at LDS and Holy Cross hospitals. From 1934 to 1949 he was governor of the Utah Region of the American College of Physicians, and he served as president of the Utah State Medical Association, 1943–44.

Dr. Viko, like his close personal friend Dr. Richards, was a slight, wiry, quick-moving man. He was keenly analytical and perceptive, yet soft-spoken, modest, humble, and a devoted family man. Drs. Viko and Richards were highly ethical practitioners. When they were asked to see a patient as a consultant, each insisted that the attending physician introduce them formally to the patient. They had an agreement that if a patient left either of them to be attended by the other, each would report to the other so they would know if anything had been missed. They insisted that patients notify the current physician of their intention to change doctors.

Dr. Fuller B. Bailey was a handsome, distinguished-looking man, born in Imperial, Nebraska, in 1896. He attended Hastings College in Nebraska and graduated from Rush Medical College in Chicago. After postgraduate training in internal medicine at Presbyterian

Hospital in Chicago, he took more postgraduate training in Vienna. He started his practice in Salt Lake City in 1923 and was a member of the staff at Holy Cross Hospital. He served as governor of the Utah Region of the American College of Physicians from 1949 to 1954; was regent of the ACP from 1954 to 1962 and second vice president in 1963–64.

Dr. James Rex Miller was born in Price, Utah. He attended the University of Utah two-year medical school from 1932 to 1934, then transferred to Northwestern University School of Medicine, graduating in 1936. He served an internship at St. Luke's Hospital in Chicago until July 1937, when he came to Salt Lake City to serve a preceptorship with Dr. Gill Richards at the Salt Lake Clinic. In 1939 he began a fellowship in internal medicine at the Mayo Clinic, where he associated until April 1944, when he was called to active duty in the Navy. After serving for two years he returned to the Salt Lake Clinic and the LDS Hospital staff in 1946. From 1967 to 1973 he served as Governor of the Utah Region of the American College of Physicians.

Dr. Wesley E. Peltzer was the first post-war Mayo Clinic–trained internist on the St. Mark's Hospital staff. He became chairman of the interns' committee and played an important role in the teaching program. Dr. Robert M. Dalrymple, a graduate of Cornell and a resident in internal medicine at the University of Utah and VA hospitals, began his practice in 1949. Dr. John F. Waldo, the first specialist in infectious disease and a faculty member at the University of Utah School of Medicine, moved to St. Mark's Hospital in 1956 to become the part-time director of medical education.

Dr. Roy E. McDonald spent his early life in Erie, Pennsylvania. He attended Pennsylvania State University and was graduated from Temple Medical School. After his internship in Erie and two years of military service, he served a residency in internal medicine at the Veterans Administration Hospital in Maryland. There he met Dr. John Bowers, who invited him to come to the University of Utah Medical School. In 1950 he joined the faculty, performing research on radiation injury in dogs. Dr. McDonald joined the medical staff of St. Mark's Hospital in 1953, serving periods as chief of the medical service, medical education director, and president of the staff. In his early days at St. Mark's, working part time in the psychiatry division of the new Ft. Douglas VA Hospital, he was involved in drug research with psychiatric patients. He established the climate for the first therapeutic patient government in Utah. While previously the average length of hospital stay had been seven years, he was successful in discharging long-term hospitalized patients at the rate of two per month. He also did research with calcium-47 in renal stone formers and had a lifelong interest in hyperparathyroidism.

Internists began to practice in Ogden in the early 1940s. Dr. J. G. Olson opened his practice there in the mid-1940s after special training in internal medicine at Northwestern University and in Vienna and London. He died in 1975.

Drs. Drew Peterson and Donald Moore, who arrived in Ogden in the later forties, were instrumental in establishing a one-year residency in internal medicine at the Dee Hospital. Dr. Floyd W. Seager was the first resident in internal medicine under this program, which he completed in 1949. Dr. Seager later became a charter member of the Ogden Clinic. Other early internists at the Ogden Clinic were Drs. W. P. Daines and Don Dee Olsen. Dr. Daines became president of the American Society of Internal Medicine and was the medical director of the McKay-Dee Hospital in Ogden.

Many excellent internists played a major role through the fifties into the seventies as primary care physicians and diagnosticians, but also as consultants in the entire area of medicine. They formed the mainstay of most of the clinics and served as the major source of referrals for specialists in their organizations. They took a very personal interest in their patients and many were known to make house calls. Some distinguished themselves as outstanding teachers, such as Dr. Alan Lindsay, especially in cardiology and electrocardiography, or Dr. Alan Nelson, who became only the second Utah physician elected to the national presidency of the AMA.

The increasing subspecialization that started in the sixties changed medicine from a thinking to a doing field, and the number of residents remaining general internists dwindled. Unfortunately it has been increasingly difficult to find internists in the cities who will provide primary care, and the family practitioners have had to step into this void.

Special tribute is due a group of physicians in many specialties who were able to involve themselves in academic pursuits with significant scientific output while working full time in the three major private hospitals — LDS, Holy Cross, and St. Mark's — as well as Primary Children's Medical Center in conjunction with the Medical School and University Hospital. Some of these held full-time University appointments and some clinical appointments; some were on full-time or part-time salaries at the respective hospitals, and some were entirely dependent on their own private practices. The enormous contribution of this dedicated group to medical teaching and research is inestimable.

CHAPTER FOUR

Cardiology

HIROSHI KUIDA, MD

THE APPROXIMATELY FIFTY-YEAR HISTORY of cardiology in Utah owes its rapid and significant expansion to the arrival of Dr. Hans H. Hecht at the new four-year College of Medicine, but it began with Dr. Louis E. Viko. Dr. Viko had been practicing cardiology at the Intermountain Clinic in Salt Lake City for thirteen years when Dr. Hecht arrived in 1944. Dr. Viko obtained his medical education at Harvard Medical School (1920) and his postgraduate training in cardiology at the Massachusetts General Hospital, where he worked under Dr. Paul White, the acknowledged dean of American cardiologists; in London, under the legendary Sir Thomas Lewis; and in Vienna before returning to Salt Lake City in 1931. Everyone recognized Dr. Viko as the dean of Utah cardiologists and accorded him the honor and respect that were his due. A warm and congenial friendship existed between Viko and Hecht throughout Hecht's twenty-year stint in Utah.

This spirit between town and gown is nowhere more evident than in their collaborative effort with Dr. William Ray Rumel in launching the Utah chapter of the American Heart Association in the early fifties. Significantly, Dr. Viko was elected its first president. Dr. Hecht was instrumental in establishing the L. E. Viko Chair of Cardiology at the Medical School, which was sponsored by the Heart Association through its research grant program and was a fitting honor to Dr. Viko. Dr. Hecht was its first occupant, from 1957 to 1964, and the chair provided an important source of support ($10,000 per year) for his academic position in the Department of Internal Medicine. It permitted Utah to stay abreast of and contribute to the explosion of cardiologic knowledge, technology, and manpower requirements following World War II.

Dr. Viko was a staunch supporter of the establishment of the four-year Medical School. As one of the three senior members of the clinical faculty of the Department of Medicine in its early days (with Drs. Gill Richards and Ted Bauerline), he was a consistent and enthusiastic participant in its clinical educational programs. When Dr. Hiroshi Kuida was chief medical resident in 1957–58, he had occasion to arrange Professor's Rounds with the junior ward clerks, and Dr. Viko often substituted when Dr. Wintrobe was out of the city. The cordial town-and-gown precedent continued to be important. An example of this legacy is the late Dr. Alan E. Lindsay, a former internal medicine resident and Dr. Viko's associate at the Intermountain Clinic. Few clinical faculty members demonstrated a commitment to clinical teaching to match Dr. Lindsay's throughout his long and distinguished professional career.

During the forties and early fifties many internal medicine specialists, such as Dr. Lindsay, began focusing on areas of special interest. In so doing, they became de facto subspecialists without the formal training that was only then becoming commonly available in academic centers. Among those in cardiology can be counted Dr. Harold Brown, associate chief of medicine at the Salt Lake Veterans Administration Hospital and a faculty member in internal medicine. One reason for Dr. Brown's interest in cardiovascular disease was the inordinate commonness of both acute rheumatic fever and rheumatic valvular heart diseases in the veteran population that expanded rapidly after the war. Not only was rheumatic fever endemic in the Intermountain region, an epidemic of the disease had occurred at the Navy boot camp at Farragut, Idaho, during the war.

Other formally trained or de facto cardiologists of this era in private practice were: Drs. Kenneth Crockett of the Salt Lake Clinic, James Orme and Wally Sorenson of the Memorial Medical Center, Wesley Peltzer, George Curtis and Irving Ershler in Salt Lake City,

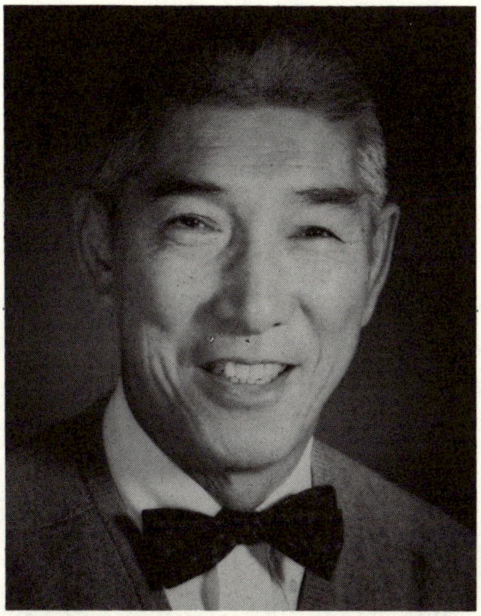

Hiroshi Kuida.

Drew Peterson of Ogden, and John Rupper of Provo. Most of these leading internist-cardiologists served terms as president of the Utah Heart Association in its early years.

Dr. Orme spearheaded expansion of cardiology at the Memorial Medical Center by recruiting several newly trained cardiologists, including Dr. Wallace Jenkins (Utah 1955), a Hecht trainee; Dr. David W. Richards (Utah 1951), who received his cardiology training at Massachusetts General and preceded Kuida as one of Dr. Wintrobe's chief medical residents; and later Dr. William Vincent, a trainee of the program who came to Utah with Dr. J. A. Abildskov.

At the Salt Lake Clinic, Crockett and Dr. Ernest Wilkinson were rapidly followed by Dr. Alan Barker (Utah 1952) and, later, Dr. Michael Preece (Utah 1969).

Dr. Hecht's boundless energy, deep devotion, natural talent, and productivity in basic and clinical research quickly resulted in his achieving a national and international reputation as an academician, scientist, and clinical cardiologist. His achievement netted the financial support for establishing the first modern cardiac catheterization laboratory in the western U.S., for creation of the first cardiac microelectrode laboratory in the world, for doing basic and clinical studies in pulmonary hypertension, for continuing studies in basic and clinical electrophysiology (with the late Dr. Lowell Woodbury) and electrocardiography, and for establishing cardiology training programs at both the undergraduate and graduate levels under the aegis of the National Heart Institute.

Many students of the early four-year Medical School were made aware of cardiology as an important and rapidly growing subspecialty of internal medicine, which influenced their careers. Most notable among these were two Utah alumni, Drs. J. A. Abildskov (1946) and Homer R. Warner (1949), who worked with Hecht at different phases early in their training and who later achieved world-class status as scientists and academicians equaling that of their former teacher. Both returned to Utah, where they replicated his model of academic achievement with their own large-scale programs.

Other students or residents who caught the cardiology bug deserve recognition. While they are now scattered all over America, and a few foreign countries, many remained in Utah. One of the earliest Hecht trainees in this category is Dr. Merrill C. Daines (Utah 1943), the first cardiologist to settle in Logan, in the fifties. Likewise, the first trained cardiologist in Ogden was Dr. C. Basil Williams (Utah 1956). Ogden cardiology took a quantum leap forward when Dr. Farrell Calton, a later Hecht trainee, set up the first cardiac catheterization laboratory outside the confines of Salt Lake City at McKay-Dee Hospital in 1965. The first formally trained cardiologist in Provo, Utah, was the late Dr. Leland Briggs (Utah 1958), the first trainee following Kuida's appointment in 1964.

Hecht's role in the development of pediatric cardiology in Utah deserves to be chronicled. Pediatricians of Hecht's early days at Utah obviously had a long and abiding interest in acute rheumatic fever (ARF). In fact, the commonness of the problem in the pediatric inpatient service at the Salt Lake General Hospital (SLGH) led to the appointment of Dr. Vincent C. Kelley, an ARF specialist, to the pediatrics faculty in 1948. New and exciting developments in pediatric cardiovascular surgical procedures, such as patent ductus arteriosus ligation (PDA) and so-called "blue-baby" operations, stimulated interest in congenital heart disease. The advent of pediatric cardiac catheterization as pioneered in the late forties and early fifties by Dr. André Cournand at Columbia, Dr. Rudolph Bing at Hopkins, Drs. Lewis Dexter and Alexander Nadas at Harvard, and Dr. Earl Wood at the Mayo Clinic was also decisive.

Hecht was intrepid. With no particular prior clinical experience or training in pediatric cardiology, beginning in the early fifties he dedicated his cardiac catheterization laboratory at the SLGH to the diagnosis of pediatric as well as adult cardiovascular disorders. One of his early colleagues, Dr. Harry Stoeckle of the pediatrics department, left Utah to head up the pediatric cardiology program at the University of Missouri, Columbia.

Dr. L. George Veasy (Utah 1946) was the next pediatric cardiologist. Having received his formal training at the University of Minnesota, he returned to Utah to work with Hecht in 1952. Later Veasy was to set up pediatric cardiac catheterization at LDS Hospital, working with Dr. Homer Warner, and also at the Primary Children's Medical Center (PCMC), where he has had a distinguished career as its medical director.

Dr. Lorin Ainger followed Veasy as the pediatric cardiologist in Hecht's lab at the SLGH. Dr. Ainger left Utah to accept a position at St. Jude's Hospital in Memphis, Tennessee. Dr. Douglas Heiner succeeded Dr. Ainger in 1960 and was the pediatric cardiologist when Kuida succeeded Hecht in 1965, but Heiner decided on a career change and left Utah for training in pediatric immunology. Pediatric cardiology became a fully independent subspecialty with the appointment of Dr. Herbert Ruttenberg as its chief in 1969 and the amalgamation of the cardiology programs at the PCMC and University of Utah Hospital. Thus Hecht's interests, concerns, and impact extended beyond adult cardiology.

Cardiology in the Community Hospitals

No account of Utah cardiology can be complete without a description of developments at LDS, Holy Cross, and other Utah hospitals.

Although Dr. Homer Warner is widely recognized for his contributions in biomedical computing science (now Medical Informatics), his first major accomplishment was establishing the cardiac catheterization laboratory as well as the computer center at the LDS Hospital in 1954. While not trained primarily as a clinical cardiologist, Dr. Warner acquired cardiac catheterization expertise during his studies with physiologist Dr. Earl Wood, whose Mayo Clinic laboratory was world renowned. Warner brought the Wood oximeter technology to Hecht's laboratory in 1953 before moving to LDS Hospital.

Demand for a second and independent catheterization laboratory at LDS Hospital was dictated by the rapid escalation of adult and pediatric cardiovascular surgical procedures there owing to a growing cardiologic and cardio-thoracic surgical staff. Warner was recruited from Hecht's staff to satisfy this demand. Drs. Ray Rumel and Preston Cutler had pioneered surgical developments in the early fifties (PDA closure, mitral commissurotomy), but procedures and surgeons grew rapidly in number, making a diagnostic facility a necessity. Drs. Alan Toronto and Veasy did most of the procedures in the early days. Application of computer technology to these catheterizations, as well as physiological studies in animals, led to Warner's growing recognition as a computer specialist and biophysiologist par excellence. The ever-increasing number of qualified "invasive" cardiologists, more CV-thoracic surgical groups, and the advent of coronary artery bypass graft surgery resulted in the lab's being expanded and made accessible to all appropriately trained staff.

The cardiologic service at LDS Hospital continued to grow rapidly. When echocardiography was emerging as a clinically useful diagnostic procedure, Dr. Douglas Ridges (Utah 1964) was recruited from Stanford to head up the new laboratory. In rather quick succession, Dr. Marshall moved over from Holy Cross, Dr. Arthur Hagen was recruited to lead the cardiology section, and in 1982 Dr. Michael Vincent (Utah 1967), a Hopkins-trained cardiologist from the University staff, was appointed chief of medicine. Dr. Frank Yanowitz, a former fellow of Dr. Abildskov, was recruited to head a preventive cardiology program. When Dr. Hagen resigned in 1985, Dr. Jeffrey Anderson from the University of Michigan took his place. Many newly trained cardiologists joined the staffs of virtually all major Utah hospitals during the seventies, primarily as a consequence of technological developments in the management of every aspect of coronary heart disease.

The third Salt Lake City–based cardiac catheterization laboratory was established at Holy Cross in 1962. A friend of Dr. Warner's from the Mayo Clinic, Dr. Hiram Marshall, was recruited to direct this facility. Thus all three Salt Lake City labs shared similar Wood oximetric technology. Dr. Marshall subsequently (1971) joined Dr. Warner at LDS, and the Holy Cross lab was headed by Dr. Thomas Keith from the Utah program.

Expansion and modernization of other private centers followed quickly, including new labs at the Utah Valley Medical Center headed by Dr. John Frischknecht, new St. Mark's Hospital Medical Center, and the Cottonwood Hospital Medical Center — a prodigious expansion of cardiologic resources in Utah.

A federal initiative which had an impact on cardiology in Utah was the Cancer, Heart Disease and Stroke program, formally entitled Regional Medical Program (RMP). As a facet of his Great Society campaign, President Lyndon Johnson decided to try to conquer these common major disorders through education and demonstration projects. The RMP was separate from basic and applied research budgets but directed by the National Institutes of Health (NIH). A lot of money was spent during the late sixties, and Utah was in the thick of that spending, due in no small part to the aggressive vigor of the local leadership provided by Dr. Hilmon Castle, then a faculty member in cardiology and internal medicine at the Medical School. The Intermountain Regional Medical Program (IRMP) was among the most successful in the country and received liberal funding for its multifaceted programs. The RMP accomplished rapid dissemination of physician, nursing, and paramedical education and training in the state-of-the-art diagnosis and management of myocardial infarction, or heart attack.

The RMP was instrumental in the setting up of acute coronary care units in hospitals large and small throughout the country, including the IRMP region. This was most certainly the beginning of heightened public as well as general medical awareness of intensive care technology, hypertension, and coronary heart disease. Dr. Alexander Schmidt (Utah 1954), another cardiologist and internist at the University, was recruited in 1967 by the national director of the RMP to assist in directing the federal program. This experience eventually led to his appointment by President Gerald Ford as Food and Drug Administration (FDA) Commissioner. This Utah cardiologist, who had been dean of the Abraham Lincoln School of Medicine (Chicago), later became vice chancellor (CEO) for medical affairs at the Chicago campus of the University of Illinois.

Dr. Castle went on to become the first chair of the Department of Family and Community Medicine at Utah. Having succeeded at this as well, Castle has since retired from academia to an active cardiology practice. It should be noted that Castle, also as a consequence of his IRMP role, was the director of the Salt Lake component of the landmark VA Cooperative study on treatment of hypertension and of the community-based Hypertension Detection and Follow-up Project in Utah. These population-based epidemiologic studies, with the IRMP Cancer Registry and prior human genetic studies in Utah kindreds (hereditary nephritis, hemochromatosis, and cancer), provided the general framework for more ambitious population-based human genetic studies.

During the 1963-64 academic year, Dr. Hecht spent a sabbatical in Europe. As the senior member of his staff, Kuida served as acting chief of cardiology during his absence. On his return, Hecht was vigorously and successfully recruited for the chair of the cardiology division at the University of Chicago, where major expansion was planned. Not long after he had accomplished this expansion, he was elevated to the chair of the Department of Internal Medicine.

About the time Hecht left Salt Lake City in the late fall of 1964, Dr. Wintrobe offered, and Kuida accepted, the position as Hecht's successor. While he was acting chief, Kuida had been involved in difficult and complex negotiations with Dr. Wintrobe, Dean Castleton, and others concerning the problem of the academic cardiovascular surgery program following the departure of Dr. Russell Nelson to private practice at the Salt Lake Clinic. The staff was in the middle of moving the operation to the new University Hospital, and Kuida was actively recruiting both Dr. Arthur M. Brown (another former Utah medical resident and cardiology fellow) to head up a new physiologic research laboratory and Dr. Theofilos Tsagaris (also a former fellow) to lead a new cardiology section at the Salt Lake VA Hospital. Dr. Schmidt, in the midst of setting up his new and modern cardiac catheterization laboratory at the University Hospital, decided to stay in Utah rather than go to Chicago with Hecht. Dr. Tsagaris returned from Marquette University in Milwaukee, Wisconsin, in 1965 and set up a cardiac catheterization laboratory at the VA Hospital in 1972. He established an outstanding cardiology section in which, over the years, he has personally trained nearly a hundred cardiologists. During his tenure, cardiologic care at the Salt Lake Veterans Administration Medical Center has been second to none in the entire country, and Dr. Tsagaris is legendary as a teacher.

Dr. Ramon Lange, a Wisconsin native and graduate of Duke University School of Medicine, came to Utah for medical residency training, stayed on as a cardiology fellow, and continued on the faculty in 1953 as one of Dr. Hecht's first full-time colleagues. Intrigued by inquiries being made in the mid-fifties by Dr. Joseph Thorne (at that time a veterinarian at Utah State University), Drs. Lange and Hecht embarked, with Thorne's help, on their famous hemodynamic studies of so-called Brisket or pulmonary hypertensive heart disease in Utah cattle. Dr. Thorne, stimulated by this experience, subsequently entered medical school (Utah 1961), completed both medical residency and cardiology training at Utah, and eventually joined the cardiology faculty himself. Dr. Lange left Utah in 1961 to assume the chair of cardiology at Marquette University School of Medicine in Milwaukee.

During the year before he left Utah for Washington in 1967, Dr. Schmidt headed an institutional planning effort (as an associate dean under Dr. Castleton) to examine the feasibility of establishing an interdepartmental cardiovascular center of excellence under the aegis of another NIH initiative. Dr. Wintrobe, who had stepped down as department chair, took over the planning effort. Dr. Abildskov, re-recruited by Dr. Wintrobe, brought two senior cardiology faculty members — Drs. Mary Jo Burgess and C. Kay Millar — to establish the Cardiovascular Research and Training Institute, into which Dr. Brown's laboratory was amalgamated. This major, multifaceted research enterprise grew, flourished, and was a huge and enduring success by every measure. Eventually, with major funding from the Nora Eccles Harrison Foundation, a new research building was dedicated in 1983 to house expanding operations and staff. Dr. Stephen M. Prescott, another former Utah medical resident and cardiology fellow, had returned in 1982 from Washington University in St. Louis, where he had been sent by George Cartwright expressly to obtain specialized biochemical training with Dr. P. W. Majerus. Prescott quickly became a nationally recognized biochemist and academician in his own right.

Another outstanding back-to-Utah recruit in 1976 was Dr. Roger Williams (Utah 1971). Dr. Williams had gone to Duke University Hospital for internal medicine residency training and then to the NIH in Bethesda, Maryland, where he was involved in epidemiological research and acquired expertise in computer technology. Dr. Williams became head of the Cardiovascular Genetics Research Center, which would utilize computerized LDS Church genealogical data for pinpointing study populations. He was enormously successful in garnering some of the largest NIH research grants in the history of the University, and he has earned a worldwide reputation in the field of epidemiology and genetics of hypertension and coronary heart disease.

Dr. Cartwright resigned as chair of Medicine and was eagerly looking forward to devoting himself to research and teaching. Dr. Kuida was planning to step down himself after fifteen years as cardiology head, having survived a heart attack and emergency coronary artery bypass graft surgery three years earlier. While he was on a trip in the east in 1980, Kuida learned with shock and horror of

Dr. Cartwright's sudden and unexpected coronary death. The shockingly premature deaths of three of Kuida's closest academic associates (Drs. Cartwright, Hecht, and Lange) in a brief time span produced a sense of loss from which he has yet to recover.

When Dr. Odell took over the reins of the department in 1981, Kuida's stepping down (in 1982) seemed timely, natural, and appropriate. It set the stage for the subsequent recruitment of Dr. Jay Mason from Stanford, who, with the large and strong cadre of cardiologic associates he recruited, in a mere half-dozen years has lifted academic and statewide cardiology to new heights of excellence. The history of that accomplishment undoubtedly will be written elsewhere. Drs. Wintrobe, Viko, and Hecht deserve to be proud of what they spawned here.

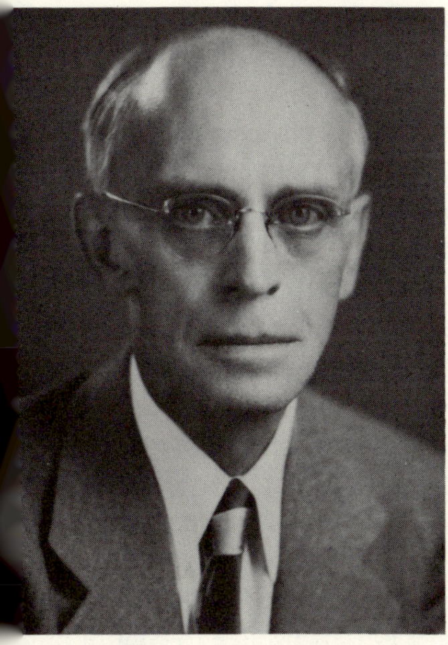

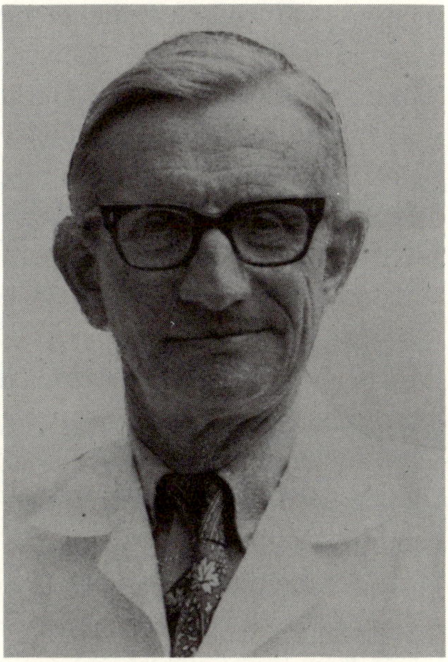

Louis E. Viko, MD, left, was Utah's pioneer cardiologist from 1931 to 1966. One of two physicians on the University of Utah Board of Regents asked in 1942 to draw up plans for the four-year Medical School, he became one of its strongest supporters. Dr. Viko died in 1968 at the age of seventy-one. Hans H. Hecht, MD, right, was recruited from the University of Michigan in 1944. Utah's premier academic cardiologist, investigator and teacher, Dr. Hecht was director of the heart station and was appointed the first Louis E. Viko Professor, 1957–64.

CHAPTER FIVE

Infectious Diseases

CHARLES B. SMITH, MD

THE HISTORY OF MEDICINE is for the most part a history of infectious diseases. Even before the recognition of microbial causes of disease in the mid-nineteenth century, the syndromes of many common infectious diseases such as influenza, diphtheria, smallpox, malaria, and the plague were well recognized, and every physician was obliged to spend the majority of his practice providing symptomatic therapy for fevers, diarrheas, and other manifestations of infectious diseases. The sense that illness was due to invasion of the body by a foreign disturbance was well developed before specific infectious agents were identified, and many of the common curatives were attempts to rid the body of these toxic invaders by using purgatives, emetics, and bleeding. That some diseases were communicable was recognized by the ancients, and the Hebrew advice to isolate lepers and avoid unclean foods was the beginning of control of infectious diseases by public health measures.

Some effective infectious disease control practices were developed during these years before microbes were identified, for example smallpox immunization by Jenner in 1796. Its use led to control of the disease in Western countries by the end of the nineteenth century, long before the virus particle had been demonstrated by light microscopy and the virus successfully cultivated in the laboratory. A distressing outcome of advancing knowledge about the communicability of smallpox occurred in the American West as the settlers came into

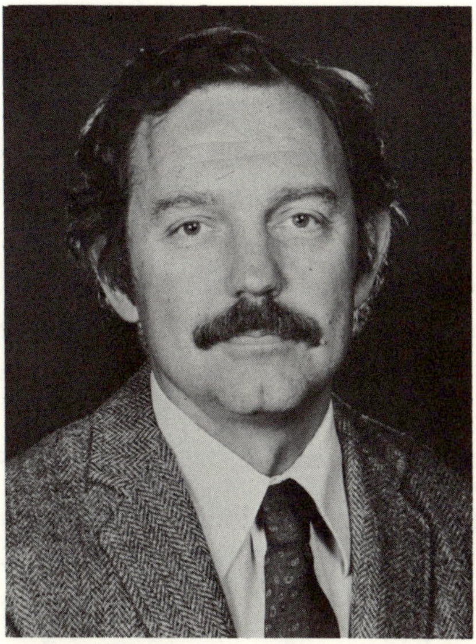

Charles B. Smith.

conflict with the native Indians. Because smallpox was a European disease and native Americans had not been previously exposed, genetic selection of resistance traits had not occurred in the Indians as it had in Europeans over many centuries. The Indians were thus exceptionally susceptible to smallpox, and mortality rates were so high that entire villages, even entire tribes, were wiped out by the disease. Historians tell us that the settlers were aware of the susceptibility of native Americans to this infection and that on occasion blankets contaminated with the virus were deliberately given to Indians with the intention, and effect, of starting epidemics.

The settling of Utah in the mid-nineteenth century coincided with a major event in the history of medicine; the discovery of the microbial etiology of disease. In the 1840s Ignaz Semmelweis was arguing that childbed fever was communicated by the dirty hands of physicians, and the association of cholera with contaminated water from the Broad Street pump was described by John Snow. However, the bedrock observations, techniques, and methods that characterize the science of microbiology came later in the century, primarily through the insights and diligence of Pasteur, Koch, and their associates as they discovered and characterized major bacterial causes of diseases, e.g., anthrax, tuberculosis, pneumococcal pneumonia, typhoid fever, and cholera. These remarkable discoveries led to some improved control of infectious diseases by application of good public health practices and by the development of antisera and vaccines. However, infectious diseases continued to dominate the medical practice of most physicians until the late 1930s, when the development of antimicrobial agents finally permitted physicians to cure them.

Introduction of the Subspecialty in Utah, 1946–1954

The formal specialty of infectious diseases, interestingly, did not develop until after the end of World War II, when most of the common infectious diseases were coming under control because of effective antimicrobials, and it was no longer expected that every physician would be an expert in them. A generation of medical students and physicians was developing who had never seen smallpox, diphtheria, and other classic infectious diseases, and some academicians argued that there was a need for specialists who were expert in these, now-rare, diseases and in the application of new chemotherapeutic agents. On the other hand, the remarkable curative effects of penicillin, tetracyclines, streptomycin, and the sulfonamides led some to question the need for infectious disease specialists. Selman Waksman, the co-discoverer of streptomycin, predicted in 1954 that control of all infectious diseases of man and animals was now within sight, and using this reasoning some argued that infectious diseases was a transient specialty which would likely die out in a few years for lack of patients. As we near the turn of another century it has become apparent that microbes have been able to adapt to the pressures of new antimicrobials at a rate somewhat faster than physician scientists can develop new remedies, and the field of infectious diseases is now one of the most rapidly growing medical specialties.

John Waldo was the first specialty-trained infectious disease physician to practice in Utah. A Utah native, he trained in medicine at the University of Rochester in New York. It is likely that his interest in infectious diseases was kindled by his own bout with tuberculosis during medical school. He attributed his infection to the practice of his pathology professor, George Whipple, of insisting that medical students learn the smells of disease and get their noses down next to diseased organs during autopsies. Waldo lost two years from his medical training taking the rest cure at Pottenger's sanatorium in California. His eastern professors had strongly recommended the Saranac Lake sanatorium, but his Western roots led him to reason that the sun would shine more regularly upon him in California than in upstate New York.

After medical school, Waldo continued his studies in the microbiology laboratory with George Packer Berry at Rochester, and upon completion of his training in 1946, he accepted the offer of Maxwell Wintrobe to return to Utah to join the newly developing Department of Medicine at the Medical School. His research interests were focused on the new miracle antibiotic, penicillin. Then, as now, antibiotics were often overused, and Waldo was concerned about this practice. Medical students were quick to pick up on Waldo's concerns about excessive use of penicillin, and at one of their graduation banquets, they parodied him with a song and dance entitled "Penicillin is now part of the diet." In collaboration with his colleague Val Jager, he studied the pharmacokinetics of penicillin in patients on the venereal disease ward at the County Hospital (Salt Lake General — SLGH), and they were among the first to show that probenecid was effective for increasing the blood levels of penicillin. At that time, clinical research was a new concept, and these physicians struggled, as we do today, with the ethical issues of human research. Both Waldo and Jager were described as unusually caring physicians who exhibited utter kindness for the indigent patients on the VD ward.

Because infectious disease specialists have the pleasure of dealing with all other specialties, including pediatrics and surgery, they have traditionally been very active in postgraduate medical education programs. Waldo exhibited this trait and was instrumental in obtaining Kellogg Foundation support for postgraduate medical education in

Utah. A program Waldo developed entitled "Modern Medical Show" was presented at meetings of local medical societies throughout the Intermountain West and became the progenitor of a larger federally funded Regional Medical Program established in the 1960s.

In the post–World War II era, veterans returned to Utah with exotic infectious diseases acquired abroad. Malaria was common, and Drs. Waldo and Wintrobe had a busy practice in treating it. A notable patient who came under their care was the journalist William McDougal, who had been a prisoner of the Japanese. He had promised himself that if he survived the ordeal, he would become a priest. After his malaria was cured by Drs. Wintrobe and Waldo, McDougal went on to become a prominent Catholic priest in Utah.

In 1954 Waldo's tuberculosis was determined to be no longer an adequate reason for military deferral, and he was drafted into the Army, spending two years in Germany. On returning to Utah in 1956, he decided to go into private practice in Salt Lake City. He continued to maintain a primary interest in infectious diseases and was an active leader in public health immunization campaigns. A 1963 photo in the *Salt Lake Tribune* shows Waldo administering Sabin polio vaccine-

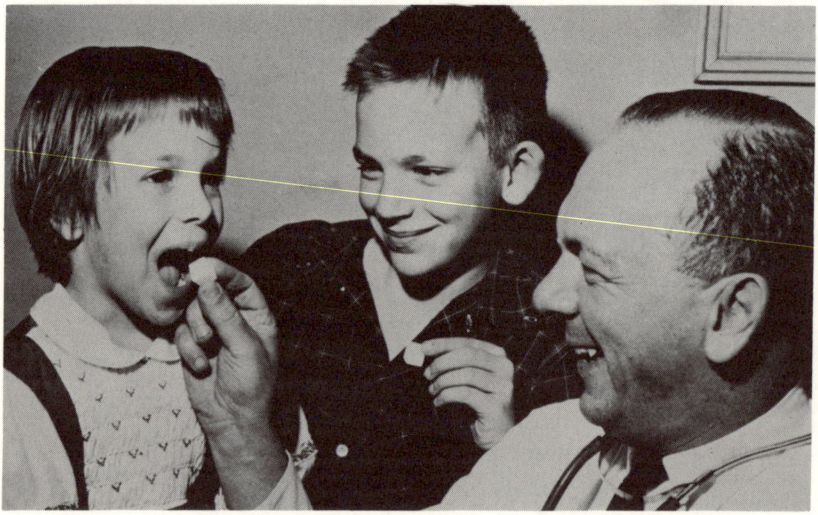

John F. Waldo, MD, Utah's first infectious disease specialist, giving a polio vaccine sugar cube to a young patient in 1963.

laced sugar cubes to his two children as part of the advertising for the statewide vaccine campaign. Waldo was a highly respected leader among Utah physicians; he served as president of the Utah Medical Society and was the first part-time director of Medical Education at St. Mark's Hospital.

Training and Research, 1957–1967

With Waldo's departure from the Medical School, Wintrobe, searching for a new chief of infectious diseases for the Department of Medicine, followed the traditional pathway in those days: he recruited Paul Hoeprich, a bright young academician from Johns Hopkins Medical School. Hoeprich was just finishing his training with Ivan Bennett at Hopkins (following residency at Yale with Paul Beeson) and was anxious to apply the new sciences of microbiology and chemotherapy to the clinical field of infectious diseases. The salaries and physical facilities at the Salt Lake General Hospital were meager. However, the enthusiasm of Wintrobe, Hecht, Athens, and Perkoff for the future of the expanding Department of Medicine at Utah, and the typical Western advantage of being able to "develop your own program from scratch" were attractive to Hoeprich. In December of 1956 he drove his family through Midwestern ice storms and Wyoming blizzards to begin the year and a new Division of Infectious Diseases at Utah.

The clinical consulting and teaching load was heavy since Hoeprich developed his program as the sole faculty person in the division during his decade in Utah. Encouragement was provided by Glen Leymaster and Lyman Fulton in the Department of Preventive Medicine; they were primarily interested in epidemiology, however. Thomas Good in the Department of Pediatrics took care of pediatric problems of infection until he left Utah around 1961. Nevertheless, the Hoeprich decade saw publication of forty-two original articles, seven book chapters, and a monograph written with John R. Ward, *The Fluids of Parenteral Body Cavities*, that won first prize in Grune and Stratton's 1959 competition.

William Carnes, chairman of the Department of Pathology, asked Hoeprich to supervise the diagnostic microbiology laboratory at the SLGH in 1958, and this support allowed Hoeprich to initiate a productive research program in diagnostic microbiology. Important contributions in this area included the use of phage typing to characterize epidemic strains of staphylococci, a new method for differentiating the *Haemophilus* species, and a practical method for quantitative culture of the urine; the latter two are still in daily use in clinical laboratories.

With support from the expanding National Institutes of Health (NIH) and from the pharmaceutical industry, Hoeprich established a vigorous program of research in antimicrobials. He demonstrated the importance of alanine antagonism with the anti-tuberculosis drug cycloserine and reported on the efficacy and toxicities of the new aminoglycoside antimicrobials. Hoeprich was particularly adept at combining laboratory with clinical research, a valuable result of his combined roles as clinician, teacher, and investigator. One of his most valuable contributions was introducing the anesthesiologists' technique of transtracheal aspiration into clinical medicine, documenting its usefulness to obtain uncontaminated lower respiratory tract secretions for culture. His first trials of the technique were on Utah medical students, and the story is told that one of the first volunteers developed mediastinal and subcutaneous emphysema with swelling of the neck and face before Hoeprich realized the need to insist on bed rest following the procedure.

Hoeprich was successful in obtaining NIH funding for a training program in infectious diseases in 1960 and trained five fellows. One, Richard Parker, is now on the faculty of Howard University Medical School, and Richard Kalinske went into academic medicine, then practiced, and recently went into the Department of Clinical Investigation at the Upjohn Company. Burton Janis, a veterinarian who went on to medical school, followed his fellowship with Hoeprich with a year at the Scripps Research Foundation, with Karl Habel, doing rabies research. Janis subsequently returned to join the faculty at Utah, where he continued his research on the effect of interferon on rabies. Renowned for his skiing, mountain climbing, and superb clinical skills, Janis recently moved to Anchorage, Alaska, to practice infectious disease medicine and nurture his love of the wilderness.

In 1967 Hoeprich was recruited away from Utah to help start a new University of California Medical School at Davis. Shortly after his move he published his textbook *Infectious Diseases*. Now in its fourth edition, it remains the standard work in the field.

Ernest Runyon, PhD, is another Utahn who made very important contributions to the field of infectious diseases during this period. Originally trained as a botanist-microbiologist at Chicago, he became interested in the mycobacteria while working at the Saranac Lake sanatorium, New York. In 1958 he moved his mycobacteriology laboratory to the Salt Lake Veterans Administration Hospital, and over the next fifteen years his laboratory became the world's leading center for identification and taxonomy of the various species of mycobacteria which infect humans. The "Runyon Classification" for mycobacteria became the international standard, and although he officially "retired" in 1973, he continued his work for several more years and is still an active and recognized contributor to this important field. Runyon's successes are also testimony to the valuable contributions the Veterans Administration has made through its consistent support of medical research and teaching.

Expansion of Training and Research, 1969–1981

The next phase of growth at the Medical School began in 1969, when Charles Smith was recruited by George Cartwright to become chief of the Division of Infectious Diseases in the Department of Medicine. Dr. Smith had trained in medicine and infectious diseases with Maxwell Finland at the Harvard Service of the Boston City Hospital and then had done research with respiratory viruses at the NIH. Dr. Attilio Renzetti, then chief of pulmonary diseases, had been successful, with Hoeprich's help, in applying for research grant support from the NIH for a long-term study of the role of infection in the pathogenesis of chronic bronchitis; Dr. Smith fulfilled the need for an infectious disease investigator. The two physicians, with Dr.

Richard Kanner, had a very productive collaboration over a ten-year period investigating chronic bronchitis. The disease is characterized by recurrent exacerbations of acute productive bronchitis, and these investigators showed that respiratory viral infections were the initiating factor in most exacerbations and that secondary bacterial infection often followed the viral infection.

When Dr. Smith first arrived in town, the only other practicing infectious disease specialist was Dr. James Mason, who was based at the LDS Hospital. He had been attracted to Utah from a position at the Communicable Disease Center in Atlanta because of the recurrent problem of unusually high rates of rheumatic fever in the Intermountain West. Not surprisingly, given the unpredictability of nature, the epidemic fizzled out shortly after his arrival. Rheumatic fever didn't return until the late 1980s, by which time Dr. Mason's career had included directorship of the Utah State Health Department and the National Centers for Disease Control!

Dr. James Wilfert was the first person to join Dr. Smith at the Medical School. He had been trained in clinical infectious diseases and in diagnostic medical microbiology at Harvard and immediately filled a serious void in laboratory microbiology. Few of the Intermountain hospitals had adopted the new Kirby-Bauer technique for determining antimicrobial susceptibilities, and Dr. Wilfert, with the support of Dr. Hilmon Castle and the Intermountain Regional Medical Program, set up a regular training program for laboratory technicians throughout the Intermountain area. Within a year the laboratories had all adopted this standardized test, and it was possible to evaluate patients and provide telephone consultations about serious infections using consistent and reliable laboratory data.

As might be expected, the concept that a clinically trained microbiologist could move into the territory of the classical pathologist was disturbing to the community of pathologists. Dr. Ernst Eichwald, chair of the Department of Pathology, had his hands full mediating the conflicting demands of the clinicians and pathologists. When Dr. Wilfert left the Medical School in 1974 for private practice in the community, Dr. John Matsen, a pediatrician and infectious disease specialist with experience in managing the microbiology laboratory, came to direct the laboratory at the University Hospital. Matsen is a highly energetic and creative academician who immediately expanded the laboratory and its training program for technicians, as well as for physicians, and established a large program for evaluating new antimicrobials in the laboratory and in clinical trials. It happened that Matsen had exceptional managerial skills, and soon he was appointed director of all laboratory functions at the University Hospital; then he accepted the position as chair of the Department of Pathology. In recent years Matsen has established a large University-owned company for providing clinical pathology services (ARUP) and symbolically demonstrated the acceptance of clinically trained laboratory directors by being elected president of the American Society of Clinical Pathologists. Matsen's contributions as a scientist were also recognized in 1988, when he received the Becton Dickenson Award from the Infectious Disease Society of America.

Dr. Harry Hill was a pediatrician–infectious disease specialist who joined the Medical School community in 1974. Hill had special training in immunology and in 1976 established a separate Division of Clinical Immunology based in both the departments of pediatrics and pathology. His studies of the abnormalities of leukocyte function that characterize the newborn period of life, and the role of these transient deficiencies in the pathogenesis of group B streptococcal infections in neonates, have achieved international acclaim. In recent years Hill has assumed responsibility for directing the clinical microbiology, immunology, and virology programs of ARUP.

The notion that hospital-acquired infections were a serious cause of morbidity and mortality was gaining recognition, and an expert in this field, Dr. John Burke, was the third person to join the expanding Division of Infectious Diseases in the early 1970s. He had trained in medicine with Paul Beeson at Yale and then in infectious disease epidemiology with the Centers for Disease Control (CDC) and at the Channing Laboratory at Harvard Medical School. Burke set up shop as the chief of Infectious Diseases at the LDS Hospital and was soon successful in obtaining NIH funding for his studies of hospital-acquired infections. Working with three dynamic fellows who later joined the faculty of the Medical School — Jay Jacobson, Dick Garibaldi, and Mike Britt — Burke made major contributions to our understanding of the importance of urinary catheters and other risk factors for nosocomial (hospital-acquired) urinary tract infections and the host determinants for nosocomial pneumonias. In recent years, Burke has made use of the world-class clinical computer database at the LDS Hospital to define the importance of timing of administration of prophylactic antimicrobials during surgery.

Spotswood Spruance was another CDC-trained epidemiologist who continued his training in infectious diseases as a fellow in the Utah program and who then joined the faculty of the Medical School. While assigned to the Utah Department of Health, Spruance made several important contributions to the understanding of two infectious diseases which are unusually common in Utah: Colorado tick fever and echinococcosis. With the collaboration of Ferron Anderson from the Department of Zoology at Brigham Young University and several physicians from the CDC, Spruance followed up several anecdotal reports of echinococcal disease in Utah ranchers. The first demonstration in the U.S. of the full cycle of infection from sheep to dogs to man was made by this group from their studies of an outbreak which occurred in a small sheep-raising community at the southwest corner of the Salt Lake Valley. Subsequent studies showed an extraordinarily high incidence of human disease and infected dogs in Sanpete County, Utah, and control measures, such as preventing the feeding of sheep viscera to dogs, have been shown to be effective.

Colorado tick fever (CTF) is a viral disease common in the mountainous areas of eastern Utah and western Colorado. It is characterized by severe muscle aches, fever, and a peculiar bi-phasic course with associated neutropenia. Frank Tyler describes his own case and that of his wife as being acquired when they were bitten by a tick while camping in the Wolf Creek Pass region in the Uinta Mountains in 1955. Their convalescent sera contained such high titers of antibodies that the Rocky Mountain Laboratory in Hamilton, Montana, used them as national reference testing sera for several years. Spruance was the first to document the importance of this infection in Utah when he screened for CTF antibodies in several hundred sera that had been submitted to the State Department of Health for testing for possible Rocky Mountain spotted fever (RMSF). A high percent of the sera tested positive for CTF, while the more famous RMSF was rarely detected. That the CTF virus is endemic to the Salt Lake foothills was demonstrated by a puzzling outbreak among several patients at the VA Medical Center. A search for ticks in the hospital was unsuccessful, and the explanation was not apparent until one patient mentioned that he had joined a whole busload of VA patients for a fishing trip to the lake behind Fort Douglas in Red Butte Canyon.

Toxic Shock Syndrome (TSS) is another infectious disease that led to publicity for Utah. Smith saw the first case in 1980; a young woman college student presented in shock with what looked like atypical scarlet fever. The unusual aspects led him to consult with James Overall, the chief of pediatric infectious diseases, and Overall suggested that the illness resembled a new staphylococcal disease described in children by James Todd from the University of Colorado. Smith called Todd in the early hours of the morning to find out that he was just beginning to get reports that TSS was occurring in young women and that they were often menstruating at the time. The Utah patient was, in fact, menstruating, and staphylococci were isolated from the tampon that she was using. Over the next few weeks many Utah physicians reported seeing patients with TSS, and the opportunity to determine the pathogenesis of the disease became apparent.

At this time in the history of toxic shock, the association with tampons was not at all clear, so a case control study was designed to explore the association of a large variety of exposure, such as sexual practices, use of antibiotics, and use of catamenial devices, such as tampons, with risk of disease. Several physicians and epidemiologists from the State Department of Health, including Mark Kehrberg, Bob Latham, and Craig Nichols, collaborated with the University physicians on this important study, which was one of the first in the U.S. to document the critical role of tampons as risk factors for TSS. The association of TSS with the Rely brand of tampons was particularly supported by the Utah data, because Utah had been a national test marketing site for these "super" tampons before they were generally available elsewhere. The Utah data are now often mentioned in courtrooms, as the legal aspects of this illness have become a large industry.

The collaboration between Smith and Overall in taking care of this TSS patient was typical of a strong association that developed between the infectious disease programs in medicine and pediatrics during the 1970s. Dr. Overall was recruited in 1970 by Dr. M. Eugene Lahey, chair of the Department of Pediatrics, to build a pediatric program in infectious diseases. He had a strong background in virology and established a vigorous research program which looked at the role of interferon and interferon inducers as antiviral agents. Animal models for important human viral diseases such as herpes simplex virus and cytomegalovirus were established, and these became important testing systems for a large variety of antiviral agents in addition to interferon. In collaboration with Dr. Spruance, Overall developed a clinical program in the evaluation of antiviral compounds which pioneered clinical antiviral study methodology and earned Utah a national and international reputation in this field. In recent years Overall has directed the diagnostic virology laboratory at ARUP.

Overall and Smith shared a training grant for both pediatric and adult infectious diseases, and fellows and faculty enjoyed the opportunity to see both adult and pediatric infectious disease patients and to share common research and clinical conferences. Several graduates of this program have gone on to distinguished academic careers, including Val Hemming, who is chair of the Department of Pediatrics at the Uniformed Services Health Sciences Center in Bethesda, Maryland; Howard Faden, professor of pediatrics at the Buffalo Medical School; José Santos, chief of pediatric infectious diseases at the prestigious Hospital Infantil in Mexico City; Jim Cook, associate professor of infectious diseases and medicine at the University of Colorado; Don Granger, associate professor of medicine at Duke Medical School; and Alan Barbour, professor of medicine and chief of infectious diseases at the University of Texas Medical School in San Antonio. This program also graduated distinguished clinicians who include Tom Kurrus, a busy practitioner of infectious diseases at St. Mark's Hospital and a very active clinical professor at the Medical School.

Because Utah is a small state with limited resources for higher education, the unusual degree of interdepartmental collaboration that developed in the Medical School has enabled a critical mass of investigators and scholars to produce high-quality science and education. In the field of infectious diseases, this collaboration is further illustrated by the strong ties which have developed between the clinical infectious disease faculty and the Department of Microbiology. These ties were greatly strengthened in 1970, when Lowell Glasgow, a pediatric infectious disease specialist who had been working with Overall at the University of Rochester, was recruited to chair the Department of Microbiology. The selection of a clinician for this position reflected a trend of the times for greater clinical "relevance" in basic science departments. Glasgow immediately set out to fulfill this need by recruiting the members of the pediatric and medicine infectious disease faculty to join in the teaching and research aspects of the department. Glasgow established an exciting research program in viral immunology, and his research accomplishments earned him the coveted Squibb Award of the Infectious Diseases Society of America in 1977. In 1973 Glasgow decided that he was unhappy with his decision to give up his clinical role for a basic science department chairmanship, and he accepted the dean's offer to become chair of the Department of Pediatrics. He was similarly successful in building up the department following this move and was in high gear as a researcher, teacher, and clinician when he suffered an untimely heart attack and died in 1982.

When Glasgow stepped down as chair of the Department of Microbiology in 1973, the whole field of microbiology was advancing rapidly. It was increasingly apparent that the research tools of the bacteriologist and virologist were valuable not only to the clinicians for better understanding the pathogenesis of infectious diseases, but also to medical biologists in general. The bacteriologists and virologists were now using their techniques to explore the genetic and biochemical functions of cells, and these techniques were important for the entire medical school research community. With this need in mind, and because a large group of infectious disease specialists were now available to teach the classic microbiology course to medical students, the search committee recruited Don Summers from Albert Einstein Medical School to come to Utah to establish a new Department of Cellular, Viral and Molecular Biology. Dr. Summers did this in a grand manner, and in a few years the new department was one of the strongest in the school. With the encouragement of George Cartwright and others, Summers was influential in establishing a new, separate Department of Human Genetics. Although a basic scientist, Summers had his original training in internal medicine at the Boston City Hospital and thus has been able to interpret easily the new biology for clinicians and to enter into very profitable collaborative research projects with infectious disease clinicians. For example, Summers and an infectious disease fellow, Jeff Johnston, recently inserted a piece of the hepatitis A virus genome into a mutant enteric bacterium as part of a project to develop a new hepatitis A vaccine.

The Current Scene, 1981–1990

In 1981 Smith was recruited to the VA Medical Center to become chief of the Medical Service by William Odell, the new chair of the Department of Medicine. Zell McGee, who was chief of Infectious Diseases at Vanderbilt Medical School, was recruited by Odell to become the new infectious disease chief in 1982. McGee had a national reputation as an expert in meningitis and sexually transmitted diseases, and his recruitment was timely since the 1980s could well be described as the decade of venereal diseases. McGee, using modern immunologic techniques and electron microscopy, helped identify the pathogenic parts of the gonococcus and demonstrated mechanisms by which these pathogens invade the cells of the genitourinary tract. The goal of his research has been to identify molecular mechanisms of disease and to develop treatments which are directed against specific pathogenic mechanisms. McGee and two infectious disease fellows, Ward Robinson and Gary Gorby, have recently shown that hormone receptors may be important attachment sites for the gonococcal pathogen. McGee has been successful in obtaining training grant funds from the CDC for fellows in the field of venereal diseases, and an expanded teaching and research program was established for fellows and medical students which utilized the Salt Lake City–County Venereal Disease Clinics.

AIDS is clearly the most important new infectious disease of the decade, and the identification in 1983 of the first Utah patient with this infection was the harbinger that our "hallowed hills" would not protect Utahns from this dreaded illness. As the decade of the 1990s begins, several hundred Utahns have developed the full syndrome, nearly 100 patients have died from AIDS, and the medical system is under strain from the personal and monetary costs of caring for the several hundred infected individuals who need constant monitoring and expensive drug therapy. The initial burden of caring for Utah's AIDS patients was primarily borne by a single practitioner, Kristin Ries, who has specialized in caring for AIDS patients while also practicing general medicine and infectious diseases. Dr. Ries has also been a very active member of the Governor's Task Force on AIDS and is nationally prominent as an educator of physicians and patients about AIDS. Tom Kurrus has also carried a heavy caseload of AIDS patients and has been active in advising the legislature and the Department of Health about AIDS programs and legislation.

As these private practitioners began to be overwhelmed by the AIDS caseload, the University faculty began to get fully involved. Larry Reimer, an infectious disease clinician based primarily at the VA Medical Center, opened the first VA AIDS clinic in 1988, and the VA now cares for approximately 15% of the AIDS cases in the state. In early 1989, Reimer started the first AIDS clinic at the University Hospital, and in September of 1989, Tom Evans, a new faculty member in the Division of Infectious Diseases who has had special training in AIDS at San Francisco and Charlottesville, Virginia, took over control of the rapidly expanding University clinic.

The caseload of AIDS patients in Utah is now large enough to allow for clinical research projects, and new experimental drugs are undergoing testing in these clinics under the supervision of Drs. Ries, Evans, and Spruance. AIDS education has become a big business in Utah over the past few years, with the support of a large federal grant to the State Department of Health and the Department of Family and Preventive Medicine. In addition, the Utah AIDS Consortium, a group of six community-based agencies, recently received a large grant from the Robert Wood Johnson Foundation to conduct AIDS education in Utah. A recent report that the number of cases in Utah is now smaller than was originally projected may indicate that active education programs are effective in changing the behavior that increases risk of this infection.

In late 1989 another era began in the evolution of the infectious disease teaching and research program at the Medical School as John Hibbs replaced McGee as chief of the division. Dr. Hibbs originally trained in medicine at Pittsburgh and Oregon and then did his infectious disease training with Jack Remington at Stanford. In 1971 he was recruited by Smith to head up the Infectious Disease Section at the VA Medical Center, and Hibbs has developed a superb research program at the VA. His research has been more immunological than primary infectious diseases; he has been interested in how macrophages protect the host against cancer. Hibbs was among the first to prove that macrophages are important host defense mechanisms against cancer, and in recent years he has begun to identify the signals which activate macrophages to become killers of cancer cells and the mechanisms by which the cancer cells are killed. Interestingly, these mechanisms may also be important for macrophage-dependent defenses against infectious diseases, including some infections associated with AIDS.

Hibbs has begun to tackle the restructuring of the infectious disease program with great vigor, and it is likely that the next decade will be characterized by innovative and timely responses to the ever-changing needs of the field of infectious diseases.

CHAPTER SIX

Rheumatology

JOHN R. WARD, MD

UTAH HAS ALWAYS BEEN PROUD OF ITS ENERGETIC, competent, and caring physicians. In the late 1940s, Dr. Jack Nunemaker, chief of medicine at the Salt Lake Veterans Administration Hospital, was interested in arthritis but had no formal training in rheumatology. Prior to 1957, no physician with special training in rheumatology could be identified in the state. Until that time, care was provided by primary care physicians, internists, and orthopedic surgeons, none of whom professed special knowledge or interest in the diagnosis and treatment of arthritis. This is not surprising viewed in light of the quite recent emergence of this specialty on the national scene.

The first rheumatology units in the United States were established at the Mayo Clinic in 1926 and full-time, university-accredited programs at Harvard and Columbia universities in 1929, New York University in 1932, and the University of Michigan in 1937. The American Rheumatism Association, a professional organization of rheumatologists, was established in 1948 and had a membership of 908 physicians by 1954. In August 1950, the National Institute of Arthritis and Metabolic Diseases was established, affording funding for research and training in rheumatology.

At the University of Utah School of Medicine, Dr. Maxwell M. Wintrobe, chair of the Department of Internal Medicine, had established a small but superior faculty for his program. In the early 1950s he was extending his concept of subspecialty units. He felt it important to develop a rheumatology program to provide the best and most current training for medical students, interns, and residents to improve diagnosis and management of patients with rheumatic diseases.

In 1954 Dr. John R. Ward was a research fellow in medicine working with Dr. B. Valdemar (Val) Jager in an attempt to purify acetylcholinesterase from human erythrocytes. He had completed medical school at the University of Utah, taken a one-year research fellowship in physiology and pharmacology under the stimulating guidance of Drs. Horace Davenport, and Louis Goodman, chairs, Departments of Physiology and Pharmacology, respectively. He had also completed his internship and residency in medicine at the Salt Lake General Hospital (SLGH). After a two-year tour of Army service during the Korean conflict, he had returned to the Department of Medicine.

Dr. Ward's ultimate goals were not formalized beyond his desire for a career in academic medicine. At this point Dr. Wintrobe shared with him his desire to establish an arthritis unit in his department. After much thought and encouragement by lay leaders who were in the process of establishing a Utah chapter of the Arthritis Foundation, Ward told Wintrobe of his interest and enthusiasm for embarking on a career in "arthritis."

With Wintrobe's guidance and help, he applied for and was awarded a two-year fellowship grant and a combined clinical and research position in arthritis with Dr. Walter Bauer, Jackson Professor of Medicine at Harvard Medical School and chief of medicine at Massachusetts General Hospital, starting on July 1, 1955. His return to the University in July 1957 to establish a Division of Arthritis was rather inauspicious. He had a small office measuring about sixty square feet and shared laboratory space with whoever was willing to offer a few feet of bench space. He was soon able to obtain a National Institutes of Health (NIH) training grant, however, which helped support some research and provided stipends for training fellows.

The original impetus was to establish an outpatient arthritis clinic at the SLGH and an arthritis research and teaching program for medical students and house officers. In 1957 a regular outpatient

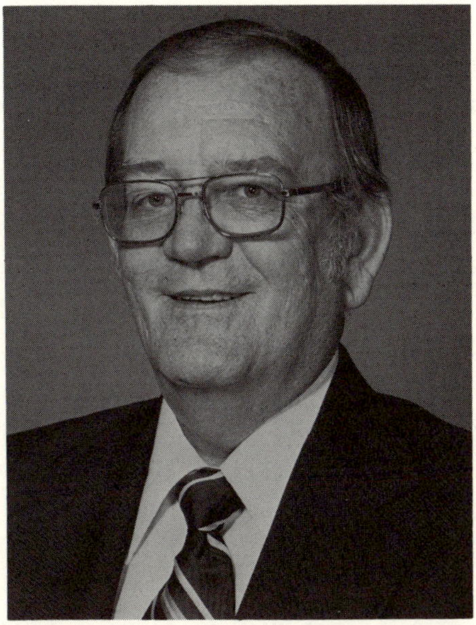

John R. Ward.

arthritis clinic for "county hospital patients" and a single weekly clinic for referred patients with arthritis were established. An active teaching program was implemented with formal lectures, and inpatient consultations at the SLGH were used as teaching exercises for house officers.

In 1958 Marlin Shields, a physical therapist, returned to Salt Lake City after completing his training at Stanford University. He teamed up with Dr. Ward to establish the first Utah arthritis/physical therapy program at the SLGH. Once this was in place, they initiated a home-based program for homebound arthritis patients with support from the Utah chapter of the Arthritis Foundation. This effort was not considered "cost effective," however, and was discontinued in 1960.

In 1965 a more aggressive arthritis rehabilitation program was implemented which included pool therapy and the establishment of a brace and splinting facility in the new University Hospital. With the assistance of two orthopedic surgeons, Robert Carson, and Robert H. Lamb, a research project to assess the value of static resting hand splints in retarding hand deformities was begun. The role of hand surgery in rheumatoid arthritis was also studied. As part of the project, the development of new foot appliances and shoes for management of rheumatoid foot problems was initiated. At one time Dr. Ward and Marlin Shields made regular visits to several communities, such as Delta and Moab, to explore the value of seeing patients with their primary care physician as a method of improving the diagnosis and management of arthritis patients in remote communities.

Dr. Ward lectured the medical students on drug therapy of arthritis during their course in pharmacology. Dr. Goodman commented after the discussion of gold treatment that "a major indication and result of chrysotherapy is to fill the pockets of the treating physicians." Dr. Wintrobe, not known for or given to humor, would often say, "John, it seems to me that you know all about the arthritides except their cause or their cure."

After these efforts were well in place, a fellowship training program was initiated. The first clinical fellow was Dr. John Baukol. After completing his fellowship in 1961, he became the first trained rheumatologist to practice in the state of Utah. At this time, thirteen rheumatologists trained at the University of Utah School of Medicine have remained in Utah. Two practice in Provo, one in Ogden, one in Logan, and five in Salt Lake City. Another four have remained in academic medicine at the University of Utah. One other faculty member was a medical student at the University who received his training elsewhere and returned to Salt Lake City. Of the two remaining practicing rheumatologists in Utah, one was recruited to be chief of rheumatology at the Salt Lake Veterans Administration Medical Center and subsequently left this position for private practice. The other received his training elsewhere before establishing his practice in Ogden. A total of twenty-eight clinical and three research fellows have been trained by the division, and three clinical fellows are currently in training.

In addition to his responsibilities in rheumatology, Dr. Ward agreed to assume the chairmanship of the Department of Public Health and Preventive Medicine in 1965. He gladly relinquished this burden in favor of Dr. C. Hilmon Castle in 1970, when the name (and emphasis) of the department was changed to Family and Community Medicine.

Research has slowly developed, and four PhDs now devote either all or major research efforts to the field of arthritis. Each has made major contributions to the field. In addition, the six clinicians in the rheumatology division have all been active in research.

In the late 1950s, the Division of Rheumatology conducted the first double-blind clinical trial which established the efficacy of indomethacin in rheumatoid arthritis. Since that time, the division has been active in clinical trials of other antirheumatic drugs. In 1976 the staff was awarded an NIH contract to conduct drug trials and has continued to obtain competitive awards. Under these contracts, a Coordinating and Data Center manages a series of extramural university participating clinics. Participating clinics are competitively recruited to conduct the studies according to protocols prepared at the University of Utah. The program has conducted pivotal studies for all of the so-called "second-line" drugs and has pioneered the use of "intent to treat" analysis, "subset of responder" analysis, and power analysis in anti-arthritis therapy trials. As a result of these trials, the division has developed an international reputation.

In addition to clinical studies which described the first patient with varicella arthritis and the initial report of "pseudoseptic arthritis," significant contributions have been made in basic research. The development of disease is a complex interaction between environmental agents such as infecting organisms, noxious chemicals, deficiencies of necessary substances such as vitamins, and/or preexisting inherited defects.

Immune response genes appear to be important in susceptibility and expression of rheumatoid arthritis, but how they operate is unknown. Rheumatoid arthritis is thought to be an autoimmune disease probably initiated by as yet unknown microbial agent(s) or virus(es). An overactive and uncontrolled immune system leads to inflammation and joint damage through a complex system of cellular responses and cell products.

The division has characterized mycoplasmas and diseases which they produce in rodents and rabbits. Careful studies using egg embryos, intrauterine mouse fetuses, and cell cultures have failed to identify an infectious agent recoverable from patients with rheumatoid arthritis. Other probes such as expression of reverse transcriptase from cells of patients with rheumatoid arthritis have been used but failed to demonstrate evidence for a viral etiology.

A recent discovery has been a unique mitogen recoverable from cultures of *Mycoplasma arthritidis* (MAM). MAM can activate all T cells which express V_B 8.1, 8.2, 8.3, or V_B 6 T cell receptor proteins. MAM shares properties with the so-called "superantigens" such as staphylococcal enterotoxins, the study of which is expected to yield important knowledge on the complex relationships between microorganisms and their hosts, the T cell repertoire, and the development of autoimmunity.

Experimental models of arthritis, especially arthritis induced by injection of type II collagen in mice and rats and by injection of Freund's adjuvant in rats, have been intensively studied. Development of the division's own genetically distinct inbred rat strains has led to the identification of a minimum of three genes which are involved in collagen-induced arthritis of rats.

To date, present animal models have not been capable of identifying disease-modifying antirheumatic drugs or their mechanism(s) of action. A recently developed experimental animal model, the passive transfer of adjuvant-induced arthritis of rats, has demonstrated efficacy of gold salts in this model and will be used to study other antirheumatic drugs, with the eventual goal of identifying and developing new treatments for rheumatoid arthritis.

A major project involves: (1) the epidemiological analysis of the distribution of familial rheumatoid arthritis in Utah; (2) a case control study to identify genetic differences between patients with "familial rheumatoid arthritis" and "singleton patients"; and (3) an extensive genetic analysis (complex segregation and linkage) of the distribution of immune response genes and rheumatoid arthritis. Investigations include: (1) the typing for three DNA polymorphisms spanning the

T cell receptor region; and (2) determining the unique DNA sequences of serologically defined HLA alleles which confer susceptibility to rheumatoid arthritis.

With the advent of better disease classification, improved drug therapy and surgical treatments, primary care physicians, internists, and orthopedic surgeons have increased their interest and skills in the management of the various forms of arthritis. The rheumatologists in Utah have been industrious and diligent in providing talks and seminars for primary care physicians throughout the state, and Utah can be proud of its physicians and specialists who manage these diseases.

CHAPTER SEVEN

Allergy

LORIMER T. CHRISTENSEN, MD

THE HISTORY OF ALLERGY IN UTAH in many ways mirrors the story of allergy as it unfolded throughout the country. Beginning with largely empirical observations, many clinicians were quick to grasp the implications of early developments in the treatment of their patients. As would be expected of any new specialty, the early practitioners were untrained, often exhibiting nothing more than a healthy interest in a newly described phenomenon.

In 1943 the Society for the Study of Asthma and Allied Conditions merged with the American Association for the Study of Allergy to become the American Academy of Allergy, which, in 1982, changed its name to the American Academy of Allergy and Immunology. In 1974 the Conjoint Board of Allergy and Clinical Immunology was established as a subspecialty of the boards of both pediatrics and internal medicine. As a rule, only physicians who are already boarded in pediatrics or internal medicine can be certified as allergists by this conjoint board. The certified allergist has a broad background in the fields of pediatrics and/or internal medicine plus another two years of specialization in allergy and clinical immunology. An allergist, then, is not just any doctor who chooses to do skin tests or Radio-allergosorbent (RAST) testing followed by allergy shots, but a physician who has interest and expertise in a variety of areas, including botany, pulmonary and respiratory physiology, pharmacology, immunology, bacteriology, anatomy, and skin diseases.

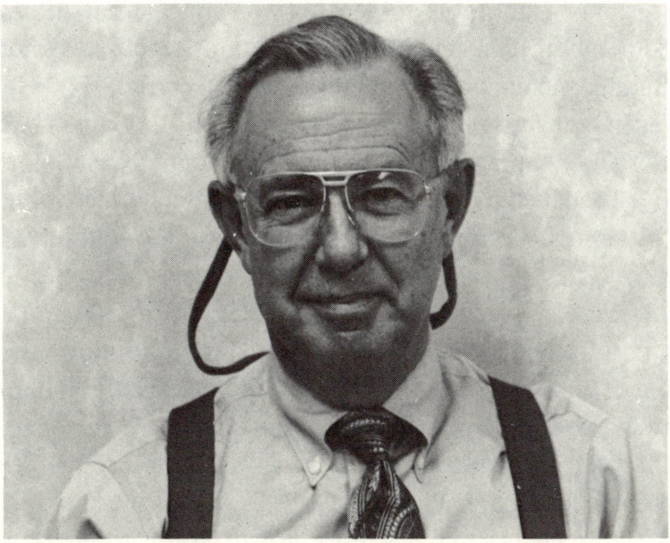

Lorimer T. Christensen.

In 1986 the Utah Society of Allergy and Asthma was formed to promote the scientific interests of certified allergists and enhance their ability to provide high-quality allergy care, as well as to provide members a forum for the exchange of new ideas, discussion of difficult patients, journal club, etc.

Since the history of the specialty in Utah is so interwoven with the development of allergy as a new science, it may be helpful to trace some of the key discoveries in the field of allergy and see how they have been applied by Utah practitioners over the past eighty years.

The word allergy was first used by Von Pirquet in 1906 to denote a state of altered reactivity which resulted from antigenic exposure and was harmful to the host. In 1923 Coca coined the word atopy (literally "out of place") to describe the hereditary, familial predisposition in a person to produce an allergic response to ordinarily harmless materials such as pollen, dust, and animal danders. This response was mediated by an antibody called reagin, which was often associated clinically with the standard allergy syndromes of asthma, hay fever, hives, and eczema. Reagin was found to be humoral or circulating in nature, able to sensitize or attach itself to skin and mucous membranes, inactivated by heat, transferable to serum, non-precipitating, and unable to cross the placental barrier. While its presence was known for many years, it was not until 1966 that Kimishige Ishisaka found that reagin was in fact IgE or Immunoglobulin E.

IgE is produced by all individuals but in greatly increased quantities by those who are atopic. The production of the antibody appears related to genes located on the #6 pair of chromosomes. IgE is responsible for anaphylaxis, hay fever, pollen asthma, and some types of urticaria, eczema, insect allergy, and drug allergy; that is, the spectrum of disease dealt with by the clinical allergist/immunologist. The discovery and demonstration of the characteristics of IgE elevated the field of allergy from the quasi-mysterious to the accepted immunologic science that it is today.

In 1911 Freeman and Noon treated successfully grass-pollen-sensitive patients with injections of grass pollen extracts. This approach, at first empirical, has been scientifically validated. It is now possible to show that several interesting immunologic changes occur during immunotherapy. In the hands of well-trained allergists, hay fever (allergic rhinitis) and carefully selected asthma patients can be successfully immunized against house dust, animal danders, and pollens.

The history of allergy and asthma treatment in Utah demonstrates in many ways the frustration of doctors and patients seeking quick and easy answers to complex and clinical diseases. For example, asthma is a chronic disease with a 5% mortality rate originally characterized clinically by the demonstration of reversible bronchospasm. Newer evidence of the importance that inflammation and inflammatory mediators play in the genesis of this disorder suggests that a better description might be eosinophilic bronchitis. While the specific biochemical and/or patho-physiologic defect still eludes identification, it is known to be of multifactorial inheritance. Afflicting some 3% to 5% of the general population, asthma is responsible for more work and school loss than any other chronic disease, and its treatment over the ages has encompassed many standard and unorthodox approaches in Utah as well as throughout the world.

For centuries asthma sufferers smoked stramonium leaves in a water pipe, a form of therapy also used in Utah during the early part of this century. Intravenous drugs of various kinds were utilized, including calcium, iodides, triple-distilled water, and even hydrochloric acid. Aspirin was noted to help an asthma attack occasionally, but it was also found to be capable of precipitating severe asthma in some patients, so its use was recommended "with caution."

Most emphasis in the early years was on the standard symptomatic treatment of allergic diseases with epinephrine, diphenhydramine, iodides, oxygen, and aminophylline. Nearly 50,000 patients worldwide, including many in Utah, had sympathetic glomectomies (glomus jugulare), and the procedure enjoyed growing popularity, particularly among surgeons, until a study compared a sham operation with actual glomectomies. No differences were seen between the two study groups in those patients who reported "benefiting" from the glomectomy. Surgical interest in asthma declined sharply.

The single most significant advance in the standard treatment of allergies occurred with the introduction of cortisone derivatives in the 1950s. Many asthmatics were spared premature death due to the addition of this "wonder" drug, which was soon found to produce significant side effects if not used with respect and caution. Cortisone added a measure of relief and control to severe asthma, hives, eczema, and allergic rhinitis not possible with any other drug.

Also popular in Utah during the forties, fifties, and sixties was the use of autogenous bacterial vaccines. Cultures of their own respiratory tract bacteria were grown, filtered, and reinjected in patients originally thought to be "allergic" to their own bacteria — a consideration which was later carefully refuted and the practice subsequently abandoned.

Skin testing, though not as traumatic as many people believe, was originally made more palatable by having the patient's blood drawn and transferring the sera to the skin of a non-allergic volunteer, who, for a fee, allowed himself or herself to be skin-tested at these passively sensitized sites. The passively transferred antibodies, reagin or IgE, attached themselves to the mast cells in the recipient's skin and remained there long enough, a few days, for scratch or intradermal testing to be done at these sites. This approach, valid in theory, lacked sensitivity and was difficult to standardize. Increased concern regarding the transmission of infectious agents, especially hepatitis and AIDS, has relegated this practice rightfully to the historical graveyard.

While selected allergens for skin testing could be ordered from commercial laboratories, many allergists, including the early pioneers in Utah, extracted many of their own antigens from flora and fauna indigenous to their own areas. In fact, allergists' children often could be seen wading through fields of weeds and grasses during the height of their pollen seasons collecting the raw material from which their physician parents extracted appropriate allergens.

Gammaglobulin use was so prevalent during the 1950s and 1960s that it was said that Salt Lake City used more than New York City. Many distraught mothers were seeking a quick solution for their children's "too-frequent colds." When examined critically, most of these children were not hypo-gammaglobulinemic, and local allergists spent considerable time reassuring the parents that their children would survive without a "gamma fix."

Another drug that was and at times still is abused is Kenalog, a depot steroid capable of relieving allergy symptoms for several weeks and suppressing the adrenal gland for several months. A growing awareness of acceptable alternatives, as well as justified litigation against physicians failing to obtain informed consent from patients regarding the multiple and at times devastating side effects, has led to a well-deserved decrease in its use.

The discovery of IgE in 1966 was followed by the development of the Radioallergosorbent test or RAST. This blood test identified specific circulating IgE antibodies directed toward allergens. While the RAST test is useful in certain clinical situations, its availability stimulated a lot of non-certified physicians to become "instantaneous allergists." Many local physicians, not realizing that the demonstration of an antibody without a suitable clinical history proves nothing more than exposure, embraced this opportunity to delve into a specialty without adequate background or training.

Pharmaceutical houses anxious to increase serum sales developed a "kit" with arbitrarily selected and limited allergens to be incorporated in the RAST testing. The distant laboratories then selected for the physician hyposensitization sera based on the RAST results, but without, naturally, an examination of the patient or, more importantly, a proper interpretation of the history. With the problems of increased costs, limited allergen selection, and temptation for abuse, reimbursement for using the RAST test kit has been limited by cost-conscious insurance companies.

Improved and standardized pulmonary function machines became available which greatly aided patient management. Basic bedside and office spirometry and emergency room peak flow meters together with sophisticated tertiary pulmonary care centers aided the allergist in assessing and managing difficult asthma patients. Intermountain Thoracic Society standards for pulmonary function testing, adopted from work done by LDS Hospital pulmonologists, became recognized nationwide as the best reference criteria available.

Theophylline, a xanthine bronchodilator with a narrow therapeutic blood range, has been a first-line drug in mild to severe asthma for generations. Oral, suppository, and intravenous formulations were commonly used, but serious toxicity and even deaths associated with only moderately higher than recommended blood levels have been reported. Concern regarding school performance of children with therapeutic theophylline levels has led to a re-examination of its role.

Allergists can now obtain blood gas determinations within minutes, which aids in deciding when patients need hospitalization, intensive care management, and/or assisted ventilation. The improved oral and inhaled beta-agonists have resulted in some decrease in side effects, a prolongation of bronchial smooth-muscle relaxation, and better control of acute and chronic bronchospasm.

The production and availability of topical steroids has greatly enhanced the management of hay fever as well as some forms of chronic rhinitis and, in particular, chronic asthma. Poorly-absorbed topically-applied inhaled steroids have aided significantly the management of asthma and reduced the necessity or temptation to use

Kenalog. Emphasis has been shifting from drugs relieving bronchospasm to those that affect the inflammatory portion of the asthmatic response.

Cromolyn was originally hailed as the end-all for asthma management, but this optimism quickly faded, as many patients did not use the preparation correctly. After a period of disillusionment, more recent research has shown Cromolyn to have some properties of decreasing bronchial reactivity, and in carefully selected patients it appears particularly effective in allergic asthma. It can also prevent exercise-induced bronchospasm, and ophthalmic and nasal formulation of Cromolyn has been particularly helpful in blocking allergic reactions of hay fever in many patients. Parasympathetic-type asthma sprays also are available that in selected patients provide an additive benefit especially for those whose asthma is complicated by vagal-reflexes from gastro-esophageal reflux or sinus disease. Standardization of allergens has contributed to the improvement of immunotherapy.

In some patients, IV immunoglobulin appears to have a beneficial effect by a process described as "networking" in which Fc fragments of the administered immunoglobulin cause a type of "down" regulation of the immune response. There is a growing feeling that immune responses, even in the absence of identifiable skin test allergen sensitivity, are a critical process in asthma etiology; pulmonologists are becoming more aware of the need for allergy evaluations in their adult asthma population.

The introduction of newer antihistamines that are relatively excluded by the blood-brain barrier provided antihistamine benefits without the sedative side effects so common with the older preparations. The concern about antihistamines causing further inspissation of bronchial mucus appears greatly exaggerated, and the newer antihistamines are being investigated for asthma management.

Interest in channel blocking agents has been high, but so far calcium channel blockers have not been impressively effective in the management of bronchospasm. Current investigations center around the use of potassium and magnesium channel agents, and IV magnesium may be found to play a role in the treatment of severe asthma.

Recent studies also suggest the possibility of a carefully defined role for such procedures as continuous beta-agonist nebulization, halothane anesthesia, intravenous terbutaline (replacing isoproterenol of the 1970s), and atropine nebulization. Much effort and interest is being devoted to clarifying the proper use of these approaches in asthma management, and someday we may smile at our current efforts.

Allergists in Utah

It appears that the first physician in Utah who showed a special interest in the treatment of allergic diseases was Dr. J. Mercer Anderson, who, following an internship, began practicing dermatology and allergy in Utah in 1928. Later associated with the Salt Lake Clinic, Dr. Anderson subsequently moved his office to the Medical Arts Building, where he practiced for nearly forty years. Utah's pioneer allergist died in 1971.

In 1949 Dr. G. Harlow Richards arrived with a special interest and some special training in allergy. Associated with the Salt Lake Clinic, he was board-certified in the 1970s and retired in 1982.

The 1950s saw the arrival of the first board-certified allergists, Drs. Dean Moffat and George Peck. They were followed in the late fifties and early sixties by Drs. John Baukol and Virginia Lanier. In 1962 Dr. Peck left for the warmer climes of Southern California, having been irritated himself by the cold Utah winters. His practice passed to Dr. Lanier. In June of 1965 Dr. Lorimer T. Christensen arrived to associate with Dr. Lanier, who died suddenly while on a tour of the new University Medical Center. Within the next three years the state's pioneering certified allergists — namely Drs. Moffat, Baukol, Peck, and Lanier — all died, leaving Dr. Christensen a "lone and weary" practitioner.

Shortly thereafter, Drs. David Burkley and Lowell Hyland arrived to purchase Drs. Moffat and Baukol's practice. Soon, however, Dr. Hyland moved out of state and Dr. Edwin Bronsky from the faculty of National Jewish Hospital in Denver took his place.

In 1971 the Intermountain Allergy and Asthma Clinic was formed by the association of Drs. Christensen, Burkley, and Bronsky. With six allergists at this time, the Clinic has been recognized as the second largest allergy group practicing in the United States. Joining the Clinic and practicing in the Ogden area were Drs. Brent Burdett and Joseph Anderson. In response to the energy crisis of the seventies, the Clinic established regularly scheduled visits to outlying areas, bringing high-quality allergy care to residents in Cedar City, St. George, Logan, Moab, Price, Roosevelt, and Vernal. Clinic members continue to serve many rural Utah citizens with weekly and monthly visits.

Drs. Charles Rogers and John Stewart are currently practicing allergy in Murray, while Drs. Lowell Jones and Henry Yeates in Provo serve the greater Utah County area. Dr. Robert Griffiths heads the allergy division at the University Medical Center, where he has been joined by Dr. Kay Walker. Dr. Craig Moffat, succeeding Dr. G. Harlow Richards, has been the allergist for the Salt Lake Clinic for a decade.

As 15% to 20% of the general population experiences allergy problems, the need for specialist care is obvious. The challenge for allergists practicing in Utah is substantial, as they must treat patients living at altitudes ranging from 8,000 feet in Alta to 2,400 feet in St. George, with indigenous vegetation that varies widely at these disparate altitudes. A growing nucleus of well-trained and properly motivated allergists has substantially raised the level of specialist care available to patients severely afflicted with allergies.

As in any relatively new specialty, there are bound to be practitioners who continue with a less-than-scientific approach to diagnosis and management. The allergy field has also been "contaminated" by non-certified physicians using unproven and unscientific methods. With the establishment of the Board of Allergy and Clinical Immunology in 1974, and with third-party payors anxious to see that health-care dollars are spent most judiciously, these practitioners may be more clearly recognized and avoided by patients and insurance carriers alike.

The future of allergy in Utah is represented best by the establishment of the AAAA Medical Research Group, a division of the Intermountain Allergy and Asthma Clinic. Actively involved in numerous FDA-approved research studies, this group is currently evaluating many new drugs; for example, attempting to clarify the proper role of gold therapy and methotrexate in the management of chronic, severe steroid-dependent asthma. Also under investigation are third-generation antihistamines in the form of nasal sprays, more effective beta-agonists, mast cell stabilizing agents other than Cromolyn, and atropine-like nasal sprays and inhalers as well as improved topical steroids.

With growing physician and public awareness of the unique role that certified allergists have in the management of allergic disorders, and with a growing number of competent specialists in the field, the future of allergy in Utah does indeed look bright.

CHAPTER EIGHT

Gastroenterology

JOHN G. MOORE, MD

THE AMERICAN GASTROENTEROLOGICAL ASSOCIATION (AGA), established in 1897, is the oldest internal medicine subspecialty organization in the U.S. However, formal recognition of gastroenterology as a major subspecialty of the American Board of Internal Medicine (ABIM) did not occur until 1940 when, for the first time, subspecialists in gastrointestinal medicine sat for oral and written certification exams. This long delay in recognition is easily understood: basic knowledge of gastrointestinal physiologic processes was extremely limited, technological advance appeared to be confined only to the development of a variety of intestinal tubes (e.g., Einhorn, Miller-Abbott), and treatment of common gastrointestinal disorders was entirely empirical. These treatments included, for example, routine use of herbs and antiphlogistics, administration of dilute preparations of hydrochloric acid, abdominal belts for "misposition" of intestinal organs, and high colonic lavage — all of which did little to inspire confidence in the specialty. Roentgenography, first employed for intestinal disorders in the early 1900s, was the diagnostic "gold standard" and remained so for sixty years.

In the late 1960s flexible endoscopy was introduced, and it revolutionized the practice, teaching, and growth of the field. Invasive flexible endoscopy, employing a multitude of increasingly sophisticated instruments to examine areas of the intestinal tract not hitherto accessible except by surgical intervention, is now the bedrock of diagnostic and therapeutic gastroenterology.

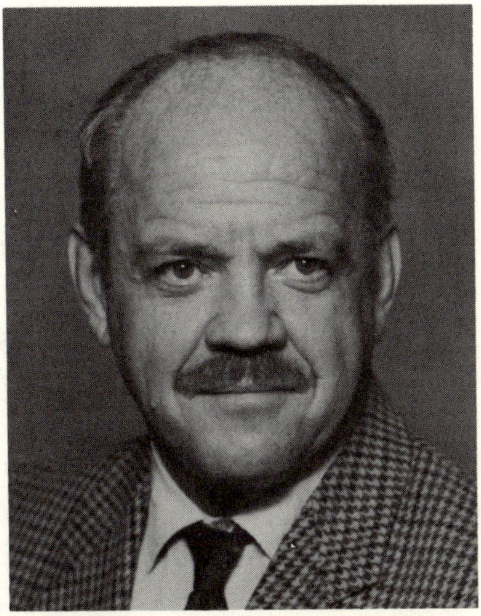

John G. Moore.

More internal medicine trainees now apply for gastrointestinal fellowship training programs than ever before, and AGA membership has risen from a few hundred in the 1950s to more than 6,000 today, including thirty-three members from the state of Utah. In 1960 there were two ABIM-qualified/certified gastroenterologists in Utah; in 1990 there are twenty-four.

The history of gastroenterology in Utah in the first half of the century was not unlike the national experience. Most specialists in internal medicine, trained in Eastern medical schools or in Europe, diagnosed and treated disorders of the intestine by clinical intuition. Radiography was the principle diagnostic test; surgery was frequently resorted to for diagnostic confirmation and/or treatment. Gastrointestinal endoscopy was limited to proctoscopic exams and an occasional stomach exam with rigid instruments. Upper gastrointestinal endoscopy, pioneered by Dr. Rudolf Schindler in the 1920s, had not achieved widespread popularity because of the hazards of rigid instrumentation use and the limited endoscopic information obtainable.

Nevertheless, Dr. Ted Bauerlein of the Intermountain Clinic in Salt Lake City adopted this then-new diagnostic modality and was the first to employ upper endoscopy in his clinical practice. He was recognized as the first specialist in gastroenterology in Utah. Dr. Bauerlein, a tall, chamber music-loving native of the Midwest, graduated from Columbia Physicians and Surgeons Medical School in 1934. He trained in internal medicine at Barnes' Hospital in St. Louis and in 1937 joined the Intermountain Clinic, where he remained for twenty-three years. In 1960 he moved to Southern California and continued an active clinical practice for fifteen more years in the San Diego–La Jolla area. Dr. Bauerlein taught his endoscopic skills to Drs. Dean Ashworth and Edwin Englert, Jr.

Drs. Ashworth and Englert were the first internists in Utah formally trained in the subspecialty. Both received their GI fellowship training in Boston in the late 1950s under the tutelage of Dr. Franz Ingelfinger, then considered the doyen of American gastroenterology and later to become editor of the *New England Journal of Medicine*. Dr. Ashworth, a native of Provo and graduate of Washington University in St. Louis, joined Dr. Bauerlein at the Intermountain Clinic in 1959. He established the first esophageal motility testing laboratory in Utah, and, for the first time, patients with primary esophageal disorders such as achalasia were accurately diagnosed. Dr. Ashworth, clinical professor of medicine at the University of Utah Medical School, still regularly contributes in teaching diseases of the esophagus to medical students, residents, and GI fellows-in-training at the University of Utah Medical Center (UUMC) and Veterans Administration hospitals. In 1987 he received the Outstanding Clinical Faculty Award of the University Department of Medicine.

Dr. Englert, a native of New York (born in 1926) and a graduate of Columbia Physicians and Surgeons Medical School, was the first gastroenterologist in Utah with a full-time academic appointment. He served for more than thirty years on the VA and UUMC Department of Medicine staffs as chief of the VA medical service (1966–70), and chief of the VA gastroenterology section (1960–80). As founder and chair of the Division of Gastroenterology at both the UMC and VA, he established the nation's first VA research and education training program in gastroenterology. Dr. Englert was known as an incisively

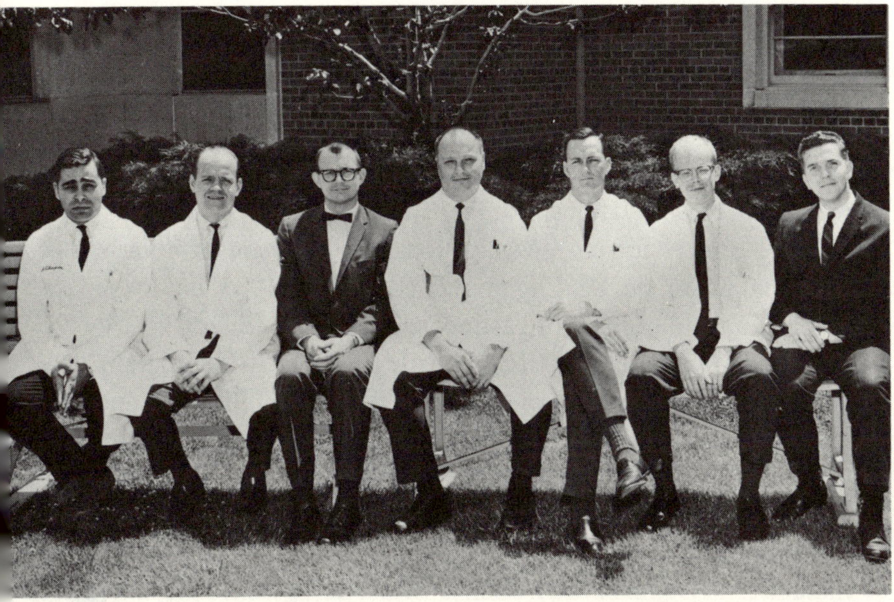

The gastroenterology staff and training fellows in 1964. Left to right: Drs. Asher Thompson, John Moore, Dean Ashworth, Edwin Englert, Jr., Jim Freston, Howard Wilcox, and Peter Midgely. Drs. Thompson, Moore, and Freston were GI fellows-in-training. Dr. Wilcox was a resident in medicine, and Dr. Midgely was then a summer research student.

critical and outspoken taskmaster, demanding of his own and others' perfection in scientific endeavors. He was also a superb and witty lecturer, especially on the subject of stools — a favorite topic among gastroenterologists — and "functional bowel disease," the bane of modern society and a still largely unsolved gastrointestinal disorder. He was also an avid fly fisherman who often regaled those around him on fly-tying techniques. He served on the editorial boards of several leading gastrointestinal journals and wrote many articles in his two major research areas of stomach and gallbladder pathophysiology.

Dr. Englert was the first to forge a lasting link with his surgical colleagues. In 1968 Dr. John Dixon, a surgeon who later became dean of the Medical School, joined the Division of Gastroenterology. Dr. Dixon established the Utah Laser Institute, adding yet another therapeutic tool to the gastroenterologist's armamentarium. Drs. Frank Moody, chair of the Department of Surgery in the seventies and early eighties, Bing Rikkers, and Jim Becker all were later to collaborate with the division in many joint surgery-gastroenterology pursuits. As a result of Dr. Englert's pioneering efforts in research and training and in forging these relationships, the University and VA hospitals have become centers for the investigation and treatment of a variety of intestinal disorders. Dr. Englert passed away in 1985, but his legacy in teaching and training of gastroenterologists continues.

Since 1961 more than fifty graduates of the Utah GI program have begun to practice in such diverse locales as the Philippines and Iran and in many states of the Union, including Utah, Idaho, Nevada, California, Oregon, Washington, Colorado, Texas, Wisconsin, Illinois, Michigan, Pennsylvania, New York, Connecticut, New Jersey, and North Carolina. Twenty-two graduates now live in Utah. These include Drs. Dennis Avner, John Bowers, Terry Box, Joseph Brown, Hal Cole, Stuart Ellington, Cliff Harmon, Wes Keller, Robert Kiyomura, Robert Miller, Kent Nelson, Robert Nielson, Keith Peterson, Dale Richey, Ray Thomason, and Lynn Wilcox — all with established GI practices on the Wasatch Front. Drs. John Moore, Malcolm Berenson, Ken Buchi, Randall Burt, and Keith Tolman remained in academic medicine and locate at the University of Utah and Veterans medical centers. Dr. Jim Freston, a native of Ogden and chair of the Division of Gastroenterology from 1970 to 1980, is now chief of medicine at the University of Connecticut. Thursday afternoon GI rounds, semiannual Utah GUT Club gatherings, and national AGA and ACG (American College of Gastroenterology) meetings afford this collegial group the opportunity to associate on a regular basis.

In 1960 GI fellows-in-training devoted most of their training time to clinical consultation, review of x-ray studies, and performance of a few simple laboratory tests. Those tests included gastric analysis, secretin tests of pancreatic function, and routine stool analysis — all of which have been virtually abandoned in training in 1990. In 1960 rigid UGI endoscopy was performed at the Salt Lake City VA Hospital at the frequency of about six per year. In 1990 flexible UGI endoscopy is performed there at the frequency of about six per day. In addition, visualization of the entire colon, small bowel, pancreatic, and biliary trees is now possible with newer flexible and "chip" endoscopic instruments, adding further to procedure-loaded daily tasks.

The 1990-trained gastroenterologist is now exposed to diagnostic and therapeutic modalities undreamed of in 1960: CT scans, abdominal and endoscopic ultrasound, laser and electro- and "heater probe" coagulation of GI bleeding lesions, esophageal variceal sclerosis, endoscopic esophageal and biliary stent placement, gallstone lithotripsy, and a host of other procedure-based tasks.

In 1960 about 75% of fellows-in-training time was spent in "cognitive" activity; in 1990, in contrast, 75% of the time is spent in procedural tasks. This transition from an intellectual ("thinking") to a semi-surgical ("doing") subspecialty with the attendant skills and risks involved has forced redirection in all GI training programs. Procedure complications — formerly the domain of surgical practice — are now a concern of the practicing gastroenterologist as well. One of the more memorable complications occurred in 1967, shortly after introduction of the new Hirschowitz fiberoptic endoscope. The instrument's flexible tip became wedged at the patient's gastroesophageal junction and required surgery for removal. The patient recovered uneventfully, but the experience served as a harbinger of future events involving increasingly invasive endoscopic procedures. Fortunately, these complications (e.g., bleeding following colonic polypectomy, esophageal and colonic perforation) are rare.

Advances in endoscopy have been paralleled by even more profound advances in molecular biology. DNA-probe and genetic-engineering technology have revolutionized the understanding of many disease processes, including those of the intestinal tract. Dr. Randall Burt has long been interested in the genetics of the common colonic polyp, a precursor lesion in the development of colon cancer. He is working in collaboration with Dr. Mark Skolnick in the Division of Genetic Epidemiology and Dr. Ray White of the Howard Hughes Medical Institute, and through their efforts inheritance patterns and polyp gene location sites are slowly becoming known. In the years to come this basic information may be employed predictively in preventing this common malignancy.

Drs. Ken Buchi and David Bjorkman are now treating tumor-bearing mice with laser-beam therapy. Dramatic reductions in tumor size are observed in rats pretreated with hematoporphyrin derivative — a heme product that localizes to tumor sites and enhances laser treatment effects. Human trials with this new cancer therapeutic modality are in progress. Dr. Bjorkman is also studying the effects of alcohol on the intestine, employing techniques that permit far more detailed scrutiny of intestinal morphology than those available in 1960.

Dr. Malcolm Berenson is engaged in several trials evaluating new drugs in old and common GI disorders: peptic ulcer disease and "heartburn" (or GERD: gastroesophageal reflux disease), for which cures have not yet been discovered. One such trial with omeprazole — a new, powerful inhibitor of gastric acid — led to the adoption of a superior dosage schedule for treatment of GERD. Dr. Berenson is also studying the metabolism of porphyrin — essential in heme formation — and its role in liver disease and gallstone formation.

Dr. Bill Hutson, in collaboration with Dean Ashworth, is studying esophageal, gastric, small-bowel, and colonic motility patterns in a variety of intestinal disorders. Dr. Hutson is also exploring a new radioisotope-based method in the study of physiological and psychological influences on gastric emptying. Dr. John Moore's interests lie in gastric emptying, examining ancient stools, and in exploring circadian rhythms of gastrointestinal function. Dr. Moore is also collaborating with Dr. Terry Clemmer of the LDS Hospital on the use of H2-receptor antagonists in a shock/trauma ward setting. Dr. Keith Tolman, chair of the Division of Gastroenterology at the University since 1983, studies the mechanism(s) of drug toxicity to the liver. Under his direction, the UUMC Drug Research Center conducts pre-marketing clinical efficacy and safety trials for new gastrointestinal drugs. These diverse activities and interests reflect the growing clinical and research subspecialization occurring within gastrointestinal medicine.

Enormous advances have been made in the field in thirty years. From the days of routine gastric analysis and reviewing x-rays, modern gastroenterologists now spend their time with a host of diagnostic and therapeutic procedures unavailable, even unimagined, thirty years ago. The future is bright with promise of even more significant advances. Video-controlled endoscopy of the entire GI tract will become routine by the year 2000. The causes of ordinary peptic ulcer disease will be better elucidated and more effectively treated. Total or partial liver and, possibly, pancreatic transplantation will be commonplace. The molecular and genetic basis for a variety of intestinal disorders will be elucidated. Genetic marker analysis will be employed as a preventive tool; indeed, the molecular and environmental basis for colonic malignancy may well be resolved by the time we enter the twenty-first century.

Training programs in gastrointestinal medicine face the challenge of keeping apace of these technological advances and meeting the demands of increasing subspecialization. In response to this challenge, gastrointestinal fellowship training programs will increase to three years — more for those pursuing academic careers. In addition, the imposition of DRG's, Joint Commission on Accreditation of Hospitals requirements and quality assurance mandates, and an increasingly competitive marketplace for the health-care dollar, have altered the teaching and practice of medicine and gastroenterology forever. All of these challenges will require a vigorous and visionary response. The revolutionary changes observed in the last thirty years are apt to be repeated in the next thirty years, and it is the challenge to our medical educators to anticipate and prepare for these.

CHAPTER NINE

Pulmonary Medicine

ATTILIO D. RENZETTI, JR., MD

PULMONARY MEDICINE WAS FORMALLY RECOGNIZED in the United States as a subspecialty of internal medicine in 1941. THE American Board of Pulmonary Diseases (ABPD) was established under the parent American Board of Internal Medicine (ABIM). At that time, and until the late 1940s, physicians who practiced this subspecialty were primarily tuberculosis specialists whose expertise naturally extended into all diseases of the chest. No board-certified pulmonary specialists practiced in Utah in the immediate post-war period. The State Tuberculosis Sanatorium in Roy was under the full-time medical direction of Dr. D. O. N. Lindbergh for many years. In private practice, patients with pulmonary diseases were cared for by general practitioners and internists. One internist with a special interest in diseases of the chest was Dr. Elmer Kilpatrick in Salt Lake City. Patients with pulmonary problems were referred to thoracic surgeons and ENT specialists because of their experience in performing bronchoscopy. Most notable among these surgeons were Drs. Ray Rumel and Preston Cutler and among the ENT group Dr. Ralph Rigby, who practiced endoscopy almost exclusively. When patients with bronchial asthma required special care, they were referred to allergy specialists.

In the immediate post–World War II period, tuberculosis was still the most common serious pulmonary disease in the U.S. However, Utah was then and still remains among the states with the lowest incidence of tuberculosis, so the need for pulmonary specialists in the

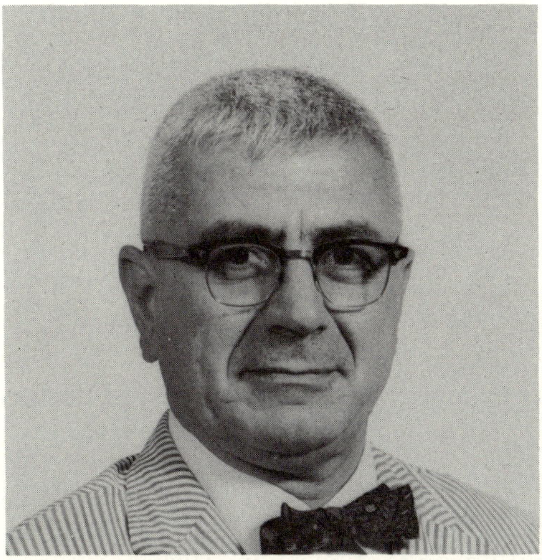

Attilio D. Renzetti, Jr.

private sector was not great. Of course, asthma was and still is very common, but it was considered the domain of the generalist and allergist. Since antimicrobial therapy had only become available in the late 1930s with the introduction of the sulfa drugs and after the war with penicillin, bronchiectasis was still frequently seen. Chronic obstructive pulmonary disease (chronic bronchitis and emphysema) and cancer of the lung were not very common in the early post-war period. In fact, the link between cigarette smoking and these conditions was only beginning to be suspected in those centers with large chest disease services. In Utah, with its extensive mining history, silicosis was among the more common pulmonary diseases; but since there was no available treatment, it was seen mostly by industrial physicians rather than private practitioners.

In the summer of 1952, the first Division of Pulmonary Diseases was established in the Department of Medicine at the University of Utah with the recruitment of Drs. John McClement and Attilio Renzetti as co-directors. Since space was not available at the Salt Lake General (County) Hospital (SLGH), the teaching base for the School of Medicine until 1965, the Pulmonary Division was located at the new Fort Douglas Veterans Administration Hospital on Foothill Boulevard, coincident with its opening. In contrast to the old VA Hospital on the north bench, which was a general hospital, the new one was designated as a neuropsychiatric-tuberculosis hospital. The Division of Pulmonary Diseases occupied all of Building 2, which had four fifty-bed wards and space for such supporting services as an operating room for thoracic surgery, a fluoroscopy and x-ray unit, clinical laboratories, and rooms specifically designed for the treatment of psychiatric patients with cold pack, hot tub, and electroshock therapies. The four patient-care wards were designated according to the type of patients housed: closed (locked) psychiatric TB, open (unlocked) psychiatric TB, non-psychiatric TB, and non-TB chest diseases. The last-named ward came into being as a condition by Drs. McClement and Renzetti of accepting their positions in the Medical School. They came to Utah from the Bellevue Hospital Chest Service in New York City, which was a teaching service of the Columbia University College of Physicians and Surgeons and considered the leading hospital in the U.S. for the training of physicians in the field of chest diseases. It was the goal of the new Pulmonary Division directors to establish a patient care and physician training program like the one at Bellevue, devoted to the broad field of chest diseases rather than to tuberculosis alone.

The beginning of the Pulmonary Division at the University of Utah brought to Utah either the first or one of the first two or three clinical pulmonary function testing laboratories in the United States. The testing techniques and methodology had been developed in large part at Bellevue Hospital in the period when Drs. McClement and Renzetti were in training, so they were in a position to establish a laboratory for both the diagnosis and management of patients with pulmonary diseases and research into their pathophysiology. Also for the first time, through rotations on the wards of the new pulmonary service, residents in internal medicine received training and experience with tuberculosis and other pulmonary diseases. Among the first of these trainees was Dr. Ted Bernhisel, who devoted extra elective time to this field and who, when he entered private practice in Salt Lake City, made pulmonary medicine his area of special interest. From that point on, physicians who received their internal medicine training at the University of Utah were exposed to up-to-date knowledge in the pulmonary field which they could bring to bear on the patients in their private practice. Some, such as Drs. John Newton and Drew Peterson in Ogden, maintained a special interest in tuberculosis; they became co-directors of the State Tuberculosis Sanatorium after Dr. Lindbergh's retirement in 1953.

Between 1952 and 1961, the Pulmonary Division underwent a number of changes in leadership while the characteristics of the patient population were changing as well. A major change was the gradual reduction in the number of patients with tuberculosis as the impact of chemotherapy for this disease became more and more decisive.

In 1953 Dr. Renzetti left Utah to become head of the Pulmonary Section at the veterans' hospital affiliated with the State University of New York at Syracuse. In 1955 Dr. McClement was lured back to New York City to become chief of the Chest Service at Bellevue Hospital, and he was replaced by Dr. H. William Harris, another Bellevue-trained chest specialist. Dr. Harris recruited Dr. Charles Pinney as assistant chief and Dr. Jerry Cohn from the Johns Hopkins Hospital to become director of the Pulmonary Function Laboratory in 1955. Between 1955 and 1960, Dr. Harris served the double role of head of the Pulmonary Division and chief of medicine at the VA Hospital until in 1960 he too was lured back East to become chairman of the Department of Medicine at the Women's Medical College of Pennsylvania.

After a year as acting head of the division, Dr. Cohn departed for the University of Kentucky, and in July 1961 Dr. Renzetti returned as division chief. By 1961 the patient population of the Pulmonary Service at the VA was entirely housed on one of the fifty-bed wards of the original four, and only fifteen to twenty beds were required for tuberculosis patients! When he returned to Utah, Dr. Renzetti was the only pulmonary specialist in the state certified by the ABPD. In fact, there were only about 400 such certified specialists in the United States at that time.

In 1961 the Pulmonary Division of the University of Utah was still based geographically at the VA Hospital. Dr. Renzetti instituted formal training for those physicians who had completed their internal medicine training and desired special competence in the pulmonary subspecialty. Training was also provided in the expanding field of applied respiratory physiology and pulmonary function testing. Dr. Renzetti also functioned as the pulmonary consultant for patients at the SLGH.

In October of 1961, Dr. C. DuWayne Schmidt returned to his native state to enter private practice at the Salt Lake Clinic. A graduate of the University of Utah College of Medicine, Dr. Schmidt, had received both internal medicine training and formal training in pulmonary medicine at the Mayo Clinic. Thus, he became the first board-eligible (later -certified) pulmonary specialist to enter private practice in Utah. As a staff member of the LDS Hospital, Dr. Schmidt also initiated the development of a Pulmonary Section there and has served as its chief since 1971, functioning essentially as a full-time faculty member.

A major development in pulmonary medicine in Utah was the first program in the United States with a declared goal of eradicating tuberculosis from an entire state. This effort, which began in 1963–64, seemed worthwhile because the United States Public Health Service (USPHS) had recently completed and reported its landmark studies demonstrating that the application of chemoprophylaxis with isoniazid led to a dramatic reduction in the incidence of new active cases of the disease. The Utah State Department of Health (G. Carlyle Thompson, Director) successfully competed for a grant from the Communicable Disease Center of the USPHS to develop and implement this program under the leadership of Dr. Elton Newman, director of the Tuberculosis Division of the Health Department (and former chair of the Department of Preventive Medicine at the University of Utah), with the aid of his tuberculosis consultants, Drs. Renzetti, Schmidt, and Newton.

The essential components of the program were statewide tuberculosis testing, chest x-rays with the aid of a mobile x-ray unit, tuberculosis referral clinics at the University Hospital in Salt Lake City and Dee Hospital in Ogden, and the administration of free antituberculosis medication or chemoprophylaxis where indicated. The major groups targeted by this program were the American Indians on their reservations and school children upon entrance to elementary school and the eighth grade. Other groups receiving special attention were elementary school teachers, LDS missionaries, coal miners, food handlers, and hairdressers. For the Indians, clinics were held four times a year on the reservations with a team of three nurses under the direction of Darlene Brian Meservy and a tuberculosis physician. When the program started, the incidence of tuberculosis among the reservation Indians was more than 400 per 100,000. Ten years later, in the early seventies, this incidence had been reduced to approximately 25 per 100,000, and the Indian children were shown to be almost uniformly negative on tuberculosis testing!

In consultation with Drs. Schmidt and Renzetti, The LDS Church instituted a tuberculin testing program for departing and returning missionaries. Another important part of the program, which was carried out with the invaluable aid of the county public health nurses and the state, was the investigation of household contacts of children entering school who were found to be tuberculin reactors and the treatment of all active cases found as a result of the various surveys. Another tangible benefit attributable, at least in part, to this pioneering effort was the closure of the State Tuberculosis Sanatorium in 1967. Finally, in addition to those mentioned above, a number of physicians gave generously of their time and effort, including Drs. Ted Noehren, Drew Peterson, Farrell Calton, and Richard Kanner. Dr. Lawrence Farrer of the USPHS, as assistant to Dr. Newman, played a major role in all aspects of the program.

In 1967, following completion of a year of training with Dr. Renzetti, Dr. Frances Beier, a trained pediatrician, brought the first pulmonary medicine to the Department of Pediatrics at the University of Utah Medical Center and then into the private practice of pediatrics in Salt Lake City. In 1967 Dr. Lowell Glasgow, then chair of the Department of Pediatrics, and Dr. Renzetti sponsored a graduating

University of Utah medical student, Dr. Dennis Nielson, for a new program at the University of California in San Francisco to train physicians for careers in pediatric pulmonology. He returned as a faculty member of the Department of Pediatrics in 1980, and in 1983 he became the first director of Pediatric Pulmonology.

Soon after the opening of the new University of Utah Medical Center (UUMC) in 1965, Dr. Renzetti established offices and laboratories for the Pulmonary Division there, while continuing to maintain the program at the VA Hospital. From that time to the present, trainees in pulmonary medicine have received their training at both institutions. Dr. Marcia Mitchell, who had trained for three years with Dr. Renzetti (1963–66), remained full-time at the VA to help maintain the clinical care and training responsibilities there. Upon completion of his training with Dr. Renzetti in 1968, Dr. Richard Kanner joined him on the full-time faculty at the UUMC, where he has remained to the present.

At the same time, Dr. Ted Noehren was recruited to join the faculty of the Pulmonary Division at the UUMC, and shortly thereafter Dr. David Scheinhorn was recruited as chief of the Pulmonary Section at the VA. The return of Ted Noehren represented an interesting twist of fate in that it was he back in 1952 who had acted on behalf of Dr. Wintrobe, chair of medicine, in recruiting Drs. McClement and Renzetti to Utah! Dr. Noehren had left the Department of Public Health and Preventive Medicine at the University of Utah in 1952 for a position at the State University of New York in Buffalo. There he developed a further interest and training in respiratory physiology and pulmonary disease which established him as a pulmonary specialist, thus preparing him to return to Utah.

In 1971 Drs. Renzetti and Schmidt decided to join forces in expanding the Pulmonary Division to the LDS Hospital. Without any written documents or formal affiliation agreements, they quietly began to build personnel and physical resources at LDS. They recruited Dr. Alan Morris in 1973 as the first full-time pulmonary faculty member to be geographically based at the LDS Hospital. Dr. Morris took over the direction of the pulmonary function laboratory there and began a long and fruitful interaction with the University's Department of Medical Biophysics and Computing (now Medical Informatics), which was also based in part at LDS. In addition, Dr. Morris established the Intermountain Respiratory Intensive Care Unit (IRICU), one of the first of its kind in the country. As one of ten collaborative units under the auspices of the National Institutes of Health, IRICU made a major contribution to current knowledge about the adult respiratory distress syndrome (ARDS) and its management, including the use of extracorporeal oxygenation therapy.

With the additional resources provided at LDS Hospital, the pulmonary training program underwent a major expansion to include rotation of trainees through the pulmonary laboratory, IRICU, and clinical services. The number of trainees entering the program increased to four per year and reached a peak of six per year in the early 1980s! The impact of this expanded training was finally felt in the community when trainees chose to remain in Utah and enter private practice. The first of these was Dr. Alfred Abaunza, who established himself at St. Mark's Hospital. He was soon joined there by Dr. Joseph Conrad. Then, after a short stay on the full-time faculty at LDS Hospital, Dr. Robert Farney joined Dr. Schmidt at the Salt Lake Clinic. Others who followed and settled in Utah (in Salt Lake City, except where indicated) are Alan Abdulla (Ogden), David Collins (Price), Tracy Hill (Provo), Martha Humphrey, James Pearl, Brad Rasmusson, Dan Rawson, William Sadler, Mark Shockey, and Donald Wilhelm. Pulmonologists who had trained elsewhere also established private practices in Utah. These include Russell Hurst (Lewiston), Ghent Graves (Logan), Joseph Schoenhals (SLC), Steven Lewis and Clark Bishop (Provo), and Gary Goucher and Jeff Abel (Ogden). The most recent additions are Drs. Kurt Francis and Nathan Dean. Most of these physicians have been appointed to the clinical faculty and thereby participate in the teaching program of the division.

An equally important impact of the expanded training program was the development of full-time faculty for the Pulmonary Division, including at LDS Drs. Robert Crapo, C. Gregory Elliott, Jim Orme, Jr., and Lindell Weaver. Drs. Guy Zimmerman, Norman Soskel,

Harold Chapman, Ralph Whatley, and Mark Elstad serve on the UUMC faculty. Some of these, such as Drs. Soskel and Chapman, have moved to other academic institutions. In addition, physicians who trained elsewhere became members of the Pulmonary Division for varying periods of time, including Drs. Jeff Simons, Kenneth Casey, and H. William Bonekat. The faculty of the division has also been enriched by the presence of individuals with PhD degrees who participate in lung research and in the training of pulmonary fellows. Drs. Reed Gardner, Adelbert Bigler, Robert Jensen, and James Walker have made important research contributions that have enhanced the national stature of the division. Finally, over the course of the thirty-nine years since its establishment, more than 100 physicians have received training in the Pulmonary Division and either practice pulmonary medicine or occupy academic pulmonary positions in Utah and throughout the nation. Support for the training endeavors of the division over the years has come from the American Lung Association and the National Institutes of Health.

Two other major developments in the Pulmonary Division occurred in 1977. Dr. Terry Clemmer, the first critical care specialist in Utah, joined the division and thereby expanded its training and patient care capabilities. He established and developed the Shock/Trauma ICU at LDS Hospital, and pulmonary trainees have rotated through this unit ever since. Those faculty members who are identified within the Pulmonary Division as both pulmonary and critical care specialists are, in addition to Dr. Clemmer, Drs. James Orme, Frank Thomas, and Lindell Weaver. In fact, with the recent addition to the faculty of Dr. Weaver, expertise in hyperbaric medicine is also a feature of the division.

The second development was the addition of Dr. William Rom to the Pulmonary Division faculty. Trained as both a pulmonary specialist and an occupational medicine specialist, Dr. Rom developed the Rocky Mountain Center for Occupational and Environmental Health (RMCOEH). The division was now able to expand its training program by providing a three-year pulmonary-occupational medicine track to train physicians for an academic future. To date, four physicians have completed this training, and one, Dr. William Sadler, has entered private practice in Salt Lake City. Drs. James Lockey and Mario Battigelli also joined the RMCOEH faculty and the division; however, all three have moved to other academic positions.

To reflect more accurately the expertise of its faculty, the scope of its clinical responsibilities, and the content of its postgraduate training programs, the division's name was changed to Division of Respiratory, Critical Care & Occupational Pulmonary Medicine (DRCCOM) in 1981.

In 1984 the Pulmonary Section at LDS Hospital established the Intermountain Sleep Disorders Center under the medical direction of Dr. Robert Farney and technical direction of Dr. James Walker. This facility has been accredited by the National Organization of Sleep Laboratories and functions as a training and research resource for the division. A sleep laboratory has also been developed at the UUMC under the co-direction of Drs. Suetaro Watanabe for pulmonary and Chris Jones for neurology.

Another important development of the eighties in which the division played a major role was the air transport services at both the LDS Hospital and the UUMC. Dr. Frank Thomas of the critical care facility directs the service for LDS Hospital, since the air service is closely integrated with the Shock/Trauma ICU there. Currently, Dr. Thomas is president of the World Organization of Air Transport Facilities.

Throughout the history of the Pulmonary Division at the University of Utah, research has been a major component of its activities. In the 1950s research projects were predominantly devoted to the chemotherapy of tuberculosis and particularly to various aspects of isoniazid metabolism and mechanisms of action. Beginning in the late fifties and continuing up through the eighties, research was predominantly in the areas of normal respiratory physiology in humans and the respiratory pathophysiology of lung diseases. In addition, long-term studies have been conducted, in collaboration with the Division of Infectious Diseases, concerning the role of infection in emphysema; and more recently the role of early intervention (e.g., smoking cessation) in the natural history of chronic obstructive pulmonary disease (chronic bronchitis and emphysema). As a result of the research projects carried out by members of the Pulmonary Division since its beginning in 1952, more than 120 articles have been published in the scientific literature. Support for the research program of the division has come primarily from grants from the National Institutes of Health.

Another major research thrust has been in the refinement and standardization of pulmonary function testing, particularly involving the application of computer technology. One outcome of this endeavor has been the publication, in collaboration with the Intermountain Thoracic Society (ITS), of a *Manual for Pulmonary Function Testing*, which has received worldwide recognition (more than 10,000 copies distributed) and which is now in its second edition. Although the *Manual* represents primarily the work of the faculty of the Pulmonary Division, special recognition is warranted for the efforts and guidance of Dr. Claude Lenfant, then director of the Lung Division of the National Heart and Lung Institute and Dr. Franklin Brough, executive director of the ITS.

Throughout the history of the Pulmonary Division, postgraduate medical education has been another important area of activity. Division members have participated in lectures and demonstrations related to the care of patients with lung diseases throughout the Intermountain area. One of the jewels of these efforts has been the Annual Midwinter Chest Conference, originally held at Brighton, then for a number of years at Park City, and for the past ten years at Snowbird. Initially, these conferences were presented predominantly by members of the University of Utah Pulmonary Division and invited distinguished faculty from national medical centers. With the growth of pulmonary expertise in the private sector, lecturers have been drawn from among the local practitioners. Attendance at this popular conference averages about 150 and is national and international as well as local.

The most recent change in the DRCCOM occurred in July 1987 with Dr. Renzetti's retirement and the transfer of administrative leadership of the division to Dr. John Hoidal, who came to Utah from Minnesota and Tennessee. As a vigorous leader he has brought research expertise in the field of molecular and cell biology and has recruited additional young faculty members with similar expertise, including Drs. Kevin McCusker, Barbara McCusker, John Michael, and Bruce Marshall.

Thus the history of pulmonary medicine in Utah since the end of World War II is inextricably linked to the development of the Pulmonary Division at the University of Utah, which has provided the training for those physicians who have entered private practice. Thereby, the citizens of Utah enjoy the availability of high-quality specialty care in pulmonary medicine.

CHAPTER TEN

The Management of Renal Failure, 1953–1988

H. ALLAN BLOOMER, MD, FACP
LAWRENCE E. STEVENS, MD, FACS

THE TREATMENT OF KIDNEY DISEASE, and particularly of renal failure, is a relatively new development both worldwide and in Utah compared to the ancient specialty of urology. A little more than forty years ago two major thrusts melded into the discipline of nephrology. The first was the influence of Dr. Homer W. Smith, not a physician but a superb basic scientist at New York University College of Medicine, who trained physiologists and physicians in renal physiology and pathophysiology over decades. Concurrently, the successful application of hemodialysis to the treatment of uremia by Dr. Willem Kolff in the Netherlands during World War II provided the first powerful tool for treating deranged kidney function. Quite naturally, Dr. Kolff's new technique was embraced by Dr. Smith's scientist-clinicians, and nephrology was born. A decade later, the addition of renal transplantation provided another powerful tool for treating renal failure.

In Utah, attempts at treating renal failure started as early as 1953. In June of that year, Drs. Keith Brown (a medical resident) and Lawrence E. Stevens (a surgical intern) performed peritoneal dialysis at the Twelfth Avenue VA Hospital on a forty-year-old man in hypertensive crisis and renal failure from polyarteritis nodosa. Dr. Stevens placed a red rubber catheter well into the peritoneal cavity and sutured it into position. Dialysate solutions were made by adding various electrolytes to standard intravenous solutions, as described a few months earlier in a report by Dr. Arthur Grollman of Dallas. The two

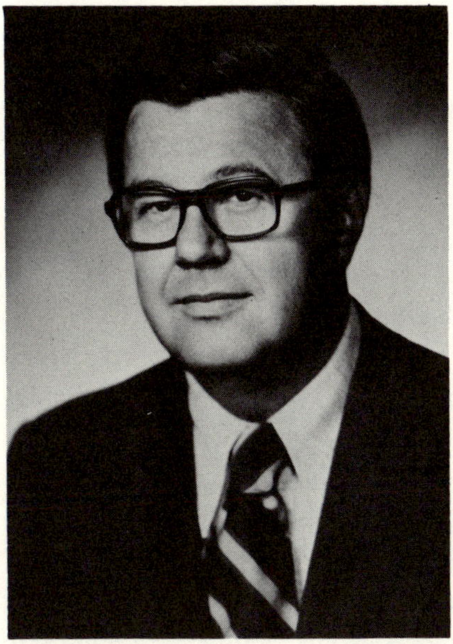

H. Allan Bloomer.

pioneers alternated twelve-hour shifts over the next four days, infusing 2-liter exchanges of dialysate solution into the peritoneal cavity, allowing equilibration, and then draining the peritoneal solution. The serum potassium fell to normal, the BUN and serum creatinine were reduced, but hypertension could not be controlled adequately and the patient expired. Dr. Brown's report of the case at Medical Grand Rounds sparked a great deal of interest and comment.

In the late 1950s, hemodialysis machines were acquired by the VA, Holy Cross, and LDS hospitals, but only a few dialyses were actually performed. None of the physicians involved in these early efforts had particular interest or expertise in the technique, and the machines were largely unused.

Then, in 1962, began one of the earliest comprehensive programs in the United States for treating chronic renal failure. Dr. Stevens, by then an instructor in the Department of Surgery at the University of Utah, excited by the early successes in human renal transplantation reported from Boston by Drs. Murray and Merrill, began transplantation in dogs. Approximately 150 kidney transplants were performed, using various immunosuppression techniques, setting the stage for eventual kidney grafts in humans.

In 1963 Dr. H. Allan Bloomer was the first formally trained nephrologist to join the faculty of the University of Utah. During the next several years, hemodialyses were performed with increasing frequency, mainly on cases with acute renal failure, at the old Salt Lake General Hospital (SLGH), the VA, LDS, and Holy Cross. But resources were scanty, and each treatment was a major event requiring the full-time attention of a small number of physicians. Dr. Bloomer recalls that at one time only one artificial kidney was in operating condition. He borrowed a pickup truck from the VA to cart the machine among the various hospitals, often in the middle of the night!

The modern day of kidney care arrived in 1965. Late the previous year, Dr. Bloomer had treated a rambunctious sheepherder with chronic glomerulonephritis and advanced renal failure. No hope was offered the man: he was considered to be rather uncooperative; there was no mechanism for regularly scheduled dialyses; Dr. Stevens was ready to transplant, but Dr. Bloomer was unenthusiastic. The patient was sent home to die.

Fortunately for the patient, he perforated a duodenal peptic ulcer one week later and was admitted to the surgical service at the SLGH. He was treated conservatively with nasogastric suction and antibiotics, and improved. He was kept in-house by Dr. Stevens until a cadaveric kidney became available. The first human kidney transplant in Utah was performed January 22, 1965, at the SLGH, and the patient survived. In fact, he is still alive and working today, still a rough-hewn character and the longest-surviving cadaveric kidney transplant recipient in the world as far as is known.

However, his postoperative course was long and difficult. He spent three months in the hospital and survived a number of complications. In this first patient, the ABO compatibility barrier was crossed unknowingly; an A kidney was transplanted into an O recipient. The diuresis was so voluminous that he required three liters of IV replacement fluid per hour at one point. He survived despite the ABO incom-

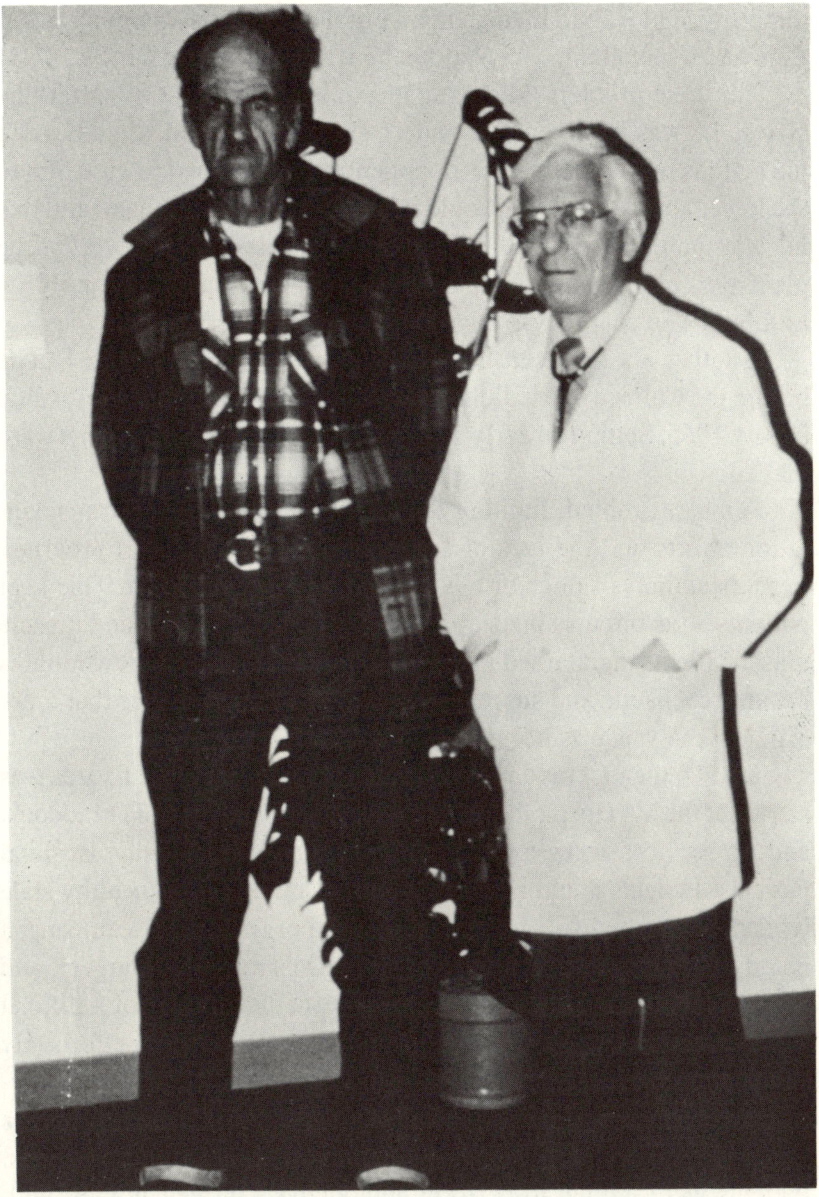

Doctor Lawrence E. Stevens and patient D. L., who received a cadaveric kidney transplant in 1965, photographed in 1988. D. L. was the first kidney transplant recipient in Utah and is now the longest surviving kidney transplant recipient in the world.

patibility, major fluid management problems, a serious wound infection, and a metabolic encephalopathy which lasted for weeks.

Yet these problems did not dampen his spirits. Shortly after discharge he was involved in an altercation and arrested. He defended his actions by stating that his opponent had threatened to kick him in the lower abdomen, which could injure his kidney transplant, and that he was defending himself. Dr. Stevens was called to verify the placement of the transplant in the lower abdomen and its susceptibility to injury. The charge was dismissed by a perplexed judge!

Another six or seven transplants were performed at the SLGH before the College of Medicine moved to the new University Hospital in July 1965. Setting an early precedent, several of these patients were diabetics.

A major problem limiting the success of early kidney transplantation efforts was the lack of an adequate dialysis support program. Peritoneal dialysis once or twice weekly was used at first. This kept patients alive but was inadequate for preserving strength and muscle mass. Patients maintained in this fashion for more than a few months became cachectic and susceptible to infection. It was clear that more efficient dialysis was necessary.

In 1966 the first modern chronic hemodialysis unit in this area was started at the VA Hospital by Dr. Bloomer and Dr. Robert K. Maddock, and its services were extended by contract to University Hospital patients. Patients could now be stabilized and kept in a healthy state while awaiting transplantation. The arrival of Dr. Keith Reemtsma, a noted transplant surgeon, as chief of the Department of Surgery, and his recruitment of Dr. Willem Kolff as head of the Division of Artificial Organs, greatly strengthened dialysis and transplantation efforts. By 1970 more than fifty transplants per year were performed.

Under Dr. Kolff's aegis, more effective dialysis support was provided and renal failure care expanded to include home dialysis. Patients were trained to perform hemodialysis in their homes, with the help of spouses or paid aides. Cost reductions resulted, but even more important was the degree of independence achieved by the home patients. They were no longer tied into dialysis center schedules but could perform their own treatments at times which would not conflict with work or family schedules. Many became more functional, and some returned to full-time employment. With the advent of home peritoneal dialysis, an aide was no longer necessary. A home patient could now be totally self-reliant. He could travel freely, provided that he carried dialysis supplies in the trunk of his car.

Some patients, for health or social reasons, could not achieve a high level of independence and remained on in-center dialysis. The "Dialysis in Wonderland" program was developed to add spice to their lives. Groups of about twenty patients rafted down the Colorado or Salmon rivers, toured Yellowstone Park in winter, lounged on the beaches of Hawaii, or traveled historic trails in Southern Utah, at minimal cost, and were dialyzed in camp!

Today, hemodialysis is provided on an urgent basis at most of the major hospitals in Utah. In addition, eleven chronic dialysis units scattered across the state serve the end-stage renal failure population. About 300 patients are on in-center chronic dialysis at all times, in addition to the home patients. The special needs of children with kidney failure are met at the University Hospital by an outpatient pediatric dialysis program developed by Dr. Richard L. Siegler.

The most exciting developments in recent years are in transplantation. Improved surgical techniques, better organ retrieval, and new immunosuppressive drugs have made kidney transplant easily available, safer, applicable to a wider spectrum of patients, and much more likely to be successful than ever before. Three transplant centers in Salt Lake City serve the state and the referral area. In a cooperative effort, LDS Hospital, the University Medical Center, and the Salt Lake VA Hospital perform nearly 150 transplants per year, with an overall success rate of almost 90%. No type of renal disease is automatically excluded. For instance, diabetic patients are about 40% of all patients transplanted. Selected patients as old as seventy-eight years of age have been transplanted successfully, as have patients with other medical problems such as severe hypertension and coronary artery disease. Complicated patients have a better long-term prognosis with transplants than with dialysis, particularly the diabetics.

In the long run, transplantation is considerably less expensive than chronic dialysis, and patient satisfaction is greater. No wonder that today in Utah more than one-half of new and end-state renal failure patients receive a kidney transplant instead of entering a chronic dialysis program.

Faces and allegiances have changed over the years. Dr. Stevens, after a stint at Columbia University, is now chief of surgery and head of the transplant service at LDS Hospital. Dr. Reemtsma is chair of the Department of Surgery at Columbia University. Dr. Bloomer is in private practice. Dr. Kolff, after receiving many international honors for his pioneering efforts in both kidney and heart replacement techniques, recently retired from the active faculty at the University of Utah. Dr. Wayne Border now ably heads a large group of nephrologists at the University and VA hospitals. But the overall program, strengthened by a close cooperative effort between the private and University sectors, flourishes and grows.

CHAPTER ELEVEN

Geriatric Care

VICTOR KASSEL, MD

IN 1909, WHEN IGNAZ NASCHER coined the word geriatrics, he identified it as a medical interest concerned with the prevention of the decrepitude associated with the later years. The cause of "old age" was not known then, or now, so geriatrics came to be identified with the sickness care of the aged.

At the time of my arrival in Salt Lake City in 1951, the idea of a medical specialty limited to the care of the aged was considered grotesque. When I applied for my state license, the examining physicians were perplexed and some derogatory remarks were made. I did receive my license, however. Later an internist criticized geriatrics as plain quackery, but I was defended by an older internist who understood the multifaceted problems presented by aged sick patients.

Geriatrics had two phases, both of which struck a negative chord in the Utah medical and lay communities: (1) prevention of "old age," actually the prevention of the diseases of later life that impair us — today known as preventive medicine; and (2) care of the aged patient using expertise in the pathology of old age. The Utahns' view of geriatrics simply reflected national attitudes.

In this troublesome intellectual environment, I accepted a part-time position with the Utah State Hospital in the fall of 1951, believing that the goal was to develop a treatment program specifically for the aged. However, since the hospital administrator considered the geriatrician simply a medical doctor and not a psychiatrist, I was to do only physical examinations on the patients. During World War II medical help was limited, and the physical examinations of the State Hospital patients had lagged. The hospital's goal in 1951 was simply to catch up on the physicals that had never been done or were too out of date. I was unable to generate any interest in a complete program based on the Troika Geriatric Diagnostic Profile, which includes detailed medical-surgical, psychiatric-psychological, and social data for each patient.

Fortunately, service at the State Hospital improved after Dr. V. M. Sevy retired from the VA and developed a geriatric program for the state similar to the one we developed at the VA during the early fifties.

Salt Lake Veterans Administration Hospital

C. H. Hardin Branch, professor and head of the Department of Psychiatry at the University of Utah, asked me to activate the Geriatric Unit of the newly constructed Fort Douglas Veterans Administration Hospital in early 1952. Building 4 had 100 beds for geriatric psychiatric patients. Medical and surgical care was rendered at the North Bench VA Hospital, and Fort Douglas was primarily for psychiatric, neurological, and tuberculosis patients.

The first patients were originally from the Intermountain West, transported from various parts of the country in order to be near their families. Since they arrived slowly, it was possible to do comprehensive geriatric evaluations. The major advantage of VA patients was the availability of their C-files, wherein could be found their complete histories, with discharge summaries from all previous admissions to VA hospitals. This comprehensive medical information enabled me to define the patients' diagnoses more accurately. It was disturbing to find how frequently they were accompanied by incorrect transfer diagnoses. Most often diagnoses were based simply on chronological age rather than past history or development of the infirmity.

Each Monday morning, rounds were made on all 100 patients. The full staff — including the nurses, the aides, the occupational therapists, the physical therapists, and the social worker — identified all the problems and made decisions concerning each patient's medi-

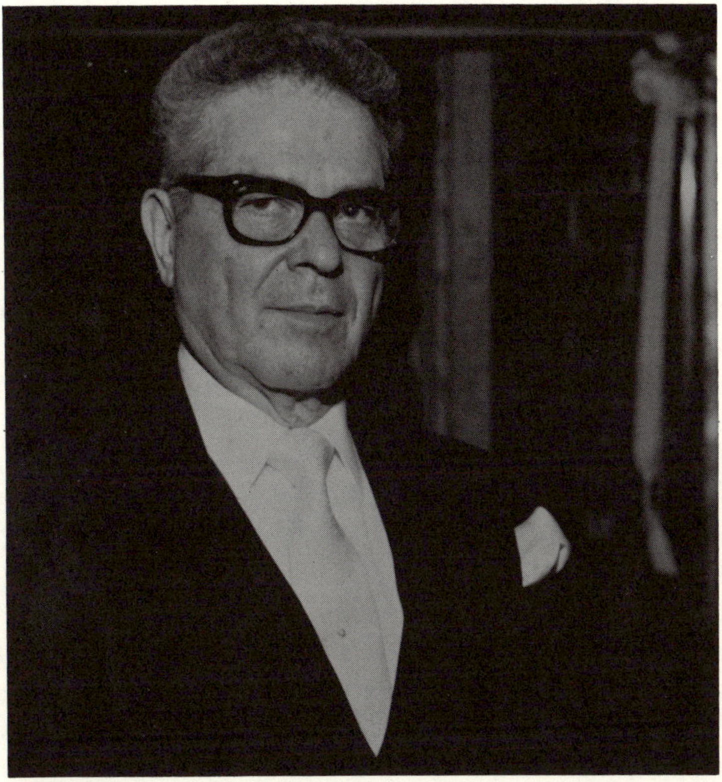

Victor Kassel.

cal-surgical, psychiatric-psychological, and social care. With this full give-and-take — with the patients' needs always the primary concern — there were never any therapeutic turf wars.

Monthly staff teaching conferences were held for the nurses and aides to discuss patients, problems, new orders, and diagnoses. Midnight conferences were also held for the night shift, as it was recognized that they generally are neglected because of the inconvenience presented by their working hours.

The Fort Douglas unit became recognized as the finest geriatric unit in the VA system. Personnel from other parts of the country came to participate and learn from our work. We were invited as a group to address other aspiring geriatric units and teach them our techniques.

An interesting result began to manifest: Patients' behavior improved. Merely the transfer of impaired geriatric patients to a treatment unit that welcomed them *because* of their age seemed to improve their morale. As time passed it became obvious that many patients did not need in-hospital care, so during 1954 we began to study alternative care.

The patients' families were horrified to learn that their relatives had improved enough to leave the hospital. They had been assured that the patients were too ill ever to leave. The social workers talked fast and furiously to assure the families that our concern was for what was best for all concerned and that we would carry the responsibility for medical, psychological, and social needs.

At that time the only other place available for the elderly veteran was a nursing home. We contacted five nursing homes in the area and explained our program. Four were willing to work with us. The nursing home administrators were guaranteed that should the placement not work out, the patient would *immediately* be returned to Building 4. The patient was on a leave of absence from the hospital, to be supervised by the social worker and visited at regular intervals. The VA would supply medication. I wanted to refer the patients to community practitioners for continued out-patient care and wrote to the Utah Medical Association for a list of interested physicians. The reply stated that the private physicians were not interested in assuming continuous-care responsibility for these old patients. Therefore I continued to follow the patients in the nursing homes without charge.

To substitute for the families, we developed a volunteer program with American Legion 40–8 ("Forty-and-Eight"). Members "adopted" the patients, seeing to it that they had companionship as well as clothing and other essentials.

Psychiatric patients on a successful leave of absence (LOA) for one year had to be discharged. We set up an LOA for eleven months, returned the patient to the VA for an annual physical examination, then reestablished the leave. Because we "bent" this VA regulation, our patients were never homeless or abandoned. They were carefully followed, and they continued to receive their medication and supervision. The cooperative nursing home administrators did excellent work as well.

The successful geriatric program continued until the early 1960s, when federal budgeting began to favor research over patient care. Personnel assigned to Building 4 were sent elsewhere, cutting the program drastically. It was decided that the VA system needed nursing homes, and Ward 18, half of Building 4, was converted into a nursing home and assigned away from the active geriatric treatment program. Over the next year, 1963, the finest geriatric program in the VA system was effectively dismantled.

Salt Lake County Infirmary

Another local government institution delegated to care for the aged, the infirm, the halt, the lame, and the incestuously genetically malconceived was the Salt Lake County Infirmary. Situated on Twenty-first South between State Street and Second East, the Infirmary housed these patients on the east side of the Salt Lake General Hospital (SLGH). The three floors of patients received a sort of nursing home care but were not overseen by a physician. Whenever a serious acute illness intruded, an intern from the Medical School side was called.

The patients were selected by the County Commissioner and admitted to the Infirmary by political mandate. In charge of the unit was a "matron," a political appointee with no medical or nursing training. When I went to her office in the early fifties to discuss the general care of these invalided geriatric patients, she considered it an intrusion.

After a conference with the powers, I was granted permission to *volunteer* my time. It was a major task trying to unravel the patients' histories. Working at the Infirmary was a political plum, and the political appointees were not going to allow an "invasion" by any outside force. The Infirmary looked like any nineteenth-century hospital back ward. Nothing deliberate was done to improve the state of these patients, and they were left to carry on as best they could with minimal nursing care.

Things did not begin to improve until a national commission found the SLGH, the teaching hospital for the University of Utah Medical School, "noncompliant" in 1954. The Medical School could not keep its accreditation as a training school unless improvements were made. The Infirmary was not included in the requirements, but it experienced a secondary gain resulting from the hiring of the hospital's first trained administrator, Kenneth Rindflesch. In correcting the hospital's defects, he also had a compassionate concern for the Infirmary residents. He encouraged rotation of house staff through the Infirmary, but the Medical School staff still saw no advantage in caring for the infirm.

As more sick patients were admitted, rather than those simply needing a home, treatment was upgraded; still the primary admissions were for those who needed long-term care. When Caroline McKean was appointed nurse in charge, a fine program ensued.

In 1965 the University of Utah built a medical center on the campus. The initial monies came from a fund from the State of Utah that was to be used for the treatment of and rehabilitation for chronic lung disease. The faculty promoters had promised that if they could use this money to start building the Medical Center, a geriatric unit would be included in the plans. When construction was completed, the Medical School moved and the Infirmary was abandoned — the patients distributed among nursing homes in the valley. The move precipitated a number of deaths among the patients. It took the University Medical School more than thirty years to fulfill its promise.

Nursing Homes

The history of nursing homes in Utah is not unlike nursing home development throughout the nation. Other than St. Joseph's Villa, established by the Sisters of Charity of the Incarnate Word in 1947, all the nursing homes at origin could be described as "mom and pop" homes. In the beginning, a daughter assumed the responsibility for the care of an older infirm parent. With the increased number of the elderly, the daughter opened the doors to infirm neighbors. The nursing home itself was a converted house.

With the cooperation of the operators of four local nursing homes — Clark and Edie Bonner, Jean Sinclair, Birdie Hara, and Edna Buckles — my work with the nursing homes began in the early fifties. After the program for the outpatient veterans was under way, the other nursing homes began to call upon me concerning the even greater number of elderly women.

Following the 1961 White House Conference on Aging, it became obvious to the "industry" that nursing homes could be a big business. A number of the "mom and pop" homes incorporated and built nursing facilities. Lay administrators took responsibility for running the homes until professional staff were hired. Very few nurses or doctors were trained to care for the long-term chronically ill person in a nursing home (a state of affairs that exists to this day).

The 1971 White House Conference on Aging found the government bureaucracy upset over the poor quality of nursing home patient care. Representatives of President Nixon announced that nursing homes would no longer be paid from Medicare or Medicaid unless they upgraded their patient care. With the cooperation of the states, the federal government introduced care regulations and legislated that skilled nursing facilities must have a medical director to oversee the quality of patient care. The nursing home administrators were naturally unhappy about this added expense. Unfortunately, far too often the job was given to a new practitioner in the area to help support him while he was building his practice or to an elderly physician who was phasing out his practice.

The problem of patient care continues today. Patients continue to be overmedicated; physicians refuse to see them in the homes, demanding that they be brought by ambulance to their offices; medical doctors do not answer their telephones or return the nurses' calls.

Most nurses have been trained for acute hospital care. In the hospital the nurse's burden is easier because the patient is seen daily by the physician. In the nursing home, the nurse may *never* see a doctor. A great burden is thrown upon the nurse, who has to depend upon her or his ability to identify problems. For a long time, nursing personnel suffered a 100% turnover each year. Many nurses' aides were hired "off the street" just to fill a slot. Recently the state has demanded that only trained aides be hired for this work.

Today, with DRGs and the demand that patients be discharged from the hospital earlier, the nursing homes are forced to administer to more acutely ill patients. The nursing homes are understaffed because of this change, and they are paid less than is needed for them to render the quality of service necessary.

Senior Citizen Centers

The first dedicated activity center for older citizens in Utah was built by L. C. Romney, Salt Lake County Commissioner. He and I selected the site at the Felt Boys Club at 440 South Ninth East in 1963. Since then many senior citizens' centers have been developed throughout the state. The importance of avocational activities for the aged has been recognized, and they have become a part of life for the elderly.

Home Health Care

About sixty years ago, Salt Lake Community Nursing Service began to offer professional visiting nurse care to the elderly. In the 1960s Eva Hancock, executive director of the Community Services Council, and myself, as president, were able to convince Maxine Thomas, director of the Community Nursing Service, to develop a homemakers' service for which we had obtained a three-year federal grant. Afton Crockett, a retired social worker, came out of retirement to direct the program. Community Nursing Service built a superb Homemakers Service to help older people stay at home rather than having to be placed in nursing homes.

The point of the federal grant was to demonstrate the viability of the service. After three years and completion of the grant, the United Fund (now United Way) had agreed to carry the responsibility.

We now had a flourishing program to help the aged and the infirm stay at home without hospital or nursing home care. Unfortunately, at the end of three years the United Fund refused to take on financial responsibility for the Homemakers Service. Instead, they added the Boy Scouts to their services, claiming that this organization was more *politically* acceptable. Without financial support, Homemakers Service died. A variety of similar services have since developed within the loop of total home health care. Still, the rejection by the United Fund of Homemakers Service as part of Community Nursing Service was responsible for a major denial of care to the aged for about fifteen years.

University of Utah

The University of Utah was exceedingly slow to recognize the needs of the elderly. In 1970, the Department of Family and Community Medicine was established. It eventually developed a Geriatric Medicine service.

Very recently, a Division of Human Development and Aging was created in the Department of Internal Medicine under Dr. Gerald Rothstein, a professor of medicine and pediatrics. The division is responsible for teaching clinical care and research in geriatrics at the University and VA hospitals, and it operates a seventeen-bed geriatric evaluation and treatment unit at the VA Hospital. It also has begun a consultation and outpatient service.

With the ever-increasing number of elderly patients, geriatrics must assume a more prominent role and attract greater funding. It is hoped that more sensitive and compassionate medical students will come forth to fill the future needs. So far, there has not arisen anyone from the University of Utah to enter the private practice of Geriatrics in the community and to have dedicated his/her entire professional life to serve the aged sick.

CHAPTER TWELVE

Endocrinology and Metabolism

FRANK H. TYLER, MD • DON H. NELSON, MD, PHD

WHEN DR. FRANK H. TYLER arrived at the University of Utah Medical School in 1947, metabolism was a component of clinical medicine. It included not only endocrinology and diabetes, as it does today, but also nephrology, genetics, and intermediary metabolism. This was a large order, but youth does not know its limitations.

The physical facility at that time was quite limited. A former hospital barrack which had housed the VD ward was the site of the basic science component. Fortunately, a large cement shower room of World War I vintage was also available. The building was anchored to the mountainside with plumbing, and work started. On the clinical scene, space for a very small metabolic ward at the Salt Lake General Hospital included four beds, an office and treatment room, and a tiny kitchen. The County continued to support this facility until the Medical School moved into the new University Hospital in 1965.

Geneticist Dr. Fayette Stephens had accumulated considerable material on genetic transmission of muscle disorders. Three major diseases as well as several others of considerably less frequency were present among these patients. The initial studies centered on facioscapulohumeral dystrophy, which was present in at least four large pedigrees in the area. A major advantage for establishing the study in Utah was these large families — a result of early polygamy — and the careful genealogic records encouraged by the Mormon Church. It was possible to establish as many as 2,000 members of an individual

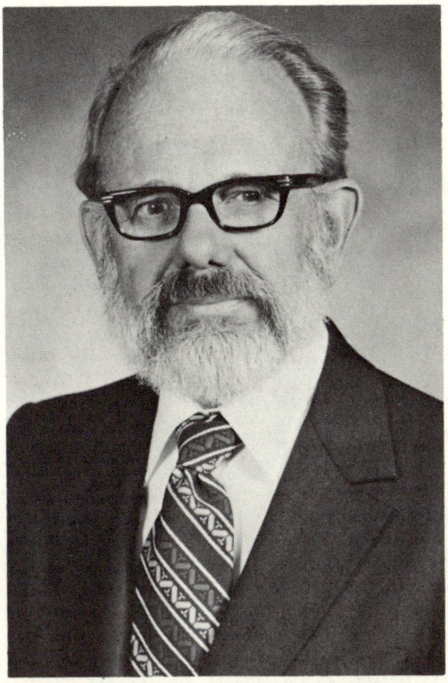

Frank H. Tyler.

pedigree. In studying such kindreds it was easy to trace an autosomal dominant trait, one of which was clearly the mechanism of inheritance of facioscapulohumeral dystrophy. Next came the study of Duchenne muscular dystrophy, the x-linked disorder which still results in early disability and death for many boys.

An early recruit to the program was Dr. Gerald T. Perkoff, who joined Tyler as the first clinical fellow in 1952–53. He helped with the muscle disease research and also studied a large pedigree in which hereditary nephritis was present. In association with Drs. Stephens and Tyler, he determined the distribution of the disease in that disorder and examined its clinical characteristics. The subsequently founded Division of Nephrology carried on this study. Very recently, in cooperation with the Howard Hughes Medical Institute at the University of Utah, members of the division were able to discover an anomaly in one of the collagen genes and to sequence that gene to identify the specific mutation which leads to these anomalies.

Among the families Dr. Stephens had interviewed were also patients in a sizable pedigree (about thirty involved persons) who had an unusual kind of periodic paralysis which did not fit the then-described "Familial Periodic Paralysis." Studies of these patients demonstrated that this was again an autosomal dominant trait and that the episodes of paralysis were precipitated by rest following activity rather than by heavy carbohydrate ingestion or insulin administration, as is the case in familial periodic paralysis. In contrast to that disorder, the patients did not develop hypopotassemia during the periodic episodes. These studies led to the publication of the first description of this condition, which is now called adynamia or hyperkalemic periodic paralysis.

Dr. Tyler had developed a serious investigative interest in endocrinology during his training at Johns Hopkins and Harvard, particularly with Dr. George W. Thorn, Hersey Professor of Physic (Medicine) at Peter Bent Brigham Hospital. On his arrival at Utah, a remarkable opportunity presented itself to continue these studies because of the presence of Dr. Leo Samuels, chair of the Department of Biochemistry, an already firmly established leader in steroid biochemistry; of Dr. George Sayers in the Department of Pharmacology and Physiology, who had emphasized the role of stress on adrenal secretions and had already established a method for the assay of ACTH by depletion of the guinea pig adrenal concentration of ascorbic acid; and of Dr. Tom Dougherty, who had arrived from Yale with an extensive background in the study of the physiological effects of adrenal cortical steroids. Dr. Horace W. Davenport and his wife Dr. Virginia Davenport were also on hand with expertise in electrolyte metabolism and technical aspects of laboratory procedures.

Only very primitive mechanisms were available for measuring the many compounds found in adrenal extracts. Crude steroid extracts of urine had some activity as reducing substances after the other reducing substances were removed from the extracts, and 17-keto steroids could be measured by the Zimmermann reaction in urine. Both of these methods were non-specific and very crude in their evaluation of adrenal cortical function. Dr. Samuels was a known authority in

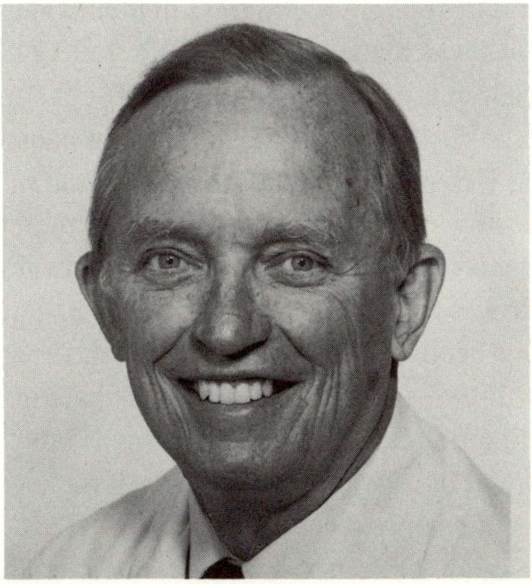

Don H. Nelson.

the field of steroid biochemistry but had not done any work with corticosteroids. He suggested to Dr. Don H. Nelson that he should attempt to set up a procedure for the measurement of corticosteroids, but he explained that the specific steroid to be measured was unknown.

Nelson and Samuels mounted an effort to isolate from blood the steroids of the neutral fraction which contained the adrenal cortical hormones. The technology was difficult and the yield small. Large amounts of blood were required, which was impractical for clinical studies. However, it was possible to demonstrate in a quantitative fashion that the delta-4-ketone structure and its ultraviolet absorption were present in these extracts, confirming that steroids of adrenal cortical characteristics were present in considerable amount. The subsequent development of the so-called Porter Silber reaction allowed Nelson and Samuels' studies to apply this technology to the extracts. This allowed the determination of 17-hydroxy-corticosteroids, subsequently identified in relatively small samples of human blood and plasma as primarily cortisol.

While Thomas Addison had described the syndrome of adrenal insufficiency usually produced by tuberculosis or metastatic tumor of the adrenal gland in 1855, little progress in identifying and producing adrenal hormones was made until the 1930s and 1940s. Drs. Nelson, H. Reich, and Samuels of the Department of Biochemistry at the University of Utah published one of the significant papers on the "Isolation of a Steroid Hormone from the Adrenal Blood of Dogs" in 1950.

The availability of the "Nelson-Samuels" method allowed the accelerated pursuit of the physiology and pathophysiology of adrenal cortical secretion. The demonstration of the capacity of ACTH to stimulate cortisol secretion, its metabolism in the body, and its pathophysiology in diseases such as Addison's disease and Cushing's syndrome led to a number of clinical advances which are still basic to the management of adrenal cortical disorders.

This method also encouraged the study of secretion of cortisol in normal subjects and the demonstration of the circadian variation in its secretion. The studies, resulting in many publications, were assisted by a series of fellows in the metabolic division, beginning with Dr. Avery Sandberg and followed by Drs. Charles Nugent, William MacDiarmid, and Gerald Perkoff, among many others. After Dr. Nelson was drafted into the Navy in 1949, he continued his research at the Naval Hospital in Bethesda before moving to Boston. Dr. Kris Eik-Nes from Norway contributed in many ways to the technology and understanding of adrenal biochemistry and physiology for a number of years. Following Dr. Eik-Nes, Dr. Claude Migeon from France worked for several years in an extremely productive fashion. After some time in Norway, Dr. Eik-Nes returned to the biochemistry department at the University of Utah and managed many investigations as well as a steroid training program for many years.

Also important in these steroid studies was Dr. C. Donald West, who obtained a PhD with Dr. Samuels after finishing his medical degree and worked with the metabolic division before his departure for Sloan-Kettering Memorial Hospital in New York City. West returned in 1957 as chief of research at the VA Hospital, where he carried out many of the steroid studies. Having had training in biochemistry and clinical medicine, he was an extremely important force within the division. He continued on the faculty for many years and was instrumental in the development of radioimmunoassay of hormones in plasma and urine. These techniques remain the mainstay of endocrinology today.

The division also pursued a number of other areas of metabolic abnormality. One of the most productive was the study carried out with Dr. Marvin Armstrong, a biochemist associated with the University's Laboratory for the Study of Metabolic and Hereditary Disorders. Phenylketonuria (PKU) was recognized as a genetic disorder rather early. More recent was the demonstration that phenylalanine accumulated in the plasma of these subjects. It was quickly demonstrated that the urinary metabolites were dependent on a phenylalanine excess in plasma and that the restricted phenylalanine diet was capable of controlling this excess. The diet was extremely difficult to manage, and much of the credit goes to the dieticians, particularly Jackie Abraham (later Mrs. Virgil Parker) and others, including the nurses who cared for these extremely difficult patients in the limited metabolic ward setting.

It was disappointing to find that these striking biochemical improvements did not result in a significant modification of the basic intellectual deficit, the prime problem in these patients. It was essential to study younger subjects, since a large part of brain development occurs in the first two years. Some babies in the first few months of life were recruited for study. By this time the diet had been improved with amino acid digest from which the aromatic amino acids had been removed and then replaced without phenylalanine, and the changes produced progressive intellectual development. Diagnosis from routine tests for newborns allows treatment from the very earliest weeks of life that results in relatively normal growth. The metabolic anomaly may persist without hampering further intellectual development.

Another area of extensive study is the metabolism of uric acid in patients with gout. Drs. Charles Nugent and Tyler demonstrated in 1959 that gouty subjects also had an anomaly in the clearance of uric acid. In a series of studies, hyperuricemia was induced in normal subjects via the administration of uric acid precursors. Their clearance of uric acid at plasma urate levels was much greater than those observed in patients with gout. An anomaly in the renal handling of uric acid in most gouty patients, including many of those who also showed evidence of increased urate production, was established.

The division grew in numbers and also sponsored the development of separate units in the Medical School related to nephrology and genetics. These separate disciplines provided the background for strong research and clinical training of a series of clinical and research fellows, some of whom have gone on to support investigations here and elsewhere in the world, including Japan and Scandinavia. Others are active in the local area as clinical practitioners in endocrinology and metabolism.

One final evolution was the development of a General Clinical Research Center Branch at the National Institutes of Health (NIH). This development, pushed by Drs. Wintrobe and Tyler as well as many others in the clinical investigation arena in the U.S., also led to the establishment of a Clinical Research Center under the directorship of Dr. C. D. West in the unified hospital and Medical School building occupied in 1965.

The Center provided for a considerable increase in clinical research at the University. Members of the metabolism group included, in addition to Drs. West and Tyler, Drs. William A. Jubiz, A. Wayne Meikle, and later Dr. Dana E. Wilson.

In 1966 Dr. Wintrobe recruited Dr. Don H. Nelson, who was born in Salt Lake City on November 28, 1925. As a student at the University of Utah Medical School, he became interested in research with Dr. Samuels. After graduating in 1947 and completing an internship at Milwaukee County Hospital, Nelson returned at Samuels' invitation to be a research fellow and later research assistant professor of biochemistry. After leaving Utah again in 1949, Nelson had completed a residency in medicine and a fellowship in endocrinology at Peter Bent Brigham Hospital under Dr. George W. Thorn. He was on the faculty at Harvard Medical School and serving as director of the Clinical Research Center at that institution when he moved to the University of Southern California as chief of endocrinology in 1959. There he established a new Clinical Research Center. Dr. Wintrobe was interested in establishing a full-time Department of Medicine at the LDS Hospital and recruited Nelson for this position. Research on many aspects of endocrinology was carried out during this period, with emphasis on steroid metabolism, application of steroid techniques to evaluation of clinical conditions, and some early work on mechanism of steroid action.

In 1980 Dr. George Cartwright, chair of medicine, died, and Dr. William D. Odell was appointed in his stead. Dr. Odell was a distinguished endocrinologist then serving as chief of medicine at Harbor Hospital (affiliated with UCLA). Dr. Tyler retired as head of endocrinology but has remained in charge of the Clinical Research Center, carrying on active research to this day as the only survivor of the original six members of the Department of Medicine. Dr. Odell asked Dr. Nelson to become head of endocrinology.

During the next ten years, many aspects of endocrinology were studied, again with emphasis on steroids. Dr. West, prior to his retirement in 1985, demonstrated significant effects of corticosteroids in the production of atherosclerosis, and Dr. Meikle increased the understanding of androgen secretion and metabolism. Dr. Nelson continued his studies on the mechanism of corticosteroid action through modifications of sphingolipids. During this time, Dr. Steven Elbein, with an interest in the familial basis of diabetes mellitus, and Dr. P. H. Iverius, an expert in lipid metabolism and lipoprotein lipase, joined the division. Dr. Odell continued his studies on peptide hormones, their secretion, and action.

The establishment of a University-affiliated Department of Medicine at the LDS Hospital was a challenging but rewarding effort for Dr. Nelson. The hospital provided funds for the recruiting of full-time physicians in cardiology, pulmonary, infectious disease, and endocrinology. Students now rotated from the University, and postgraduate training was improved. The house staff training in medicine expanded ten-fold, and it was generally agreed that patient care benefited greatly.

Dr. Nelson had been one of the first fellows in the Howard Hughes Medical Institute at Harvard University and then at the University of

Southern California. Through his friendship with Dr. William Gay, a member of the board of the Howard Hughes Medical Institute, the Institute was invited to the University and decided to establish a branch there. This branch has grown to the important status it occupies in the University's research program today.

CHAPTER THIRTEEN

The University of Utah Department of Family and Preventive Medicine

C. HILMON CASTLE, MD

IN 1969 DR. C. HILMON CASTLE was challenged by Dean Frank Ebaugh to assume responsibility for establishing a new academic department in the School of Medicine. Many of his colleagues at the University did not share his views of what was necessary to meet the needs of the community, and the development of the department is a colorful and somewhat stormy saga.

After completing four years of internal medicine training and two years in cardiology as a fellow/instructor, Castle had become a full-time member of the University of Utah faculty in July of 1959 and intended to focus on cardiology. At the same time, he planned to develop the new Division of Post-Graduate Medical Education envisioned by Philip B. Price, then dean of the Medical School, and by Hans Hecht, chair of cardiology and of the committee responsible for postgraduate education.

Castle's willingness to accept multiple responsibilities also made it possible to generate salary support for him; but even without a budget, postgraduate activities were in demand and developed rapidly, eventually becoming self-supporting. Three- to five-day courses for practicing physicians were developed. Participating faculty traveled to remote communities to lecture and conduct seminars by two-way radio between the Medical School and community hospitals. They also provided late-night, open-circuit television broadcasts of medical education programs for physicians over the University's educational television station, KUED, one of the first in the country. Such programs are common now but were rare in the early sixties.

National legislation to combat heart disease, cancer, and stroke — called the Regional Medical Program (RMP) — was passed in October 1965 and implemented by the National Institutes of Health in July 1966. Dr. Kenneth Castleton, dean of the School of Medicine during that period, appointed Castle to chair a small committee of medical faculty chosen to determine whether the University should apply for RMP support. The RMPs were designed to facilitate cooperative arrangements among educational institutions, hospitals, health-care professionals, and civic leaders in order to effectively transfer existing research and technology to the practicing community. The RMP premise was that the latest advances in treating heart disease, cancer, and stroke could then be more rapidly adopted by practicing physicians. The ad hoc committee was unanimous in its recommendation that the School of Medicine take a leading role in developing an RMP for the Intermountain region, and Castle was appointed coordinator. In July of 1966, the University of Utah received one of the nation's first four RMP grants.

As coordinator of the Intermountain Regional Medical Program (IRMP), Castle soon became acutely aware of the need for additional and improved primary care services in Utah and the surrounding states. The chronic lack of sufficient numbers of physicians practicing in small communities continued to hamper all efforts to provide adequate patient care and even became an issue among the medical students.

Late in 1969 Governor Calvin L. Rampton appointed a special ad hoc task force to consider the rural health care crisis in Utah. Dennis McCarty chaired the bipartisan group of community leaders, including Frank Ebaugh, who had just become dean of the Medical School. When the committee published their report and recommendations in November of 1969, Governor Rampton moved rapidly to obtain a special state appropriation to establish a new Department of Community and Family Medicine within the Medical School. The legislature appropriated $91,000 for the new department in February 1970

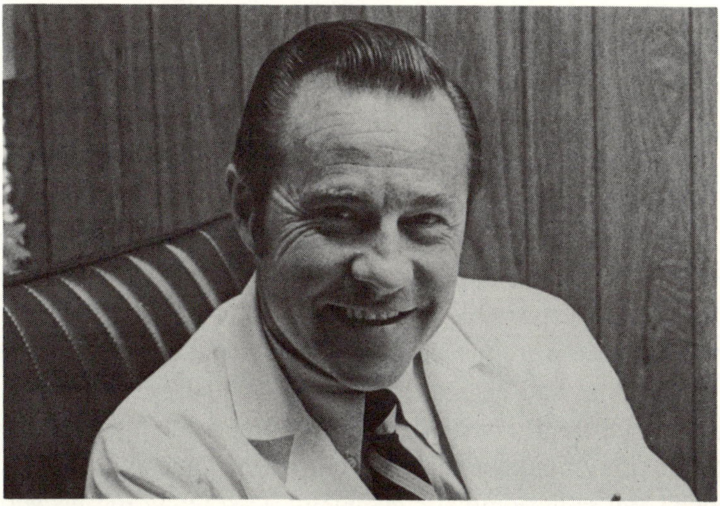

C. Hilmon Castle.

— during a period when, paradoxically, a statewide moratorium prohibited the development of any new educational programs or departments in Utah's institutions of higher education. Since the Medical School already had a Department of Public Health and Preventive Medicine, chaired by Dr. John R. Ward, Ebaugh simply went to the University's Institutional Council and asked for permission to change the name to Department of Community and Family Medicine. When they readily concurred, he asked Ward to consider implementing the recommendations of Governor Rampton's special committee. In early 1970, Ward decided instead to return to his primary duties in the Department of Medicine as chair of the Division of Rheumatology, and Castle was appointed in his place.

In 1970 Castle took a three-month administrative leave and enrolled at the Johns Hopkins School of Public Health to work with Kerr White, an internist and epidemiologist with impressive publications concerning the delivery of medical care and strategies for improving primary care services. The leave gave Castle an opportunity to explore new developments in other medical schools and to formulate his own ideas about how a new department should be developed.

Pressed by Dean Ebaugh to make a decision about assuming responsibility for the new department, Castle met with the dean and with Dr. George Cartwright, then chair of Castle's home department, internal medicine. Cartwright openly expressed his reservations about both the desirability of a new department and Castle's suitability to serve as its chair. Ironically, however, Cartwright was experiencing an additional set of frustrations in his attempt to staff and manage the University outpatient clinics, for which he and the Department of Medicine were responsible. The clinics, poorly regarded by the faculty and residents, were inadequately covered and therefore a chronic problem to him and his staff. When Ebaugh suggested that a new department of family medicine might appropriately assume responsibility for the ambulatory care and outpatient clinics, Cartwright had a sudden and rather dramatic change of heart regarding his support for the entire endeavor.

The New Department

Castle became chair of the new department on July 1, 1970. Anticipating that Dean Ebaugh might have difficulty fulfilling his agreements, Castle outlined the departmental goals and objectives, including the dean's guarantee of support, and obtained Ebaugh's signature — a move which would prove critical to the department's survival.

Dean Ebaugh departed abruptly in 1973, and Dr. Frank Tyler became acting dean. Development of the Department of Community and Family Medicine (DCFM) slowed, and there was even discussion concerning reallocating some of the space and budget originally promised. Castle met with University provost Dr. Tom King, presenting the original agreement signed by Ebaugh as the only evidence of the department's claims. Provost King made it clear that the University would live by those commitments and encouraged Castle to proceed toward the original goals.

Within a few months, Dr. John Dixon was appointed dean. He was supportive of the DCFM's goals, and in 1974 he very effectively portrayed to the state legislature the department's accomplishments and its potential for ameliorating the problems of medical care in rural communities. He also made the case that further expansion of the University Medical Center's facilities was needed desperately. His negotiations with the legislature culminated in 1975 with a $50 million appropriation; an accompanying fund-raising campaign brought in another $10 million, which allowed the expansion of the Medical Center facilities that opened in 1981.

In 1976 Dixon was promoted to Vice President for Health Sciences, and Rick Davern, PhD, a biologist, was appointed dean. Davern was primarily a scholar unfamiliar with the power structure of the Medical School, and although he expressed support for DCFM, it was difficult for him to promote progress in a specific department when sixteen chairs were competing vigorously for their own interests. A year later, Dixon resigned as Vice President to return to teaching and research in the Department of Surgery and Davern was appointed Vice President for Academic Affairs.

Richard Lee, who had worked as associate dean under Dixon, was appointed dean. Castle submitted his resignation as chair of DCFM in May of 1982, but having observed the devastating attrition that occurs in departments during intervals with either an acting chair or no chair at all, he agreed to continue as chair until a full-time replacement was available. The process took more than two years and culminated in the selection of Marian Bishop, who holds an MSPH and a PhD rather than an MD — a first for the chair of a clinical department in the Medical School.

People and Progress

Programs were developed to meet ambitious goals and objectives that were themselves hard-won:

1. To attract more medical students to enter family practice and to locate them in geographic areas of greatest need.
2. To train and certify physicians through residency training who are likely to remain in the Intermountain area to practice family medicine.
3. To train physicians and nonphysician health professionals in community medicine and occupational and environmental health.

4. To develop and apply methods for assessment of quality of care and educational needs of physicians and other health-care professionals engaged in patient care.

5. To study the delivery of patient care and common clinical problems that present to an office practice and engage in health services research and develop demonstration projects with the potential to improve health services.

Castle's original strategy was to recruit two key faculty members, one to head community medicine and the other to head family practice. Dr. Robert Kane joined the faculty in July of 1971 to head the former, and Dr. John Guyman arrived in early 1972 to head family practice. Guyman had clear ideas about what needed to be done for family practice, but some of them were considered too advanced and others anachronistic by the School of Medicine faculty. Moreover, they greatly resisted training family physicians in surgery. Frustrated by the lack of progress, Guyman accepted a position at the University of California at Davis and subsequently became chair of the Department of Family Medicine at the University of Washington in Seattle. Kane headed the Division of Community Medicine from 1971 to 1976, when he left to join the Rand Corporation and the UCLA faculty. Two large departmental divisions did not satisfy the faculty Castle had recruited, who preferred separate divisions for family practice, community medicine, biostatistics, epidemiology, behavioral science, and environmental and occupational health. Special projects such as the physician assistant (Medex) training program had also been initiated.

The accomplishments of the department's first decade were made possible by many faculty members, including John Guyman, David Feigal, John Tudor, David Sundwall, Elbert Leigh, Charles Payton, George Snell, Jerry Gardner, Clair Ellison, Richard Arbogast, Scott Sharp, David Symond, and many others in family practice. By 1980 most of the family practice faculty were being recruited from the department's own residents and fellows, for example, Cami Collett, Sue Edwards, Gerry Goodenough, Douglas Hadley, David Heaston, Konrad Kotrady, Larry Lutz, Kevin Patrick, Barbara Reed, John

Robinson, Lee Schussman, Tom Schwenk, and others. The medical student program was headed by Donna Harris and benefited for several years from David Sundwall's involvement. In behavioral science, Charles Hughes and Josephine Kasteler were recruited, then Edward Hershgold, Elaine Litton, Robert Simmons, and Oz Rothermich. The community medicine division was developed initially by Robert Kane and later maintained by James Mason and Ross Woolley. The Division of Biostatistics was fortunate to have Melville Klauber, James Reading, and Marlene Egger. Occupational and environmental health was started by Thomas Smith, who was followed by William Rom and Jeffrey Lee, Dick Johns, and others. In epidemiology, Lynn Lyon, John Gardner, and Dee West were primary faculty. The physician assistant program, developed by Bill Wilson, had Peter Caine, Bernie Asahina, Mike Hogben, Larry Reynolds, and others, and graduates of the program have later become the key staff members.

The name of the new Department of Community and Family Medicine was appropriate at the beginning. However, the subsequent emphasis on family practice eventually gave family medicine top billing. Castle formed a Family Practice Advisory Committee in 1972 to provide advice and counsel from the practicing community. The group consisted of Joseph M. Heath, Wendell Hyde, Jack Johnson, Robert Poulson, David Symond, and David Wray. A few years later, Robert Kelly, Wayne Mineer, David Garr, and Roger Lewis contributed their time and expertise. The Advisory Committee insisted that a "Department of Family and Community Medicine" was much more acceptable to the practicing community. Castle agreed, and the change was easily accomplished through a request to the Institutional Council. In 1986 department chair Marian Bishop reintroduced the term "Preventive," and the name is now Department of Family and Preventive Medicine.

Medical Student Teaching

The department's curriculum for medical students has consisted primarily of elective courses, including preceptorships in family practice, clerkships in clinical services run by family practice, and an honors program for senior medical students. In 1980 a three-hour required course entitled "Medicine and Society" was established for all first-year medical students. The course gradually evolved into one in preventive medicine that emphasizes the role of the primary care physician, especially the family physician.

Family Practice Residency

Shortly after the department was formed, Gordon Stagg, a family physician in Ogden, and William Daines, medical director of McKay-Dee Hospital, visited Castle. At that time, both McKay-Dee and St. Benedict's hospitals in Ogden operated general practice residencies (each with only two or three residents), and they had decided to discontinue them. Daines and Stagg wanted to start a new family practice residency there connected with the University of Utah. Their interests coincided with Castle's and they all moved quickly to work with the local physicians. Fortunately, George Snell, a family physician practicing in Kaysville, was willing to join the University faculty in early 1971 to direct the program at McKay-Dee. Robert Potts, a family physician from Riverside, California, also joined the faculty to direct the program at St. Benedict's. The hospitals offered the residents stipends and covered their expenses, and they provided funds for faculty to begin a class of six residents each in 1971.

Good candidates were found without difficulty to begin the program. However, an enormous amount of work was required to formulate a curriculum which met national criteria, to establish clinical services that would be suitable for training, and to organize a teaching faculty on short notice. This was an exhausting yet exciting period of development which was only possible because of the help of the many interested Ogden physicians.

In July of 1972, St. Benedict's residency component was transplanted to Holy Cross Hospital in Salt Lake City, a move made primarily because of limited resources at St. Benedict's and the hospital's inability to fund the training program adequately over time. In Salt Lake City, pediatric training took place at Primary Children's Medical Center (PCMC), and block electives in other specialties for both components of the residency were provided at the University Hospital. Since family practice residents still were not accepted within the internal medicine inpatient service at University Hospital, a general medical service was established at Holy Cross.

To their credit, the McKay-Dee Hospital staff continued to find the resources to fund eighteen residents and three full-time faculty.

Partial federal funding for residency training was secured in 1973, but support was temporarily interrupted on two occasions, causing considerable consternation and great difficulty to those struggling to maintain a stable and growing program. In 1979 a crisis in funding became imminent when federal funds were insufficient to provide further residency program stipends, despite the fact that thirty-six residents had been accepted into the program. In the Salt Lake component, funding from the various hospitals accommodated only sixteen residents. Castle approached the dean of the School of Medicine, who made a formal request that the University administration consider including family practice training in the overall budget. However, funding for family medicine was not part of the administration's budget request presented to the state legislature. When the Family Practice Advisory Committee was apprised of the situation, they took it upon themselves to approach the legislature directly to obtain line-item funding for family practice training. Such action was, of course, in direct violation of the University's policies. Undaunted, the Advisory Committee proceeded to wage a very aggressive and ultimately successful campaign to obtain legislative support in the amount of $300,000 per year for family practice residency training.

The direct-line legislative appropriation stabilized the residency for a time, and specific family practice funding soon was included in the regular budget for the School of Medicine. Gradually, however, the department's overall budget was reduced until, by 1986, funding for family practice residents and faculty was again inadequate.

Finally, both the Ogden and Salt Lake components of the family practice residency were stabilized. McKay-Dee has continued to sustain eighteen residents and three full-time faculty. Funding for residents at Holy Cross, whose program also utilizes PCMC and the

University Hospital, has been provided jointly by these three hospitals. Support income is also generated from patient-care fees and various grants.

Many of the family physicians now practicing in Utah are graduates of the Department of Family and Preventive Medicine program. For example, the family practice department is the largest staff group at Holy Cross. Approximately 90% are either graduates of the residency or came to the hospital as part of the family practice faculty. Both the Salt Lake City and Ogden components of the residency have enjoyed a large number of excellent applicants. At the end of the first decade, 1981, the department had graduated ninety-six family practice physicians from the three-year program and was capable of continuing to graduate sixteen each year thereafter. In 1990, 245 family physicians had completed three years of residency training. The vast majority have either entered practice or have joined the faculty in family medicine. To the program's credit, 50% of the residents who have graduated from the Utah program have chosen to practice in rural or other medically under-served communities in the Intermountain region.

Residency in Preventive Medicine

The department offers a preventive medicine residency which includes completion of a master of science and community medicine (MSCM) degree and achievement of Board eligibility in general preventive medicine. This residency provides preparation for the recognition, evaluation, and control of community health problems. Some physicians have also opted to take a joint residency which provides skills in both fields. To date, twenty-eight physicians have completed the preventive medicine residency.

Residency in Occupational and Environmental Health

The occupational medicine residency was initiated in 1977 and was designed to provide clinical and research skills necessary for the recognition, treatment, control, and prevention of occupational illnesses. The residency is oriented to training academicians and researchers to meet the severe shortage of human resources in this rapidly growing and important field. To date, thirty physicians have been accepted into the program.

Family Practice Fellowship

In 1978 the department developed postgraduate fellowship training in family medicine. The two-year fellowships were funded by the Robert Johnson Foundation, and the fellows consisted primarily of graduates of three-year residency programs who desired additional training and experience in research and teaching for future academic careers. This program ran through 1984 and produced twelve graduates. A shorter program of faculty development included twenty-seven board-certified physicians who were interested in making the transition from private practice to faculty positions in family practice.

Master of Science and Community Medicine

The master's degree program was approved by the University in 1974 and was accredited in 1978 by the American Public Health Association's Council on Education. In addition to training nonphysician health workers, the program served as the academic portion of the preventive medicine and occupational and environmental health residencies, as well as the long-term faculty fellowship. By 1983, within a decade, thirty-six individuals had received their masters' degrees, and since then 121 more degrees have been awarded. By 1987, the master's program had been divided into two separate degrees, a master of science in public health that required a research project and a publishable paper, and a more traditional master of public health track. By 1990 thirteen had earned masters' degrees in the latter program.

Physician Assistant Training Program (MEDEX)

The department was committed from its beginnings to increase rapidly the available primary care services in Utah and surrounding states. In the spring of 1970 Castle and the faculty began exploring the feasibility of starting a physician assistant training program to begin when the department was officially established. In February of 1971, a grant from the IRMP, combined with support obtained from the National Center for Health Services Research and Development, made it possible to initiate the program that July. At its inception, the program was twelve months in length and designed primarily around extending the knowledge and capabilities of military medical corps personnel. Currently, the major requirement for applicants is a minimum of three years of high-quality primary care experience. Most successful applicants have been nurses, military corps personnel, paramedics, technicians, and technologists of various types who possess the requisite academic skills to meet the demands of the rigorous educational program.

The program uses a biphasic, twenty-four-month curriculum consisting of didactic, clinical, and preceptorship instruction. The didactic phase consists of ten months of classroom and clinical instruction at the University. In the preceptor phase, the candidate spends fourteen months of clinical instruction and practice with a primary care physician. Each graduate is awarded a certificate by the Medical School and the Utah Medical Association. Seventy-eight hours of upper-division University credits can also be obtained by students who wish to apply them toward a baccalaureate degree.

Developing the curriculum and teaching for physician assistant training and then modifying these to meet the changing needs of the learners (as well as meeting the requirements of the national accrediting organizations, the University, and the Medical School) constituted one of Castle's most satisfying experiences as a medical educator. The faculty and staff feel great pride in 99.6% taking and passing the National Boards of Medical Examiners certifying examinations.

From its inception, the program has incorporated a deployment system which virtually assures employment of each student accepted for training. Of the approximately 300 men and women graduated since 1971, 94% are still delivering care as physician assistants. Of these, 80% remain in the Intermountain region, and more than 30%

have been placed in federally designated "primary care shortage areas." Almost 70% serve in communities of fewer than 10,000 people, and more than half have remained with their original physician preceptors.

Postscript

Fortunately, the NIH preventive cardiology academic award provided support for Castle for six years and sustained him as full-time faculty from 1983 to 1989. He then switched to part-time faculty from 1983 to 1989. While still remaining part-time in the department, he entered the third phase of his professional career, as a cardiologist practicing at Holy Cross Hospital in association with four other cardiologists organized as Premier Cardiology Consultants. Since a number of family practice residents and medical students are assigned to Holy Cross, he also has ample opportunity for teaching and clinical research in cardiology.

Castle considers his involvement in the development of the department to be his greatest challenge and most lasting contribution. His efforts, along with those of other faculty, have made a difference for family physicians, for physician assistants, for the quality and quantity of primary care in Utah, and for providing a diversity of educational opportunities for scores of health-care professionals in the Intermountain West.

Note: The author is indebted to William Wilson, PhD, not only for his assistance in developing the department, especially the physician assistant training program, but also in writing this essay. He provided many of the details, as well as making it more readable through editing the original efforts.

CHAPTER FOURTEEN

Hematology–Oncology

JOHN H. WARD, MD

THE STORY OF HEMATOLOGY AT THE UNIVERSITY OF UTAH School of Medicine is inextricably interwoven with the evolution of the four-year Medical School and the growth of the Department of Medicine because of the influence of Dr. Maxwell Wintrobe and his successor as department chair, Dr. George E. Cartwright. The emergence of medical oncology and its merger with hematology also had a profound effect on the face of the current training program and direction of the Division of Hematology–Oncology.

Dr. Wintrobe moved to the University of Utah in 1943 as the first full-time professor and head of the Department of Medicine. Dr. Cartwright was recruited as a resident in January 1944. After a year of residency and two years of service with the U.S. Army in China, he joined the faculty as an instructor in 1947 and became the first chief of the Division of Hematology in 1950.

The early years were full of innovation. In 1946 the first research grant made by the Public Health Services was obtained by Dr. Wintrobe for the study of muscular dystrophy. The initial clinical report, in 1946, of the utility of nitrogen mustard in Hodgkin's disease and other lymphomas (with Dr. Louis Goodman, head of pharmacology at the University as the senior author) evolved from studies of the effects of chemical warfare agents at several centers, which were continued by Dr. Wintrobe after his move to Utah. Programs to study the anemia of infection and nutritional anemias were developed.

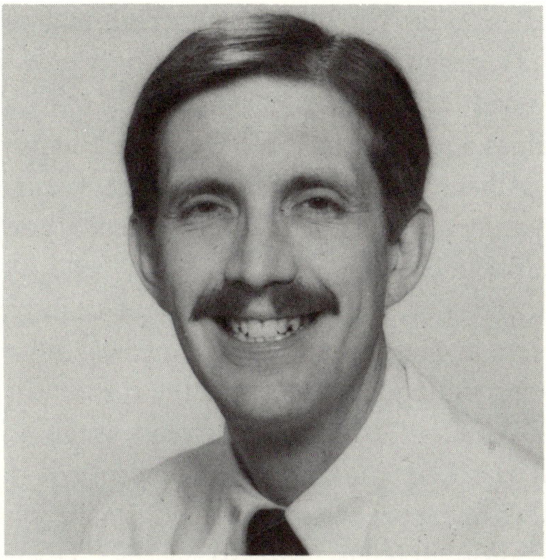

John H. Ward.

On the light side, the initial years of the division were also characterized by the traditional Wednesday noon exodus of Dr. Wintrobe, Dr. Cartwright, and the fellow to the ski slopes of Alta. Although the tradition waned in the 1970s, Wednesday afternoons were unstructured until 1982, when tradition was broken by the creation of a hematology–oncology clinic staffed by Drs. Harmon Eyre and John H. Ward.

Dr. Wintrobe resigned as department chair in 1967 and was replaced by Dr. Cartwright, who maintained this position until his untimely death in 1980. With his replacement by Dr. William Odell, an endocrinologist, the indelible association of the Department of Medicine with hematology was finally broken.

Dr. John W. Athens, born in Minnesota, arrived in Utah via a circuitous route that included a medical degree from Johns Hopkins, an internship at Peter Bent Brigham Hospital, and a brief stint as a fellow of the Atomic Energy Commission at Duke University, which included the study of radioisotope physics — to be useful in his later research. He chose to come to Utah to complete his internal medicine residency and stayed as a hematology fellow. Dr. Athens performed landmark studies on the kinetics of neutrophils and became division chief in 1967. He remained in this position for twenty years, until the reins were passed to Dr. James P. Kushner in 1987. Following his arrival in Utah as a resident in 1959, Dr. Dane Boggs participated in many of Dr. Athens' studies. After subsequent career moves, Dr. Boggs was appointed chief of hematology–oncology at the University of Pittsburgh in 1969.

Dr. G. Richard Lee, a 1956 University of Utah graduate, developed an interest in hematology during medical school which was nourished during subsequent training at the Boston City Hospital, on the service of William Castle, and two years at the National Cancer Institute (NCI). Dr. Lee returned to the University of Utah as a fellow to pursue studies of copper and iron metabolism; he joined the faculty in 1963 and was promoted to professor in 1973. His term as dean of the Medical School from 1978 to 1984 serves as another example of the pervasive influence of hematology at that time. Dr. Lee is currently chief-of-staff at the Salt Lake City Veterans Administration Medical Center.

In the 1960s two key individuals came to Utah for their training in hematology: James P. Kushner and Gerald Rothstein. Dr. Kushner, born in Brooklyn, attended medical school in Pittsburgh, where he finished his medical residency. Influenced by a former Utah hematology fellow, he came to Utah for further training from 1967 to 1970, when he joined the faculty. He developed an interest in the biochemistry of porphyria which has mushroomed into his recognition as an international leader in the field. Dr. Rothstein graduated from the University of Florida in Gainesville, taking both his internal medicine and hematology training at Utah. His studies of neutrophil production using a neonatal model, in collaboration with Dr. Robert Christensen of the Department of Pediatrics, have been widely recognized. Since the late 1960s, the names Kushner and Rothstein have been synonymous with hematology at Utah. Their uncompromising demand for excellence, in addition to Dr. Wintrobe's forbidding reputation, often engendered fear in the medical students who contemplated exposure to the specialty. This reputation persists to the present.

In the 1950s and 1960s the Department of Medicine was relatively small. Socially, the division heads were tightly knit. A collegial atmosphere, apparent to the children of these early leaders, kindled friendships and camaraderie. Diluted by the explosive growth of the department over the last twenty years, the closeness of those early years has diminished.

During Dr. Cartwright's tenure as chair, the Department of Medicine underwent a dramatic increase in faculty with the development and growth of the various subspecialties. Cartwright's somewhat elitist attitudes did little to improve community relations. Initially he also had to fight the perception that Dr. Wintrobe was still in charge. Dr. Cartwright's secretary recalls that Dr. Wintrobe had difficulty moving out of his office until Dr. Cartwright finally said, "Dr. Wintrobe, I cannot run the Department of Medicine if I can't get at the desk!" An agreement was reached whereby Cartwright was allowed to ask Wintrobe for advice when he needed it — a practice that declined in frequency as the years passed by. When Cartwright took over the department, much of the grant support went to hematology with Dr. Richard Lee. Despite the tough financial times, continued growth occurred. Internal medicine flourished in the 1970s, with the best students seeking such training. Dr. Cartwright met personally with medicine honors students and directed them to first-rate residencies at places such as Johns Hopkins, Barnes Hospital at Washington University in St. Louis, and Duke, where a tradition of interchange of excellent house officers had been established. His death, on Easter Sunday of 1980, signaled the end of an era which saw the growth and development of a first-rate Department of Medicine. Dr. Cartwright was a great believer in the idea of the internist as consummate clinician and intellectual and would be saddened to see the current exodus of bright students away from internal medicine to the "lifestyle specialties."

When the Medical School moved to the University campus in 1965, the patient population changed correspondingly. Cartwright recognized the future of solid tumor therapy and instituted plans to meet the need. Dr. Joe Quagliana was recruited as head of the new

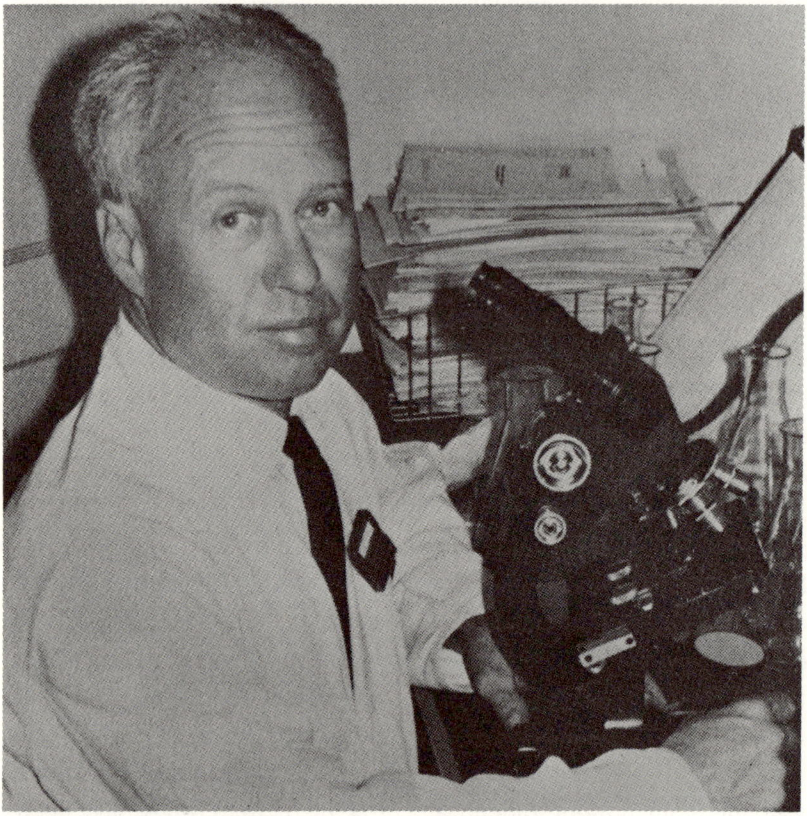

George E.Cartwright, MD.

Division of Oncology in 1968. He had been trained as a hematologist and was in private practice in San Jose, California. Quagliana took a mini-sabbatical with Dr. Richard Cooper at Roswell Park before joining the University faculty, and under his leadership medical oncology flourished. In cooperation with Drs. Hilmon Castle at the University and Stanley G. Altman at LDS Hospital, a federally supported outreach program — the Intermountain Regional Medical Program — was established, and many communities in the Intermountain West participated in cancer education. Dr. Quagliana was also instrumental in obtaining a cancer education grant from the NCI which was used to fund the training of numerous fellows in the 1970s.

He initiated membership of the University of Utah in the Southwest Oncology Group (SWOG) in about 1970, and Utah became a full member in 1972.

After three years, Dr. Quagliana was extremely busy. Dr. Albert Clarysse, a Utah-trained hematologist, joined him in 1971, but the two did not get along, and Clarysse returned to Belgium.

As it appeared that the school's class size would ultimately have to be increased, Dr. Cartwright had developed a plan (later abandoned) to incorporate St. Mark's Hospital into the University's teaching program. Dr. Harmon Eyre joined the Division of Oncology in 1972 and was assigned to teach and do clinical research at St. Mark's. A graduate of the University of Utah's Medical School, he had studied internal medicine at Johns Hopkins. He served two fellowships, one at Utah and the other at the National Institutes of Health. In 1973 he returned to the University of Utah as a full-time member of the Division of Oncology.

The first true oncology fellow, Dan Frimmer, began training after one year of a classical hematology fellowship at the University. In 1973 the first two fellows trained purely in oncology were recruited: Drs. Lou Balizet and Mary Clemmens. Over the next year oncology increased in size, and its patient load became larger than that of hematology. In addition to those with solid tumors, patients with leukemia and lymphoma were also being treated — many on experimental SWOG protocols. Dr. Cartwright could see the Division of Hematology suffering as patients, fellows, and money went to oncology. Constraints Cartwright placed on Dr. Quagliana ultimately resulted in the latter's move to private practice in Las Vegas. At the urging of Dr. Barth Hoogstraten, chairman of SWOG, Quagliana's SWOG grant was left at Utah, and Dr. Athens became principal investigator. To avoid further conflict, hematology and oncology became a single division in 1975, which changed the face of the division permanently.

Dr. Kushner moved to the University from the VA hospital, and Dr. Athens educated himself in the care of the cancer patient. With his arrival in 1975, Dr. Bruce Cheson joined Drs. Athens, Kushner, and

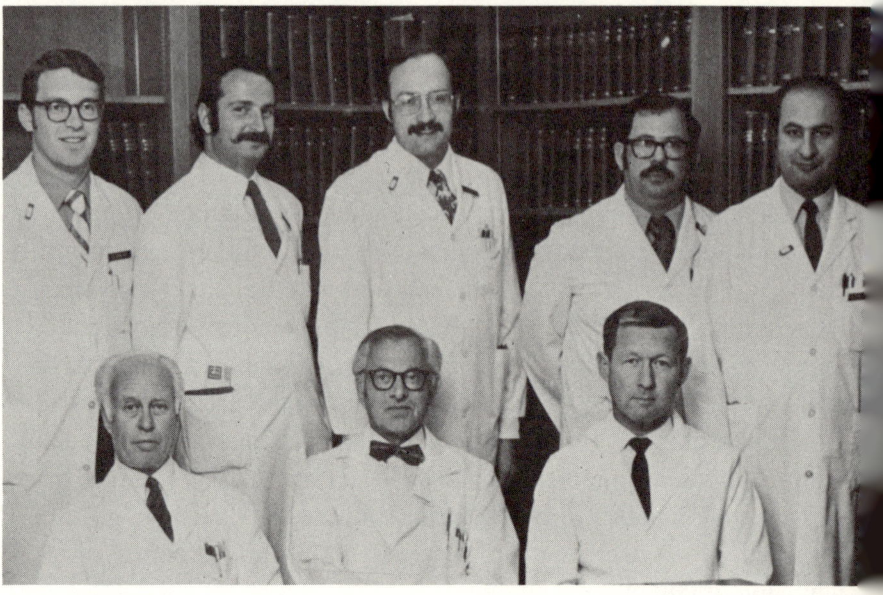

Hematology Division, Department of Medicine, about 1956. Seated, left to right, Drs. George E. Cartwright, Maxwell M. Wintrobe, John W. Athens; standing, Harmon J. Eyre, Daniel Frimmer, William Keene, Alberto Goldgaber, and Moyeen Khaleeli.

Eyre on the oncology patient service at the University Hospital. Drs. Wintrobe, Cartwright, and Rothstein maintained separate hematology clinics.

A training program in hematology was established in 1946 and expanded to include oncology in 1973. More than 200 individuals have now been trained in the clinical aspects of hematology and oncology as well as various research aspects. The list of trainees includes such distinguished leaders in medicine and hematology as Drs. Jane Fay Desforges (Tufts New England Medical Center), Wallace Jensen (Albany Medical College), Daniel Bergsagel (University of Toronto), Arthur Haut (University of Arkansas), Robert Moser (University of Pennsylvania), Dane Boggs (University of Pittsburgh, now deceased), Martin Cline (UCLA), John Forester (University of Manitoba), Darryl Williams (LSU, Shreveport, LA), Brice Weinberg (Duke University), and Gerald Roth (University of Washington).

At this juncture, separate types of clinics were maintained. Those of Eyre, Athens, Kushner, and Cheson followed a private practice model, where patients were seen and dealt with in expeditious fashion. The clinics of Wintrobe, Cartwright, and Rothstein followed a routine which was designed to maximize teaching but which could inconvenience the patient. All patients would first be seen by fellows, residents, or students. After *all* of them had been thus evaluated, the trainees would troop to a conference room, where the attending hematologist would peruse the blood smears under the ever-present microscope while he heard each case. After all cases had been discussed, the group would return en masse to the clinic and meet with the patients. Despite the fact that such a clinic could consume the whole morning, patients generally seemed pleased to receive the ministrations of the masters.

Many trainees can remember the formal nature of these clinics and the interesting responsibilities that accompanied them. For example, when Dr. Wintrobe arrived, the entourage was to be assembled, the blood films were to be at the microscope, and the chair before the microscope was to have precisely two telephone books placed on it so that Dr. Wintrobe would be at the appropriate height for the eyepieces! With Dr. Wintrobe's retirement and Dr. Cartwright's death, this leisurely and academic clinic model finally became extinct. As the oncology clinics increased in size and increasingly ill patients were managed in the outpatient setting rather than the hospital, some staff members occasionally longed for the slow pace of the academic setting of the past.

In the early 1980s, John H. Ward (at the University) and Graydon Harker (at the Veterans Administration Hospital) joined the faculty. Dr. Ward, a native Utahn, obtained his MD degree at the University of Utah in 1976. He served an internship and a residency in medicine at Duke University and from 1979 to 1982 a fellowship in hematology at Utah, after which he was appointed to the faculty in 1982 and promoted to associate professor in 1988. Dr. Harker had his internal medicine residency at Johns Hopkins and his fellowship at Stanford and was the first faculty member trained exclusively as an oncologist.

Other young faculty members recruited in the early 1980s included Drs. Charles Parker, Saundra Buys, and Wolfram Samlowski.

With the growth of the importance of medical oncology in the late 1970s, the face of the fellowship program changed. For many years, the focus had been on producing the academic hematologist. Trainees now recognized the economic realities and desired training in oncology, and a large percentage of fellows went into private practice following their training — a trend which continues to the present. The fellowship placed great emphasis on the care of patients on the busy inpatient "hem-onc" service at the University Hospital. The fellow in charge of this service put in (and continues to put in) so many hours of work that house officers often referred to the fellow as the "hematern." The fabled Grant Harrer, now in practice in Great Falls, Montana, served as the ultimate example of the hard-working fellow. It is rumored that no one actually ever saw him asleep and that he never left the hospital ahead of the interns. Dr. Ward recalls an instance when rounds were set at 7:00 A.M. on a Sunday. At the appointed hour, Dr. Harrer had already seen every patient personally and attended to all their needs — an exercise that clearly had begun several hours earlier. The University wards continue to stress the physical stamina and stretch the minds of the fellows. The ubiquitous presence of "the book," in which flow sheets, condensed histories, and progress notes reside allows immediate identification of the fellow on the inpatient service.

The weekly tumor board was the focus for rigorous review of the cases of individual patients, usually inpatients with challenging diagnostic or therapeutic problems. In addition to the responsibilities of patient care, the inpatient fellow presented about three-fourths of the cases to this conference, where attention to detail and familiarity with the literature were demanded. It has been suggested that a class in debate skills should be a prerequisite for the hem-onc fellowship. A presenter who was not conversant with the details of a case could expect to be thoroughly cross-examined by Dr. Kushner, who often assumed the Wintrobian role of the ultimate authority. The question "But what did the physical exam show?" was frequently heard, as more than one presenter neglected this time-honored part of the presentation. The tables were turned one day when Joe Volk, now in practice in Phoenix, detailed a most challenging case, specifically requesting Dr. Kushner's advice. After elaborating in excruciating detail and describing a careful exam, Dr. Volk announced that the patient was outside and requested Dr. Kushner's help with the physical exam. The patient in question was wheeled in and found to be constructed of blankets, balloons, and creatively arranged surgical gloves. Dr. Kushner had to admit that the patient was beyond his help.

Dr. Athens retired as division chief in 1987 and was succeeded by Dr. Kushner, who foresaw a division which would continue to be strong in basic sciences and which would also take advantage of Utah's unique attributes for genetic research. Dr. Rothstein left hematology to become chief of a new division: Human Development and Aging. Drs. Parker and Samlowski developed first-rate laboratories at the VA Hospital. Dr. Samlowski's efforts enabled the University to participate in clinical trials of interleukin-2 with lymphokine-activated killer cells and, in conjunction with Dr. Ward, he treated more than thirty patients with this new approach. These patients were on the Clinical Research Center Ward, where there was no house staff or fellow coverage, and the duo could often be found adjusting dopamine drips at odd hours, reminiscent of their days as residents on an ICU rotation. With Dr. Mark Skolnick, Dr. Ward developed an interest in the genetics of breast cancer.

Early in Dr. Kushner's tenure as chief, Dr. Eyre began his tenure as national president of the American Cancer Society. Though officially on sabbatical for the year, Dr. Eyre maintained his practice with the aid of Dr. Max Farver (now in practice in Yankton, South Dakota), who was completing his fellowship and who possessed the physique and personality appropriate to his past as a football player for Nebraska. Dr. Eyre endured a great deal of ribbing that year as people informed inquirers about his apocryphal second office on Concourse B at the airport and rehashed a fabled interview with investigative reporter Rod Decker concerning Eyre's smoking habits. "Frequent-flyer Eyre" survived, with his good nature and his reputation as the preeminent oncologist in the Intermountain area intact.

One of Dr. Kushner's major early efforts was the development of a bone marrow transplant program. LDS Hospital, under the guidance of Dr. Clyde Ford, had been operating a low-volume transplant unit for several years. Convinced that bone marrow transplant was here to stay but unconvinced that it should be done without a coordinated research program, Kushner recruited Dr. Pat Beatty for the University from the Fred Hutchinson Cancer Center. Since the first transplant, the demand has burgeoned and the waiting list is long. Dr. Beatty's research interest in unrelated HLA-matched transplants figures prominently in the future of the program.

Community Hematology–Oncology

LDS Hospital.* Dr. Stanley G. Altman completed his fellowship in hematology with Dr. Wintrobe at the University of Utah and in July 1956 became the first hematologist in private practice in the Intermountain area. He joined the staff of LDS Hospital and spent one-fourth of his time as hematologist to the laboratory. Dr. Altman performed most of the bone marrow aspirations, read and interpreted all bone marrows, set up a coagulation laboratory in 1957 and supervised it until 1982. In addition, he set up technology student training programs for a consortium of colleges and universities in the area until the program disbanded in 1985. He also started a hematology-oncology clinic as part of the teaching service for house staff.

In 1961 LDS Hospital was invited by Dr. William Longmeyer of UCLA to participate in the Western section of the Clinical Drug Evaluation Program. This initiated clinical anti-cancer drug research with Dr. Altman as the principal investigator. In 1970, LDS Hospital became part of the Central Oncology Group (COG), chaired by Dr. Anthony Curreri at the University of Wisconsin. In 1976, COG disbanded and LDS became a member of the Southwest Oncology Group (SWOG) through affiliation with the University of Utah. Drs. Altman, William F. Reilly, Clyde D. Ford, R. Dirk Noyes, A. Jennifer

*This section is based on Dr. Stanley G. Altman's history of hematology–oncology at LDS Hospital.

Fischbach, and William T. Sause hold membership on the GU, GI, brain, and bone marrow committees, and Sause is co-chair of the brain committee.

LDS Hospital staff took an active part in the Intermountain Regional Medical Program (IRMP) organized by Dr. C. Hilmon Castle at the University of Utah, which recruited Dr. Charles Smart from UCLA to be the first surgical oncologist in the state. A visiting cancer teaching program started by Drs. Smart and Altman in 1967 extended to many cities in Idaho and Nevada, as well as Butte, Montana. Dr. Quagliana joined this program in 1968. Numerous LDS Hospital and University physicians made regular visits to the surrounding communities and participated in tumor conferences and consultations. Drs. Altman at LDS and Eyre at the University organized physicians' assignments. This function was turned over in 1986 to the new clinical cancer center at the University of Utah headed by Dr. Robert Stewart.

The IRMP also supported computerization of the Intermountain Area Tumor Registry. Cancer was made a reportable disease in Utah, and hospital tumor registries were responsible for reporting. These activities were developed by Dr. Charles Smart, and the Utah Registry later became part of the SEER Program (Surveillance Epidemiology and End Results — a regional program under NCI tracking 9.6% of the U.S. population and 1.5 million cancer patients since 1973).

In 1974 an oncology unit was created to serve patients of the radiation oncologists. One resident and two interns were assigned to the hematology-oncology service. Dr. William R. Reilly joined the staffs of the Salt Lake Clinic and LDS Hospital in 1972 and participated in the leadership of the section. Dr. Clyde D. Ford came on staff in 1976 and Dr. Darrell G. Hensleigh in 1977. Dr. Ford organized a bone marrow transplant program to include both autologous and allogenic transplants. He also initiated a pilot program in tumor cell culture and chemotherapy sensitivity. After several moves, the oncology unit finally settled on Four North in the new hospital building in August of 1985, with a laminar air-flow unit and two functioning isolation rooms. From 1979 to 1991, seventy-five bone marrow transplants have been performed — twenty autologous, and fifty-five allogenic. The three-year survival rate in the "good-risk" patient is comparable to that of other major centers in the country, at significantly lower cost.

Holy Cross Hospital. Dr. James W. Cecil graduated from Baylor Medical School in Houston in 1963. After an internship at Philadelphia General Hospital and a residency in internal medicine at the Mayo Clinic, he completed a clinical fellowship in hematology at the University of Utah between 1969 and 1971. He became a full-time staff member of the Department of Medicine and started a teaching service in oncology at Holy Cross Hospital, with Thomas B. Keith in cardiology and Clifford Harmon in gastroenterology. One resident and two interns usually covered Holy Cross between 1971 and 1976, until Dr. Cartwright canceled the Department of Medicine's affiliation with Holy Cross.

Dr. Cecil initiated regular tumor conferences that were attended by the radiation oncologists from LDS Hospital, primarily Dr. Sause. Cecil remained a hospital-based hematologist-oncologist until April 1984, when his appointment changed to clinical assistant professor and he opened his own office for the private practice of the specialty. While some nurses were qualified for the administration of chemotherapy, no designated area for oncology was created.

In 1979 Holy Cross started a hospice ward, which was essentially an acute inpatient facility for the care of terminally ill cancer patients. This service was discontinued in 1982 because the cost for a patient on hospice was close to acute care, and Dr. Cecil did not wish to care for patients who were beyond receiving any benefits from his treatment. The patients undoubtedly received tender, loving, and expert care from the sisters and nurses.

St. Mark's Hospital. Dr. Kent DiFiore came on St. Mark's staff as the first medical oncologist in 1981. He graduated from George Washington University with his MD in 1975 and had an internship and residency at the University of Utah from 1975 to 1978 and a fellowship in hematology–oncology from 1979 to 1981. A monthly tumor conference had existed for a number of years, but it was made weekly and shortly thereafter twice-weekly after Dr. DiFiore's arrival. Radiation oncologists from LDS Hospital and the University participated in this meeting, where current tumor problems were discussed and treatment was recommended.

DiFiore was joined by two other medical oncologists, Dr. Patricia Legant in 1983 and Dr. Greg Litton in 1989; DiFiore and Litton share offices. The medical oncologists have also covered Cottonwood and Pioneer Valley hospitals. A new radiation therapy facility with a linear accelerator opened at St. Mark's in May 1991 under the direction of the University of Utah staff. Drs. Stewart, Gibbs, Hayes, and Prows rotate coverage for this service on a daily basis.

HOSPICE. In 1977 an independent group of volunteers started an outpatient service for terminally ill patients. In 1982 this group joined with Community Nursing Service to form Hospice of Salt Lake–Community Nursing Service. Professors Kathy Hardin Mooney and Vicky Slater from the University of Utah School of Nursing faculty, Dr. Arthur G. Lipman in the School of Pharmacy, Rt. Rev. Bishop Otis Charles, and Lincoln Ure, chaplain at St. Mark's Hospital, among others from the community, supported this effort.

A certified program for home care is available on request by a physician and is compensated by Medicare and Medicaid. The services include nursing care, emotional support, nutritional consultation, bereavement support, and volunteer assistance. Approximately thirty-five to fifty patients are served at any one time, for an average of one month each, for an annual total of ninety to one hundred patients. The medical adviser is Dr. Perry G. Fine of the Department of Anesthesiology at the University of Utah, who spends half a day per week in conferences concerning all Medicare patients. He and his associate, Dr. Michael Ashborn, are available twenty-four hours a day for emergency consultation.

Patients who do not qualify for federal support may benefit from funds supplied to the program by United Way of Salt Lake. About a dozen other hospice services are now scattered throughout the state providing similar services. In January 1991 the Utah Cancer Pain Initiative became effective. Affiliated with the U.S. Cancer Pain Relief Committee, the Initiative is part of the World Health Organization and cooperates closely with the American Cancer Society.

Hospice of IHC was formed in 1988 primarily to provide similar care for patients discharged from Intermountain Health Care (IHC) hospitals; an application for certification by Medicare is pending. The average caseload in 1991 has increased to about twenty-five patients at any one time. The original medical director was Dr. Clyde Ford; since Dr. Ford was called into service for Desert Storm, Dr. Kent DiFiore has served in this capacity.

Hospice has become an important service, allowing the terminally ill cancer patient to receive necessary home care from a highly skilled team of health-care professionals and volunteers to improve the quality of life.

CHAPTER FIFTEEN

Neurology

LEONARD W. JARCHO, MD

AT LEAST ONE NEUROSURGEON was in practice in Utah in the early 1930s, but formal neurology was not born for another twenty years. When the School of Medicine opened its doors, at least three nonsurgical departments shared the care of patients with disease of the nervous system: pediatrics, psychiatry, and medicine. Dr. Jean Davis, trained in epileptology by the eminent William Lennox, managed a small Epilepsy Center at the Salt Lake General Hospital (SLGH) and operated an electroencephalograph for psychiatry and pediatrics. She also maintained a largely research relationship with the Training School at American Fork. Acutely ill adults were ordinarily under the care of the Department of Medicine, while chronic cases went to psychiatry.

Minutes of the Executive Committee for October 1951 indicate a loose agreement whereby Dr. Valdemar (Val) Jager in medicine became responsible for undergraduate teaching in neurology and the relevant outpatient clinic at SLGH. Drs. Jean Davis and Frank H. Tyler, internist, "will continue their specific areas of interest" (presumably epilepsy and muscle disease, respectively); and Dr. Madison H. Thomas would be responsible for "postgraduate teaching and affiliation with the V.A., including planning for the new V.A. Hospital's neurology program." This intricate arrangement was further complicated by the remark that, "the faculty may have access to other individuals in the field of neurology as they desire"!

When Dr. Thomas returned to Utah from his training under the distinguished Dr. Russell N. DeJong at the University of Michigan in 1952, he became the first board-certified neurologist in Utah. As a staff member in the Department of Psychiatry, he served as chief of the neurology service at both Veterans Administration hospitals in turn. He also supervised electroencephalographic laboratories at SLGH and at the VA hospitals, the latter operated by Kenneth Kooi, PhD. Teaching neurology to students and psychiatry residents was another responsibility, and he also consulted at the voluntary hospitals in Salt Lake City and made occasional professional visits to surrounding states. Pursuing a major interest in epilepsy, he found time to organize and work with lay groups as medical adviser.

Thomas also appreciated the need for a residency training program to help solidify his enormous efforts in a full-scale pedagogic enterprise. Therefore, he applied for accreditation and in 1953 received tentative approval for two of the three required residency years. A grant of funds from the National Institutes of Health to increase the staff was received in 1954. Despite these successes, it was obviously impossible to produce all the elements of a full neurology unit without more personnel and funding, and the dean's office began to cast about for other answers.

In 1953 Dr. John Z. Bowers, then dean of the College of Medicine, began to explore the needs and capabilities of the entire College in the area of neurology. Little progress was made. In October 1955 Dean Philip B. Price appointed a committee to investigate all aspects of teaching, patient care, and research in neurology, which reported in February 1956. Starting with the propositions that "Neurology is an important clinical discipline in its own right" and that the elements needed for a program of high caliber were locally available, the committee recommended the establishment of "an interdepartmental division . . . responsible to the Dean." Further, the committee concluded that "the planning of the Neurology program should allow for the ultimate possibility that . . . a separate Department of Neurology might be formed."

During 1956 and 1957 a Committee on Neurology consisting of three department chairs (Drs. Louis S. Goodman, C. H. Hardin

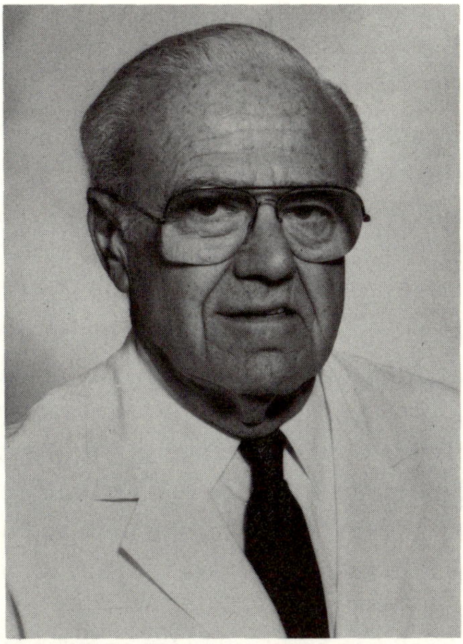

Leonard W. Jarcho.

Branch, and Maxwell M. Wintrobe) deliberated further. As a result of their work, the Executive Committee voted to establish a Division of Neurology independent of all departments and responsible directly to the dean. A search committee for a chair was to be appointed by Dean Price, who encouraged Dr. Leonard W. Jarcho to look into the possibility of becoming a candidate by completing the requirements for Board certification. Taking his previous certification in internal medicine into account, plus five years of research in neurophysiology under Drs. Philip Bard and Clinton N. Woolsey at Johns Hopkins (together with weekly outpatient clinics under Dr. Frank R. Ford and Jack Magladery), the Board required only one year of further formal training in bedside neurology. A successful application to the National Institute of Neurological Disease and Blindness (or NINDB, as it was then called) resulted in a Special Traineeship which supported eleven months of training in clinical neurology at The National Hospital, Queens Square, London, under Drs. E. Arnold Carmichael and Mac-donald Critchley and five months with Drs. Raymond D. Adams and E. P. Richardson in neuropathology at the Massachusetts General Hospital.

Meanwhile, neurologists from other universities were invited to become candidates, wisely declining, considering the paucity of facilities and funds. Witnessing to this last remark is an excerpt from the minutes of the Executive Committee of the College of Medicine for March 16, 1959: "In the face of the budget shortage, fresh consideration was given by the Executive Committee to our Neurology problem. After lengthy discussion, it was unanimously agreed that, inasmuch as there is no immediately foreseeable way to meet the $40,000 budget figure needed to establish the proposed Neurology Division, this whole matter should be deferred until after Dr. Leonard Jarcho returns (about May 1), at which time he and others interested in this problem will be asked to consider [it] anew and come forward with a recommendation . . . ."

An ingenious solution appeared in the minutes of May 11, 1959: "Upon recommendation of the Dean's Committee [the body of College of Medicine department chairs in charge of professional matters at the VA Hospital], Dr. Leonard Jarcho has been appointed Chief of the Neurology Service at the Veterans Hospital."

At the sweep of a pen neurology was rich, owning two professional salaries (Dr. Jarcho's and Dr. E. T. Ajax's), a marvelous secretary (Marcia Monaghan of blessed memory), a forty-bed ward (all adult males), a resident already hired by Dr. Thomas (Dr. Daniel Nussbaum), and the obligation to produce in- and outpatient care at the VA Hospital and SLGH, a residency program and student curriculum, plus the research program and administrative service expected of all quadruple-threat department chairs. At the June 8 meeting Dean Price announced the recommendation of "Dr. Jarcho as Chairman of the Neurology Division in the College of Medicine," with the title of assistant professor of neurology since it was the wrong month for promotions. He also donated a sheet of postage stamps with which to recruit staff and apply for grants, since it was considered inappropriate to use the VA's franking privilege for University business.

Dr. E. T. Ajax was appointed assistant chief of neurology at the VA Hospital in 1957 and joined the Division of Neurology as instructor when it was created in 1959. He brought a particular interest in cortical function and a most felicitous ability in bedside care and teaching, repeatedly acknowledged in student awards.

Special note should be made of the very important assistance of Dr. James Rex Miller, internist of Salt Lake City, in the first steps of the division. With two years in neurology at the Mayo Clinic (in addition to his training in internal medicine), he happily gave his time to assist with teaching and patient care wherever and whenever he was needed. In his footsteps have followed, in later years, a number of practicing neurologists from the community, including Drs. William R. Schmidt, Garth Myers, Wayne Hebertson, Gerald R. Moress, Robert M. Satovick, and Alvin J. Wirthlin.

At this point it may be well to describe the state of neurology at the time in the country at large. At the end of World War II neurology was more often regarded a part of psychiatry than related to medicine or neurosurgery, as witness the Divisions of Neuropsychiatry in the Armed Forces and the Veterans Administration (ordinarily headed by psychiatrists), and even the name of the American Board of Psychiatry and Neurology. At the same time, a general increase in popular interest in attacking the problems posed by organic disease of the nervous system was signaled by the formation of a number of voluntary agencies, such as The National Foundation for Infantile Paralysis, The National Multiple Sclerosis Society, The National Epilepsy League, and others, in the late 1940s and 1950.

Public pressure also produced the NINDB in 1950. In early meetings of this organization's administration it was recognized that research in neurology was unlikely to blossom in the absence of well-trained neurologists, and a series of surveys of the population of neurologists ensued. In 1952, 250 qualified neurologists were certified in the U.S. Seventy-nine medical schools mustered only fifteen accredited programs in neurology organized to graduate a total of thirty trainees annually. Research was lagging because of the paucity of trained investigators. Moreover, "as the training of clinical investigators in neurology developed, it became increasingly clear that in order for them to be effective teachers and researchers, they must master the broad principles of several basic neurologic sciences, and should have thorough knowledge of at least one basic science discipline."

To the University this meant that neurology, however organized in the catalogue, would need to pay attention to opportunities for its trainees in already strong areas like neuropharmacology (Drs. Louis S. Goodman and Ewart Swinyard, dean of the College of Pharmacy), neurophysiology (Drs. Carlton Hunt and Carlos Eyzaguirre), and psychiatry (Drs. C. H. Hardin Branch, Eugene L. Bliss, *et al.*) while trying to help develop related disciplines in other departments. Thus, a home was made for Dr. Kenneth Brizzee, a neuroanatomist whose work was unrelated to the rest of anatomy's program at that time. When he left, the department was fortunate enough to attract PhD's O. Eugene Millhouse and Suzanne Stensaas, two superb teachers who introduced the nervous system to first-year students for many years. Dr. P. A. Cancilla started a most successful tradition in neuropathology. For a few abundant years the department enjoyed a second neuropathologist, Dr. A. N. D'Agostino, as well, and the needs of two departments and two hospitals were particularly well served. Dr. Margaret L. Grunnet followed from 1969 to 1981. Dr. Jeannette J. Townsend has ably filled the slot since the change of department administration in 1982. One of neurology's grants brought the first full-time neuro-ophthalmologist, Dr. Henry J. L. VanDyk, and his recent successor, Dr. Kathleen Digre. Neurology also helped to recruit Dr. Robert Anderson, the first full-time neuroradiologist, and Dr. Petter Lindstrom, the first full-time neurosurgeon.

Breaking ground in all of these areas as a response to the department's needs brought new learning and attitudes to the practice of neurology in the state. The division became a full department by vote of the Utah Coordinating Council on Higher Education on June 28, 1965.

Throughout the years a major portion of this effort has been supported by the NIH in the form of Training Grants in both adult and pediatric neurology, research grants, and fellowships of various sorts. Evidence of the great effect of this federal program is the continuing growth of the population of qualified neurologists in the U.S. from 250 in 1950 to 5,745 in 1989. To this number Utah's small department has contributed more than 100 graduates in thirty-one years and is also pleased to take credit for most of the growth in the population of neurologists in Utah, from 1 to 39 over the same time span. Of these 20 are currently in private practice, 18 on the full-time University staff, 1 in the State Department of Health. Three others are more or less retired.

Because this volume is primarily devoted to the clinical practice of medicine, the Department of Neurology's efforts in research are intentionally left to the end, despite the fact that all members of the senior staff have been regularly engaged in investigation. The first research laboratories were those of Edward C. Beck and Robert Dustman, PhD's in physiological psychology at the VA Hospital. Their major effort was in the field of evoked cerebral potentials, but the clinical service in psychological testing under Thomas Schenkenberg, PhD, has been a most successful outgrowth. As noted above, the electroencephalographic laboratories are older than the department and have grown along with experimental work in the pharmacological and surgical therapy of epilepsy.

The names of Drs. Patrick F. Bray, Jack A. Madsen, and others in pediatric neurology and of the late, much-lamented Huntington Mavor, as well as Donald R. Bennett and Fumisuke Matsuo are associated with continuing growth in electroencephalography.

Electromyography was brought to Utah by Dr. Jarcho as both a clinical and a research tool subsequently expanded by the work of Drs. Mavor and Jack H. Petajan and recently Kathryn Alderson. Dr. Petajan has also been involved for many years in research on multiple sclerosis and a number of years ago introduced the therapy of plasmapheresis to Utah. Drs. Jarcho, Ajax, and Nathaniel Nord took part in the first country-wide study of the use of levodopa in Parkinson's disease. An extensive genealogical library of Huntington's disease cases has been collected by Dr. Jarcho, and with the expert labor of

Keith E. Johnson, BS, films of this and other movement disorders have been amassed for research, teaching, and clinical purposes. Dr. Bray has long been associated with work on the immunology and virology of multiple sclerosis. Dr. Fred A. Ziter's work has been in skeletal muscle disease, largely the dystrophies. Dr. Gregory K. Call has taken over major responsibility for work in cerebrovascular disease.

Since the appointment of Dr. J. Richard Baringer to succeed Dr. Jarcho as department chair in 1982, the major focus of departmental research has been in virology and immunology, in which he is involved with Drs. John Greenlee, J. B. Burns, and John W. Rose. An important addition is Dr. Kurt A. Jaeckle, whose research interest in brain tumor therapy bodes well for the future.

It is not only important but a pleasure to recognize that the department would have gone nowhere without the incomparable devotion of administrative assistants Donna Saunders, Ann Rokich, Mary Alm, Alice Reis, and Terrie Larsen. Research would have foundered long ago without Keith E. Johnson, BS, Research Specialist, who has carried a heavy load in the laboratories for thirty-six years.

Graduates of the University of Utah Department of Neurology

NEUROLOGIST	UNIV.	U.HS	U.FT	PVT. PRAC.	LOC.	NOTES
Alderson, M. K.		x	x		SLC	
Ajax, E. T.	x		x		SLC	
Andrews, J. M.				x	Provo	
Banta, C. A.		x		x	Ogden	NPeds
Baringer, J. R.			x		SLC	
Bray, P. F.			x		SLC	NPeds
Burns, J. B.			x		SLC	
Call, G.		x	x		SLC	
Digre, K. B.			x		SLC	NOphth
Fillioux, F. M.		x	x		SLC	NPeds
Foley, J. F.		x		x	SLC	
Goldstein, M. L.				x	SLC	NPeds
Greenlee, J. E.			x		SLC	

NEUROLOGIST	UNIV.	U.HS	U.FT	PVT. PRAC.	LOC.	NOTES
Hebertson, W. M.		x		x	SLC	
Houts, T. D.		x		x	SLC	
Jaeckle, K. A.			x		SLC	
Jarcho, L. W.			x		SLC	
Jones, C. R.		x	x		SLC	
Lynn, R. B.				x	Ogden	
Madsen, J. A.	x	x	x		SLC	NPeds
Matsuo, F.			x		SLC	
Meyer, J. G.				x	Provo	NPeds
Moress, G. K.		x		x	SLC	
Morley, G. K.				x	Provo	
Myers, G. G.				x	SLC	NPeds
Nord, N. M.	x	x	x	x	SLC	
Petajan, J. H.			x		SLC	
Reichert, W. H.	x			x	SLC	
Rose, J. W.			x		SLC	
Satovick, R. M.	x	x		x	SLC	
Schmidt, W. R.	x	x		x	Ogden	
Smith, D.		x		x	SLC	
Tait, V. F.		x	x		SLC	NPeds
Thoen, D. D.		x*		x	SLC	Fellow*
Thomas, M. H.			x	x	SLC	
Thompson, J. A.		x	x		SLC	NPeds
Thurman, D. J.	x	x	x	x*	SLC	MPH
Ziter, F. A.		x	x		SLC	NPeds

LEGEND

Univ.:	Student, University of Utah School of Medicine
U.HS:	University of Utah Hospitals house staff
U.FT:	Dept. of Neurology, Univ. of Utah, full time
*:	Utah State Board of Health
NPeds:	Pediatric Neurology
NOphth:	Ophthalmic Neurology
MPH:	Master of Public Health

CHAPTER SIXTEEN

Dermatology

LEALAND L. CLARK, MD

THE SKIN IS THE LARGEST organ of the body and provides the first avenue of its defense against disease. However, a disease of the skin that produces an unsightly rash or weeping, reddened, and raw skin, can provoke feelings of disgust in onlookers and within patients themselves. Psoriasis is said to be one of the leading causes of suicide among young women. Indeed, there is almost a cultural bias against skin disease — Job with his boils, lepers with their bells, syphilitics with their madness. Ancient writers often associated skin lesions with moral impurity, internal disharmony, and evil. Skin disease can cause some of the greatest of physical agonies — great pain, intense itching and burning, and impairment of physical activity. Two to four percent of all nonobstetric and nonaccident civilian hospital admissions are for skin disease. About one in ten persons in the United States has a skin disorder. Eighteen percent of the patients in a family or general practice are dermatological. During World War II, more evacuations from the South Pacific were for skin disorders than for battle casualties. The leading cause of hospitalization in the Vietnam War was skin conditions. Acute and chronic skin diseases account for more than half of all workmen's compensation cases in some states and constitute the most common of all occupational diseases.

Since earliest times the human race has been plagued with various skin disorders, and the ability to diagnose systemic disorders by means of cutaneous signs has always fascinated some physicians. But

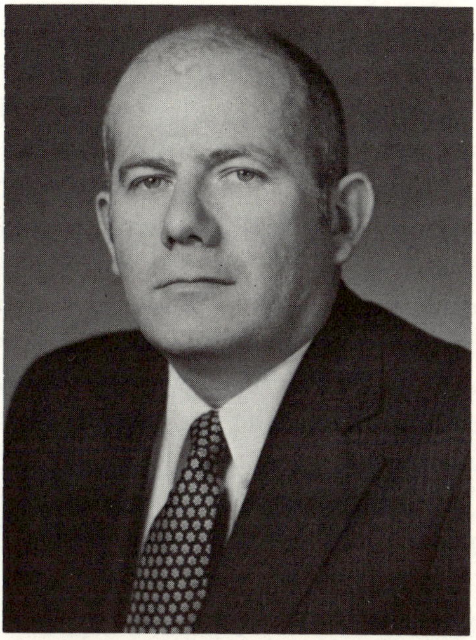

Lealand L. Clark.

until the eighteenth century, most physicians were little concerned with the skin itself, apart from the exanthematous eruptions of acute fevers. From 1775 until about 1928, investigations of the skin led to contributions to experimental pathology, beginning with the concept of chemical carcinogenesis initiated by Percival Pott's recognition of scrotal cancer in chimney sweeps. By the mid-nineteenth century an Austrian physician, Ferdinand Von Hebra, emphasized an approach to skin disease based on microscopic examinations of skin lesions.

Dermatology began to change in the mid-twentieth century from the art of description and cataloguing to a science that seeks causes and mechanisms underlying skin diseases. Stephen Rothman emigrated from Hungary, joined the University of Chicago in 1938, and fathered modern dermatology, utilizing biochemistry and physiology. A brilliant investigator, Rothman made dermatology a science through his book *Physiology and Biochemistry of the Skin*, which led to the development of more sophisticated and effective treatments and diagnoses.

Basic studies of the skin emphasize its constantly changing structures and chemistry as it adapts to its role and environment. Better understanding of the ecology and protective function of the skin, its role in immunity, and the mechanisms involved in such cutaneous processes as pigment formation is necessary before the clinician embarks upon the evaluation and treatment of disorders of this vital organ.

The explosive increase in fundamental information has made immunology an independent branch of science, with the identification of the Langerhans cell as a microphage and its "look alike" dendritic T-cell as a natural killer cell. The skin assumes its rightful place as *the* primary organ of the immune system. Additionally, growth of basic research funding, mostly from the National Institutes of Health, has had enormous impact on dermatology.

Since World War II the expansion of all scientific knowledge has assumed almost astronomical proportions. Dermatologists are being challenged to think in terms of the most advanced scientific knowledge and are supported by a score of well-staffed and -equipped dermatological clinical and research units worldwide. The three most outstanding are Yale University, the Mayo Clinic, and Harvard Medical School. In the last thirty years the character of dermatology has changed, and the work of the dermatologist now embraces every aspect of the biology of the skin, normal and abnormal.

The problem in dermatologic diagnosis is largely related to the examiner's ability to recognize specific lesions. A medical student can only be introduced to skin lesions and usually can catch only fleeting glimpses; he or she can hardly gain enough familiarity with various lesions to allow recognition of even the most common types. Not recognizing the lesions, the physician develops the habit of disregarding the skin. The identification of skin lesions requires neither a detailed history nor long contemplation but simply a "trained eye." Treatment is based on diagnosis; if the diagnosis is incorrect, treatment is likely to be ineffective.

Many diseases of the skin may be diagnosed with accuracy on inspection as surely as the pathologist recognizes a characteristic cytologic picture. Others are more obscure and require further study, utilizing all the resources of general medicine and special laboratory procedures. The disorders have been grouped in various ways: by pathogenetic mechanisms; by organ systemic involvement; by categories of disease, and on the basis of mutual, characteristic physical signs. These divisions reflect in part the types of broad clinical problems that physicians often face: i.e., cancer, angiitis, sarcoidosis, lymphomas, connective tissue diseases, and so on. At the present time dermatology is one of the most "general" of the specialties and is no longer considered a very insular subspecialty of internal medicine. The dermatologist cares for all age groups, is usually more skilled in the diagnosis of pathology of the skin than most general pathologists, and utilizes more specialized plastic surgery procedures than do most surgeons. Penicillin, griseofulvin, cortisone, topical chemotherapy, and retinoids have made life much more comfortable for millions of patients.

Although skin disease has been with the human race always, as a medical specialty dermatology is a relative newcomer. Board certification was established in 1932, and the American Academy of Dermatology was formed in Detroit, Michigan, in 1938.

The first dermatologist in the state, Dr. Clifford J. Pearsall, trained at Rush Medical School–Presbyterian Hospital in Chicago and arrived in Salt Lake City in 1923. The first Utah member of the American Academy of Dermatology was C. O'Neal Rich in 1942, followed by William J. Morginson in 1947, William L. Kirkman in 1951, Manley Utterback in 1953, John M. Coletti in 1955, Arthur N. Burton in 1957, Joseph A. Aaron and Robert G. Thompson in 1961, and Lealand L. Clark in 1962. After 1962 a steady increase continued not only in Salt Lake City but in other communities in the state.

The 1949 Utah Medical Society directory lists four dermatologists: Drs. Pearsall, Rich, Morginson, and Ynez D. Eskelson. Many of the early dermatologists used x-ray machines in their offices for various benign conditions such as acne and psoriasis with good initial regression of lesions but sometimes very damaging effects when treatment was repeated. The lack of awareness of the effects of radiation and the complete absence of physicists to calibrate the output of machines produced a number of disasters.

Dr. Morginson in particular used x-ray therapy widely in the treatment of skin cancers — without any failures, according to him, using a standard dose of 3,000 r. Even radiation therapists don't claim to have better than 90% success with excellent cosmetic results, and they vary the dose, energy, and treatment schedule according to the size and depth of the lesion.

Surgical excision has been widely used by dermatologists and surgeons with excellent results in small lesions, but in larger tumors the cosmetic results are better with radiation therapy.

Used as a last resort in basal cell carcinoma is Mohs' chemosurgical technique, involving (1) serial application of zinc chloride paste, which results in escharotic fixation of fixed tissues; (2) scalpel removal of successive layers of fixed tissue; (3) microscopic examination of frozen sections of the undersurface of each specimen removed; and (4) reapplication of zinc chloride paste to sites which have histologically been shown to contain tumor until an absolutely tumor-free specimen from all sites is obtained. This therapy is extremely time-consuming (i.e., expensive) and very painful. It causes scarring, sometimes requires lengthy skin grafting to correct wound contraction, and causes occasional hemorrhaging due to weakening of the blood vessel walls, which is both frightening and potentially life-threatening. In addition, occasional recurrences may still follow all this agony and expense. All these appear to be excellent reasons for using other forms of treatment.

Laser surgery seems to be the new treatment of choice for most basal cell carcinomas. This method of surgery is relatively pain-free for the patient, usually eliminates bleeding, is very quick, and results in very little scarring. However, it is expensive because of the cost of the equipment and the skill required in its application.

Most patients and their insurance companies seem to feel the cost is justified by the results. And for any dermatologist and his staff who have attempted to excise dozens of warts from the hands of a screaming four-year-old, the laser is nothing short of miraculous. Children especially are utterly fascinated by this application of space-age technology and actually enjoy the procedure.

Accutane, a vitamin A derivative, has a seemingly miraculous ability to cure one of the most heart-breaking of skin problems — severe cystic acne. Indeed, it is the first *cure* for acne in human history. Although the patient must have a blood test once a month to check on lipid increases, this problem can almost always be controlled with good counseling on diet; i.e., one high in fresh fruits, vegetables, and complex carbohydrates and low in refined sugars, alcohol, and fatty foods. (In other words, all the snack foods beloved by almost all Americans.) However, most patients whose acne cannot be cleared by more traditional methods of antibiotics, contraceptive pills, or topical chemotherapy to cause drying and peeling, are happy to forego the pleasures of the dinner table to achieve cure. Accutane must be continued for at least three months and sometimes, in a small percentage of patients, must be prescribed for another period of three months. Conception by female patients during this period of treatment is absolutely contraindicated.

One dermatological advance that has made headlines around the world is the discovery that retinoic acid, or Retin-A, a cousin of Accutane, has the wonderful ability to reverse sun damage or aging of the skin. Although many people, weary of the overblown, largely untrue claims of cosmetics companies over the years, were reluctant to believe the media coverage, they were forced to believe their own eyes upon seeing the new, young-looking skin of many of their friends. As a result, millions of healthy but aging consumers called dermatologists for appointments to obtain prescriptions for what really must be termed a "miracle drug." Pores shrink, wrinkles vanish, sagging and puffiness decrease, and skin tone and color improve. The application has to be very carefully controlled as the cream, unless very lightly and sparingly applied, causes burning, peeling, and cracking. Both men and women are delighted with this therapy, which is very successful if (1) small amounts are used *sparingly*, (2) followed by *generous* amounts of moisturizers, and (3) adequate sunscreens are used to protect against sunburn on ski slopes, tennis courts, and beaches, as some very painful sunburns have resulted when proper precautions were not taken. Morphogens (Retin-A) are information-bearing molecules that tell cells where to go and what to do. They control limb bud growth in the fetus, for example. The development of this drug promises a Nobel Prize for the five Harvard students who did this work, which will eventually lead to more medical wonders.

Dermatology at the University of Utah

Dr. Gerald Krueger was the first dermatologist to join the faculty in 1972 as an assistant professor in the Department of Medicine. After completing a residency and research training at the University of Colorado, he started a new division, which he headed until 1987. Dr. Krueger's major interest has been psoriasis.

Dr. John J. Zone joined the division in 1978 as assistant professor after training at the State University of New York at Buffalo. He is now an associate professor and has been chief of the division since 1987. Dr. Zone is currently involved in the study of bullous immune-mediated skin disease.

Dr. Michael W. Piepkorn received a PhD in experimental pathology at the University of Washington, where he also completed his residency in dermatology and a fellowship and residency in pathology. He joined the University faculty in 1980. Other members (assistant professors) of the division are Lynn K. Pershing, PhD, Laurence J. Meyer, MD, PhD, Marta J. Peterson, MD, and John W. Gerweis, MD, associate professor.

CHAPTER SEVENTEEN

Psychiatry

JACK L. TEDROW, MD, JD

OF ALL THE MEDICAL SPECIALTIES, psychiatry is by its nature the most sensitive and responsive to social changes. The best example is the creation in the last thirty years of drug treatment programs for the victims of illicit drug use. Additionally, psychiatrists have enjoyed the availability of new medications on a par with insulin for diabetes and digitalis for certain cardiac disorders. Witness the development of chlorpromazine for psychosis, lithium carbonate for manic–depressive (bipolar) disorder, the benzodiazepines for anxiety, including Xanax for phobic disorders and Anafranil for obsessive-compulsive neuroses. We can therefore state that progress in the last forty years in this specialty has been spectacular. Major changes in the way psychiatry is practiced have resulted from these developments. The psychiatrists in Utah, as in other states, have responded well.

The Utah State Hospital in Provo, Utah, dates from 1885, when Utah was a territory. It was then referred to as an insane asylum. As in other states, care was largely custodial, with emphasis on hydrotherapy and wet packs for their sedative value as well as use of bromides and other sedatives. In the thirties insulin coma therapy and electro-convulsive therapy (ECT) appeared. At that time Dr. Garland Pace, the superintendent, was responsible for emphasis on treatment. He was replaced in the late forties by Dr. Owen Henninger, who introduced the therapeutic community model of Maxwell Jones for which the hospital later received national recognition and awards. The patient population of the State Hospital declined as mental health centers were established throughout the state and as psychiatric wards were opened in the large hospitals. However, some patients still required longer-term care and needed admission to the State Hospital, which has about 325 available beds. A Forensic Unit was also established in the late seventies for those criminal offenders who require either psychiatric evaluation or care not available in the state penitentiary or in the various facilities treating antisocial adolescents.

Involuntary commitment of certain patients by the courts (i.e., those who are a danger to themselves or others) provides the largest number of patients treated at the State Hospital — usually patients requiring prolonged care, including those who have refused or not responded to medications. According to Dr. Louis G. Moench, who compiled figures on that population, the advent of new treatment modalities reduced the numbers from around 1,350 to those of the present time. Usually about twenty-five patients are waiting for admission.

Prior to World War II, psychiatry in Utah was essentially state hospital psychiatry. After the war ended, several psychiatrists went into private practice at about the same time (1945–48), including Drs. Roy Darke, William Pace, and Jack Tedrow.

The Department of Psychiatry was established in the University of Utah College of Medicine in August 1948, with Dr. C. H. Hardin Branch as its first chair in the old Salt Lake General Hospital (SLGH). Under his capable leadership a residency program in psychiatry was soon established, as well as lectures to the medical students, including the freshman class. Dr. Branch gradually built a staff of professionals, including Drs. William Brown and Agi Plenk, clinical psychologists, and Dr. Leonard H. Taboroff, child psychiatrist. Later Eugene L. Bliss, MD, and Ija Korner, PhD, psychologist, came on the scene. Bliss and Branch coauthored a book on eating disorders (anorexia) now considered a classic in the field. Dr. Branch and his wife, Erma, were very active in community affairs and very helpful in "selling psychiatry" to the citizens of Salt Lake City.

The psychiatric residents rotated through the Utah State Hospital, the new VA Hospital built in the early 1950s, and various clinics in

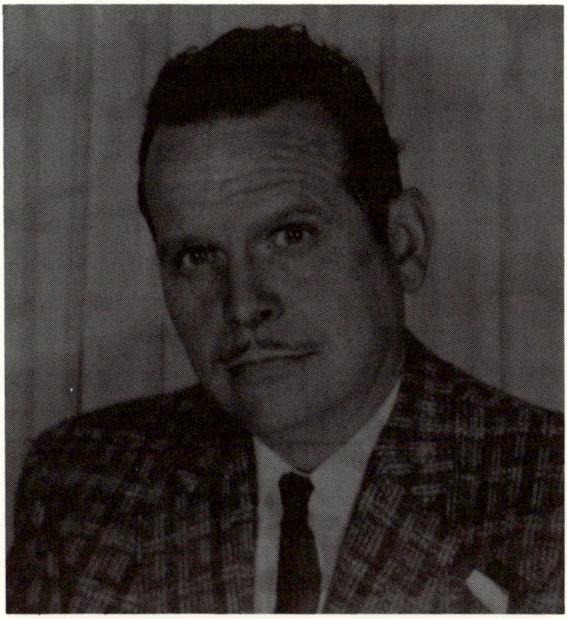

Jack L. Tedrow.

small towns scattered throughout Utah. A great effort was made to educate family practitioners in the Intermountain West. Dr. Branch gave considerable credit to the National Institute of Mental Health (NIMH) for the success of these programs. He became president of the American Psychiatric Association in 1962. When he left Utah in 1970, Dr. Bliss became chair of the department until Dr. Bernard Grosser assumed the post in 1982. Dr. Bliss has done considerable research in the chemistry of aggression. Recently his interest has been in multiple personality, and he has written extensively on the subject.

With its Grand Round lectures one or more times per month, the Department of Psychiatry has brought in outstanding psychiatrists as speakers from all over the United States to update social workers, psychologists, psychiatric nurses, and medical students as well as Utah psychiatrists. The Utah Psychiatric Association has sponsored at least one of these programs each year, sometimes in conjunction with the yearly meeting of the Utah State Medical Association. The

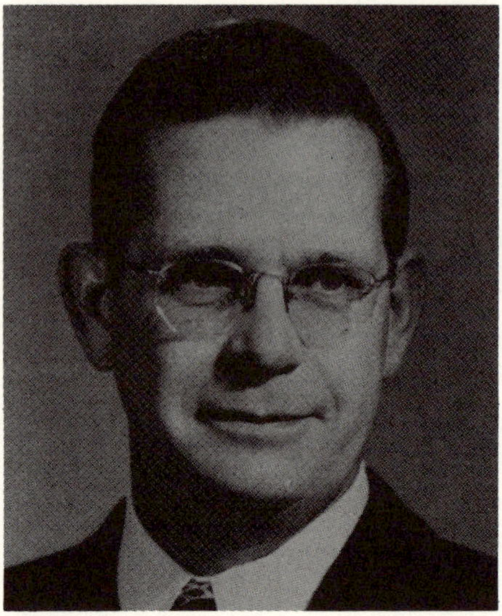

C. H. Hardin Branch.

latter programs are aimed at an audience of family practitioners and members of other specialties.

The first meeting of the Utah Psychiatric Association (UPA) was held in the fall of 1949. It was at first composed of just seven members. At that time the American Psychiatric Association (APA) had about 3,000 members. In the early sixties the UPA became a district branch of the APA, which now comprises more than 33,000 members. The Utah branch presently consists of 135 members. It is a close-knit and friendly organization mostly on a first-name basis. There are no "bad apples." Hard-working elected officers and a council that meets monthly resolve problems and promote its public image. Representatives lobby the state legislature and are active on the national scene through the APA.

Dr. Darke had established the first psychiatric ward at St. Mark's Hospital in 1946. A psychiatric ward at the old County hospital (SLGH) followed in 1948. A similar unit at the LDS Hospital opened in 1959 under the able leadership of Dr. Louis G. Moench. The new VA Hospital built in 1952 emphasized mental health care and had a separate building devoted to the treatment of psychiatric patients. During the fifties the various mental health centers were established in an effort to relieve the burden on the State Mental Hospital and to permit the healthier mental patients to remain near their families and homes, being treated as outpatients when possible. This trend followed the appearance of the first antipsychotic drugs, including Thorazine and Mellaril.

The first "all open ward" psychiatric unit was established at Holy Cross Hospital in 1961 with Dr. Jack Tedrow in charge. By this time several excellent medications were available for milder symptoms of nervous disorders, including meprobamate, Librium, and Dexamyl. Electro-convulsive therapy was used extensively for severe depression on an outpatient basis. Emphasis was now on outpatient psychotherapy.

During the sixties some remarkable social developments changed the types of patients psychiatrists were treating as well as the methods of treatment. The "drug scene" was slowly developing, first including mainly the use or abuse of marijuana, speed (the amphetamines), LSD, and in some cases, (sniffed) glue. This required a major shift on the psychiatric units to the treatment of adolescents. It is significant that the number of juvenile court judges in Utah increased from one in the fifties (Judge Rulon Clark) to twelve at the present time.

During the fifties quite a few transorbital lobotomies were performed on psychiatric patients in Utah, with questionable success. Dr. Petter Lindstrom introduced prefrontal sonic treatment at the University of Utah Medical Center, which seemed to produce less postoperative organic brain syndrome. Most of the psychiatric community considered these approaches to mental illness far too radical, and as second opinions became required by the hospitals involved, the procedures passed into history.

In the early fifties Dr. Agi Plenk began her clinical work with normal, then mentally handicapped and disturbed preschool children at the Holladay Community Church. In 1962 she moved her operation to Sugarhouse and in 1970 to the present Children's Center adjacent to the University Medical Center at Fort Douglas. This treatment program has made an outstanding contribution to the welfare of thousands of Utah's children.

Child psychiatry has grown by leaps and bounds in Utah. Part of a resident's training in the Department of Psychiatry is experience in treating the psychiatric problems of children. For many years Dr. Paul Whitehead chaired this department at Primary Children's Hospital, now headed by Dr. Richard Ferre. In the clinical area the concept of autism in children is relatively new. Additionally, the number of children who have been abused physically or sexually has increased.

Psychiatrists used to be called upon to assist the courts in determining the mental state of defendants charged with murder. The role has now expanded to many other aspects of criminal and civil law, i.e., competency of defendants to stand trial, rehabilitative potential of offenders, and custody of children, to name just a few. As crime has worsened in Utah, psychiatrists have been increasingly involved in legal matters, and two psychiatrists in Utah now hold law degrees. Jails are now required to appoint visiting psychiatrists to prescribe for mentally ill inmates.

The mental health centers required the services of many social workers and psychologists, and by 1970 they were doing a great deal of the group therapy and individual psychotherapy in those facilities. As the only psychoanalyst, Dr. Norman S. Anderson did an outstanding job in heading the Granite Mental Health Clinic in Salt Lake City. By this time a considerable number of residents had finished their training and set up practice in Salt Lake City, Ogden, and Provo as well as in the surrounding states. By the seventies the number of psychiatrists in the area had made private practice very competitive, so many hired on part-time in the mental health centers. Several psychiatrists make scheduled visits to nursing homes to treat elderly patients.

In the seventies and eighties antidepressant medications appeared and rendered electro-convulsive therapy a last-resort measure for severe depression. Emphasis on genetic factors developed, especially in the area of manic-depressive illness (bipolar disorder), and with the advent of lithium carbonate these patients could be helped as never before. Dr. Paul H. Wender arrived at the Department of Psychiatry with his interest in attention deficit disorder, and Ritalin became the medication of choice for many of the victims of this disease. Additionally, certain forms of schizophrenia were labeled as genetic in origin. Other disorders such as phobic states and obsessive-compulsive neurosis have also been identified as having a chemical basis, and medications have been developed to assist in their treatment.

In the eighties considerable ongoing research in the neuronal synapse made pharmacology the centerpiece of much of the treatment of the major psychiatric disorders. However, research indicates that patients do better when such medications are combined with psychotherapy. People obviously need help with problems unrelated to their synapses. Mental health organizations have focused the attention of the public on understanding nervous and mental disorders so that afflicted people are handled with increasing patience and compassion.

Psychiatry has always been a specialty which included many theories of psychodynamics and causation of various forms of mental disorders. Currently many schizophrenics do not fit the genetic explanation, just as there are depressed patients who do not respond to the antidepressants currently available. One of the most debated phenomena in present psychiatry is multiple personality. Dr. Eugene Bliss is a true believer. Others in the profession believe such cases are purely iatrogenic (that is, physician-induced). Dr. Wender is currently researching what happens to attention deficit disorder children when they become adults — a fascinating field. Better explanations of the factors causing certain personality disorders, particularly the antisocial ones, are still required, and society is greatly in need of better treatment modalities for all of the so-called personality disorders.

The history of psychiatry in Utah tends to parallel the developments not only in neuropharmacology but also in the changes in society, necessitating new approaches to adolescent problems, homosexuality, drug abuse and addiction, inmates in jails and prisons, ever-increasing criminality, and the emptying of the patients of state mental hospitals into mental health centers and related treatment programs. In addition to Alcoholics Anonymous, organizations for sexual addicts, gay alcoholics, etc., have sprung up.

Five hours per week on the psychoanalytic couch for three years gave way to weekly, or fewer, visits for a six- to twelve-month period as society tightened its economic belt. The use of group therapy increased at the expense of individual psychotherapy. The main change came about as a result of the development of drugs that helped depression, psychotic breakdowns, manic-depressive disease, and phobic conditions.

Some time ago the APA developed Board certification for child psychiatrists, later for forensic psychiatrists, and it is presently creating Board examination for geriatric psychiatrists due to the aging population and the need for psychiatric specialists in this area. Another good example of response to societal needs is the development of the pain clinics. Dr. Robert Burgoyne is responsible for founding and overseeing a short-term inpatient pain clinic at LDS Hospital dating from 1979. Yet another example is the much-emulated twelve-step program of Alcoholics Anonymous with its emphasis on solving life's problems with a set program rather than depending on medication, although Antabuse has helped many.

As economics has increasingly permeated every aspect of human life, emphasis on outpatient care in psychiatry has grown since it is cost-effective. Although in the last twenty years there has been some health insurance coverage of inpatient care for psychiatric patients, it is much less than that provided for patients with other types of illnesses. Currently very little economic help is provided for outpatient care for psychiatric patients, even though it has been demonstrated to be more cost-effective than hospitalization at $400 to $1,000 daily.

Computerization of records and accounts has required that every diagnosis and procedure in medicine be coded with a specific number, which led to the development in psychiatry of the *Diagnostic Statistical Manual*, now *DSM-III-Revised.* Currently *DSM-IV* is being formulated. The *DSM* attempts to list the symptoms for each psychiatric disorder so that a diagnosis can be established. The underlying personality disorder is also taken into consideration, plus any physical disease and the person's reaction to stress. While it is most useful for insurance carriers, the legal system, and Medicare and Medicaid, the manual of course provides no suggestion for what treatment should be provided.

The drug problem continues to escalate, and the increasing number of addicts has changed the face of psychiatry in Utah. Methadone clinics have been developed for the treatment of heroin addicts. Free-standing for-profit units have opened for the treatment of alcohol and drug addiction. Many of these programs are for a thirty-day period and are very expensive. They have not been in existence long enough to judge their success in treating these difficult patients.

As to the future of psychiatry in Utah, the handwriting is on the wall for the private practitioner. Medications are now sufficiently developed that the family physician or internist can prescribe Prozac, Xanax, Haldol, Valium, and other medications which help to some extent with the handling of everyday problems in our drug-dependent, pill-taking society. Psychologists and social workers are "counseling clients" and are depending on physicians for such prescriptions. The typical Utah psychiatrist is salaried by a mental health center or free-standing psychiatric hospital or general medical clinic. Insurance companies pay little for outpatient psychiatric care, and the Utah economy is of little help to the uninsured middle-class psychiatric patient. Therefore, even though it is probably one of the most-needed specialties in our complex and frustrating society, psychiatry is drifting toward paid positions much as it was prior to World War II, when almost all psychiatrists were salaried in the state mental hospitals.

As our highly competitive society grows in complexity and technological sophistication, at least twenty percent of our population will feel completely inadequate and lost in the work place. This will increase the need for psychological help much beyond the demands of the present. Anyone in the mental health profession who is adequately trained and sufficiently devoted will be as busy as he or she wishes. How psychiatrists will serve in the future cannot be predicted, especially if a universal insurance program is introduced. We can accurately predict that they will be in great demand to serve their fellow human beings.

CHAPTER EIGHTEEN

Child Psychiatry

PAUL L. WHITEHEAD, MD • MERRITT H. EGAN, MD

CELEBRATING ITS ONE HUNDREDTH ANNIVERSARY in 1985, the Utah State Hospital in Provo was the major focus of psychiatric treatment in Utah until the late 1940s. A small facility for the severely mentally ill had been founded in Salt Lake City in 1869 and operated until 1885, when the Provo facility opened. During the past four decades, psychiatry in Utah, as elsewhere, has flourished and taken an increasingly relevant role as a medical specialty. In 1948 Dr. C. H. Hardin Branch organized the Department of Psychiatry at the University of Utah College of Medicine. He was joined later by Dr. Norman S. Anderson and by Dr. Eugene L. Bliss in 1950, followed by Dr. Lincoln D. Clark in 1955.

Child psychiatry was introduced to Utah in 1949 with the arrival of Dr. Leonard H. Taboroff. Recruited by Dr. Branch, Dr. Taboroff had completed child psychiatry training at the Menninger Clinic in 1948 and remained an extra year for psychoanalytic training, the first psychiatrist with such training in Utah. With a joint academic appointment in psychiatry and pediatrics, he directed the Children's Psychiatry Service in the Department of Psychiatry at the old Salt Lake General Hospital. He also established the Utah Child Guidance Clinic, an outpatient treatment program for children and adolescents. Dr. Taboroff initiated children's services in traveling clinics servicing rural Utah and started a consultation-liaison program with the University Department of Pediatrics. The first pediatric resident rotated through his program in 1949. He published research on psychotherapeutic play

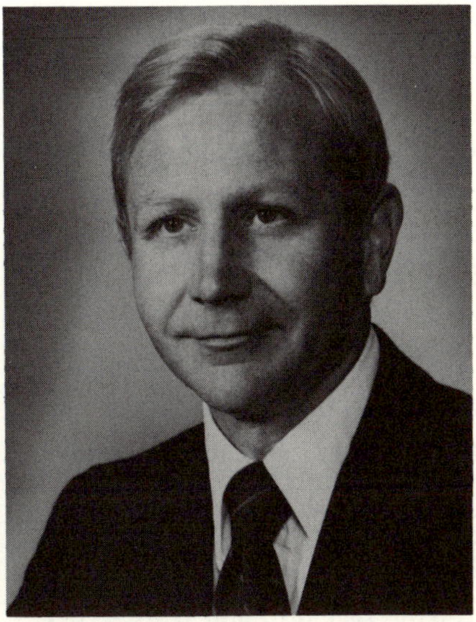
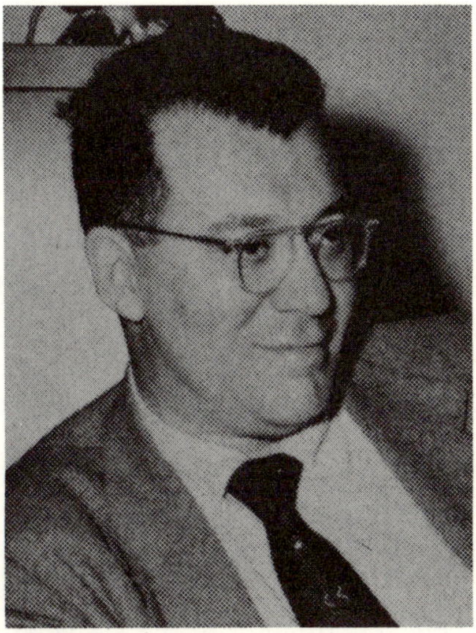

Paul L. Whitehead, left, Leonard H. Taboroff, right.

techniques and personality patterns of children and adolescents with peptic ulcer. In failing health with atrial valve disease from childhood rheumatic fever, Dr. Taboroff died in 1955 at the age of forty-one.

Dr. Frank T. Rafferty had joined Dr. Taboroff early in 1955 as assistant director of the Utah Child Guidance Clinic. Trained in child psychiatry at the University of Colorado Hospital in Denver, he was appointed director of child psychiatry following Dr. Taboroff's untimely death. Dr. Rafferty obtained accreditation for training from the American Association of Psychiatric Services for Children, a goal he had shared with Dr. Taboroff, and Utah offered the only accredited program between Denver and San Francisco. He continued the outpatient clinics and initiated an exemplary Adolescent Treatment Center in Salt Lake City, funded by the Salt Lake Junior League and a demonstration grant from the National Institute of Mental Health (NIMH).

Dr. Rafferty also acquired a training grant from the NIMH. The first child psychiatry career fellow was a former pediatrician, Dr. Merritt H. Egan, who had been the first pediatric resident to rotate through the child psychiatry program with Dr. Taboroff a decade earlier. Dr. Rafferty had a joint appointment in the departments of pediatrics and psychiatry, and for several years he directed the Well Baby Clinic. Several local psychiatrists, including Drs. Jack L. Tedrow and Louis G. Moench, supported child psychiatry training and assisted in supervision. The first physician staff member employed by Dr. Rafferty was Dr. George W. J. Smith, who joined the staff in 1957. He had completed general and a year of child psychiatry training at the University of Michigan Affiliated Hospitals in Ann Arbor.

In 1956 Drs. Branch and Rafferty initiated the Dr. Leonard H. Taboroff Memorial Lecture to honor Dr. Taboroff's contributions. Addressed to child psychiatrists, pediatricians, and allied mental health professionals, this lectureship has provided a continuous series of illustrious and informative speakers since 1957.

Following Dr. Rafferty's departure to Maryland in 1961, Dr. Egan became director of the University Division of Child and Adolescent Psychiatry in July 1962. He obtained additional federal grants which permitted considerable expansion of training programs for both career child psychiatry fellows and allied mental health professionals. The consultation-liaison program with pediatrics was further strengthened, firmly shaping the direction of child psychiatry in Utah. Dr. Egan was also a major force in encouraging child psychiatry services and training at Primary Children's Hospital.

In July 1967, Dr. Paul L. Whitehead, having completed general and child psychiatry training at the University of Cincinnati Medical Center and Cincinnati Child Guidance Home, joined the University division and became the first full-time director of child psychiatry at Primary Children's. An outpatient mental health program had been started there in 1965 under the medical direction of Dr. Robert H. Burgoyne. Formal child psychiatry programs were started with the support of the LDS Church (which owned the hospital until 1974), the University, and Primary's dedicated staff.

A formal affiliation between the University of Utah Medical Center and Primary Children's in 1968 was a monumental event for child psychiatry in Utah. Spearheaded by Dr. Whitehead, a variety of clinical and training programs was developed rapidly. Outpatient treatment was continued and expanded, and a day hospital for latency-age (seven to ten years of age) children, including a therapeutic school program, was started in 1968. Although highly successful in helping thirty-five to forty children each year, the day hospital was closed in 1976 due to lack of funding. At this time charity funding for the hospital was temporarily curtailed because of the LDS Church divesting its hospitals, including Primary, to a private corporation, Intermountain Health Care, late in 1974.

The area's first residential treatment program for eight emotionally disturbed latency-age children was opened at Primary Children's in 1969. A parent-education program promoting parenting skills, the Family Living Seminar, began a year later. In early 1972 the Intermountain West's first acute inpatient treatment program for children and young adolescents, initially an eighteen-bed unit, was opened with phenomenal success. Directed by Dr. Whitehead for the first fifteen months, this unit was subsequently directed by Dr. Cantril Nielsen from 1973 to 1975 and expanded to twenty-four beds in 1976.

During these years medical students and all general psychiatry residents and child psychiatry fellows rotated through Primary Children's psychiatry programs. Scores of other University of Utah students in social work, psychology, recreational therapy, psychiatric nursing, and special education were also trained. Clinical research was encouraged, resulting in many masters' theses and published studies. In 1975 the psychiatry program, then known as Children's Psychiatric Center of Primary Children's Medical Center (PCMC), was awarded full departmental status at the hospital at the same time as medicine and surgery. The program received one of the country's first separate accreditations by the Joint Commission on Accreditation of Hospitals, climaxing a decade of effort. With a spectrum of services annually provided to more than 1,500 children and parents, this program has made a major contribution to clinical services, training, and research in child and adolescent psychiatry. During the past five years, inpatient beds increased from twenty-four to fifty-five. A new state-of-the-art residential facility located in the University of Utah Research Park opened in August 1988, expanding the capacity from eight to twenty children.

Dr. Egan resigned late in 1976 and Dr. Whitehead became director of child psychiatry in January of 1977. He resigned from that position a year later, and Dr. Claudia K. Berenson was appointed as acting and training director of the division. Dr. Whitehead left PCMC in 1981 to pursue full-time private practice.

Dr. Thomas A. Halversen was appointed acting director of the division and acting chair of PCMC's Department of Child Psychiatry, serving in these positions until 1986. Dr. Halversen, who had practiced pediatrics in Bountiful for four years, completed his training in general and child psychiatry and became a member of the division faculty in 1968. He joined the Primary Children's staff in 1973 as director of special services in the Department of Child Psychiatry. During the late 1970s Dr. Halversen also served as chair of the Committee on Indian Affairs of the American Academy of Child Psychiatry. In 1986 University department chair Dr. Bernard G. Grosser became acting director of the University division.

Between 1962 and 1988 the Division of Child and Adolescent Psychiatry trained about forty child psychiatrists for Board qualification. One hundred percent of the child psychiatry fellows trained at the University of Utah Medical Center passed the adult and child Boards; the national average at that time was about fifty percent.

Child psychiatry in Utah came of age during the latter half of the 1960s and through the 1970s. In addition to Primary Children's program, other major efforts were being expended as well. The increase in the number of children and adolescents at the Utah State Hospital during the sixties resulted in the decision to develop a youth program. Unsuccessful efforts to recruit a child psychiatrist delayed these plans, and it was finally determined to use existing hospital personnel. Dr. Eugene J. Faux, a staff psychiatrist at the hospital, established the Youth Center in 1964, following a winter fellowship in child psychiatry at UCLA. In 1968 a ward in the hospital was provided for latency-age children. A vocational-educational wing for adolescents was added in 1972, which also provided school facilities for the younger children.

Another significant development during this time was The Children's Center. Founded in 1960 by Agnes M. Plenk, PhD, at the

Holladay Community Church, the program was initially a service to normal and then to mentally handicapped preschool children. In 1962 the program moved to Sugarhouse, and since that time The Children's Center has focused its efforts on emotionally disturbed children ages two to five years, including parent counseling. The Children's Center Group Home, a residential facility for seven emotionally disturbed preschoolers, was opened in 1967. A new facility adjacent to the University of Utah Medical Center was opened in 1970, which serves seventy-two preschool children in day treatment and many more in outpatient groups. The Kearns Center, treating a similar number, opened in 1975, and the Agnes M. Plenk Group Home, caring for nine children, ages two to seven, was completed in 1983.

Dr. George W. J. Smith served as chief consultant to Dr. Plenk for many years. Dr. Whitehead was a consultant to the first group home in 1967, and Dr. Thomas A. Halversen served as medical director and psychiatric consultant for both Centers from 1968 until 1987. When child psychiatrist Dr. Kristina F. Hindert became medical and executive director, Dr. Plenk resigned after twenty-five years of service as executive director. She continues as psychology consultant. From 1987 until his retirement in 1991, Dr. Halversen limited his activities to the Kearns Center. Dr. Frances L. Burger is now The Children's Center consultant in child psychiatry.

Child psychiatrists trained in the division have made major contributions to the mental health of children and adolescents in Utah and elsewhere. Dr. Denise C. Quinn was the first child psychiatrist trained by Dr. Egan. Completing her clinical fellowship in 1966, Dr. Quinn joined the division faculty and provided training and supervision to child psychiatry fellows, psychiatric residents, and medical students. As training grants diminished in the early 1970s, Dr. Quinn expanded her division responsibilities to the Salt Lake Community Mental Health Center and the Salt Lake City public school system. She subsequently left the division and has continued her private practice in Salt Lake City.

The Intermountain Association of Child Psychiatry held its first official meeting on May 24, 1968, and met regularly until 1983.

Reactivated in 1987 as the Intermountain Academy of Child and Adolescent Psychiatry, the group meets on a quarterly basis for educational, social, and child-advocacy functions.

During the 1970s, child and adolescent services by community mental health centers were initiated by Dr. Claudia K. Berenson, trained in general psychiatry at the University of Pittsburgh and at Utah. She completed child psychiatry training in 1972 and became the first director of children's services in the Salt Lake Community Mental Health Center. Dr. Berenson helped to develop a day hospital program for junior high school age patients. Children attended the public junior high school in the morning and spent the afternoon at the Children's Behavior Therapy Unit. In 1976 Dr. Berenson was appointed training director for the University Division of Child Psychiatry and associate dean of the College of Medicine, and she also served as acting director of the division from 1978 to 1981. During the late 1970s, with support from academic pediatrician Dr. Esther H. Wender and several division child psychiatrists, Dr. Berenson obtained a large federal grant for consultation-liaison between PCMC and the University. She continues as training director for the Division of Child and Adolescent Psychiatry.

Dr. P. Brent Peterson, who completed his training in Utah in 1976, succeeded Dr. Berenson as director of children's services of the Salt Lake Community Mental Health Center. This Center includes the Adolescent Residential Treatment and Educational Center, Adolescent Day Care, the Children's Behavior Therapy Unit, and outpatient programs. All county mental health centers were integrated into one. Dr. Peterson also held the position of assistant director of inpatient services and subsequently director of the outpatient services at PCMC's Department of Child Psychiatry. He served in that position until leaving the hospital in 1980.

After two years of general and one year of child psychiatry training at Emory University, Dr. Richard C. Ferre finished his child psychiatry training in Utah in 1976. He became director of psychiatric inpatient services at Primary Children's and joined the division faculty. He has also directed PCMC's Residential Treatment Program since the late 1970s. Dr. Ferre was appointed chair of the Department of Child Psychiatry at PCMC in 1987.

Dr. Robert H. Burgoyne, a general psychiatrist with an interest in child and adolescent mental health, developed outpatient psychiatric services at Primary Children's Hospital in 1965 and worked with Dr. Whitehead until the early 1970s. As chair of the Department of Psychiatry at LDS Hospital, he established the area's first acute psychiatric inpatient and hospital-based day treatment program for adolescents in 1975 and was the program's medical director.

A rapid increase in the number of mental health practitioners in Utah, including social workers, psychologists, psychiatric nurses, and child psychiatrists has helped to meet the mental health needs of children and adolescents. Of about 150 psychiatrists in Utah, 25 are child and adolescent specialists. Even with the other mental health practitioners, the number needed is far greater for a state in which children and adolescents comprise almost half the population.

Many other psychiatrists have made important contributions in Utah, including Drs. Delbert T. Goates, Joy M. Ely, C. Craig Nelson, and Nyla J. Cole. Dr. David E. Reiser was trained in general psychiatry at the University of Utah from 1951 to 1954, one of three residents in the first group trained in the Department of Psychiatry. He spent six months with Dr. Taboroff and then completed child psychiatry training at the Boston Children's Hospital and Judge Baker Guidance Clinic. Following several years on the staff at Boston's James Jackson Putnam Children's Center, he became its director from 1959 to 1967. In 1970 he returned to Utah and worked with Dr. Norman S. Anderson in children's services at the Granite Community Mental Health Center, a major training resource during the 1960s and 1970s. From 1971 to 1981 Dr. Reiser directed the Well Baby Program there.

Dr. David A. Tomb completed child psychiatry training at the University of Utah Department of Psychiatry in 1978. In 1988 he was appointed director of the Division of Child and Adolescent Psychiatry at the University. A prolific and gifted writer, Dr. Tomb is the author of several excellent books, including the nationally popular *Psychiatry for the House Officer*.

The past fifteen years have provided much new information, particularly biological knowledge, relating to psychiatric illnesses of children. Dr. William M. McMahon completed child psychiatry training and joined the staff at PCMC in 1979 as assistant director of inpatient services. He was co-founder, with Dr. Esther H. Wender, of the Learning Problems Clinic at PCMC, which meets the unique needs of learning disabled and hyperactive children and their parents. Improved understanding and treatment for such conditions as Attention Deficit Hyperactivity Disorder, stress-related illnesses, eating disorders, including anorexia and bulimia, learning disorders, depression, conduct disorders, and substance abuse have enabled mental health professionals to play an increasingly important role in helping children, adolescents, and their families.

Since his return from NIMH in 1973, Dr. Paul H. Wender has been in the forefront of research in Attention Deficit Disorder and hyperactivity. His wife, Dr. Frances L. Burger, a child psychiatrist trained in Great Britain, has made valuable contributions as a member of the University faculty and as a clinician.

In 1985, following the expiration of the Utah "certificate of need" law controlling construction of additional hospital beds, nine new free-standing private psychiatric hospitals were built along the Wasatch Front. While a significant need for additional child and adolescent beds existed, more than tripling the total bed capacity clearly exceeded identified needs.

As the last decade of the twentieth century begins, child psychiatry in Utah is healthy, strong, and growing. With studies indicating that more than 15% of children and adolescents are in need of treatment for emotional and behavioral problems, Utah has at least 100,000 children and youth in need of help. Only one of every five children who needs help receives it. The highest birthrate in the nation, the recent major expansion of psychiatric inpatient and residential resources, rapidly expanding knowledge and technology, significant shifts in insurance coverage, and changes in cultural attitudes toward mental illness present a future with a rigorous challenge and salient opportunity for child psychiatry in Utah.

PART THREE

•

SURGERY
AND
SURGICAL SPECIALTIES

CHAPTER NINETEEN

General Surgery

WALLACE S. BROOKE, MD, PHD

PERHAPS NO MORE IMPORTANT figure in Utah's surgical history exists than Philip B. Price, who was recruited by Dean Cyril Callister to head the new Department of Surgery in the University of Utah Medical School in 1942. A quiet, dedicated visionary, unselfish and without personal monetary ambitions, he responded to Dr. Callister's offer in November of 1942:

> While the new school has been fortunate in securing the use and facilities of the Salt Lake County Hospital, the present arrangement should be viewed as a temporary expedient. I feel strongly that if the Medical School is to fulfill its high destiny, it must have a University Hospital. This institution would facilitate carrying on the highest grade of scientific work; it would require no apologies to visitors, and by the quality of its reputation and clinical work would attract patients from the whole Mountain Region irrespective of their economic status; by its standing it would attract the best physicians and surgeons of the city to join its visiting staff. I do not think it is too early to begin planning and working for such a hospital. In my humble opinion, it is more important for your medical school than any other one thing—even an endowment. Briefly then, if you can assure me that the income of the Medical School will be in the neighborhood of $170,000 a year and that there will be $25,000 to $30,000 a year available for the Department of Surgery, and that the idea of an adequate University Hospital, or its equivalent, will have your interest and support, and at least the sympathy of President Cowles, I will gladly accept your invitation to the chair of Surgery.

One is intrigued and sadly amused to read this paragraph, written in the early days of World War II, and thereby to revisit the value of money in 1942 as well as the financial distress of the times and its implications for Utah's pioneering medical spirit.

Philip Price brought Dr. Wallace S. Brooke to Utah as his chief and only resident when he left Johns Hopkins to assume his professorship in surgery in March of 1943. The surgical department was rudimentary indeed. The physical plant of the hospital, administered by the Salt Lake County Commissioners, was deplorable. Most patients were older people, emergency cases, and almost all indigent. The residency program was not yet founded, but a group of interns were available to help for a few months. Visiting surgeons from Salt Lake City's private practice, Drs. Kenneth Castleton, Phillip Howard, Ralph T. Richards, and others, supervised the clinics.

In July of 1943, Dr. Price created a ladder of assistant residents. Drs. Steven Hatch, Robert Thomasen, Richard Clay, and Bruce Franz of Johns Hopkins had short periods of service before and after joining the Armed Services. Dr. Ralph C. Richards, an early resident who remained with the surgical faculty until his death in 1980, was a great teacher and pioneer clinician at the School of Medicine. He rose to the rank of professor and was acting head of surgery for some months.

The old Salt Lake General Hospital consisted of a group of buildings that included two operating rooms with no air conditioning and somewhat unreliable electrical and plumbing systems. As chief resident in 1943–44 and as chief resident and instructor after the war, Brooke operated hundreds of times with a nurse anesthetist or giving his own spinal or local anesthesia. Only rarely, in big cases, did Dr. Scott Smith or an MD anesthesiologist from one of the local hospitals supervise the procedure.

Once during a common bile duct operation the lights went out and the nurses were holding flashlights. Brooke called frantically to the circulating nurse, "Get Chris!" — the man-of-all-trades who alone knew the electrical circuits. Then the terrible realization came — Chris was the patient on the table! Nevertheless, the procedure was completed, with excellent results.

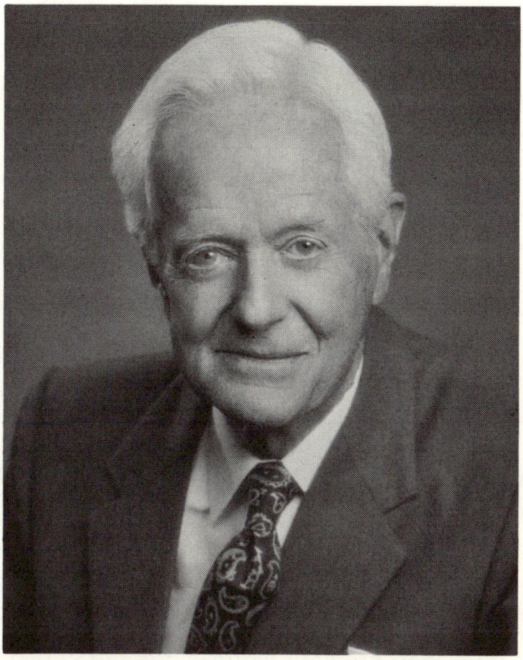

Wallace S. Brooke.

The ancillary divisions of the hospital so necessary to good surgery, such as x-ray and laboratory, left much to be desired. Both operated without full-time MD supervision. Despite these deficiencies, good surgical care was available because of dedicated hard work, and, for this time and environment, the results were satisfactory.

In the 1943–48 period, the department was truly a *general* surgical unit. The staff did abdominal, breast, neck, and ambulatory surgery and also assisted in or handled many orthopedic cases, amputations, open urological cases, and some ENT work. The residents assisted with the few chest cases performed by Dr. Ray Rumel, the first well-trained local chest surgeon. He was a true pioneer, bringing to Salt Lake Dr. Scott Smith, who introduced closed-circuit anesthesia, better anesthetic agents, and newer techniques.

Dr. Vincent Rees, a fine addition, arrived in late 1943 from the University of Michigan's surgical division as assistant professor of surgery. Classes in surgery began thereafter, with lectures, clinical-pathological conferences, grand rounds, and clinics, the latter usually run by busy clinicians from Salt Lake's private practice group. In orthopedics, Drs. Alfred M. Okelberry and Lawrence Ossman were of great help; in urology, Drs. Anthony Middleton, Sr., and later Robert Weaver ran the clinics and did the major surgery. Neurosurgery operations, except for a few trauma cases, were sent to Dr. Reed Harrow at LDS Hospital.

In July 1947, Dr. William Moretz arrived from the University of Rochester to replace Dr. Rees, who left for private practice at the Salt Lake Clinic. Until Moretz's departure in 1955 to become professor of surgery at the University of Georgia in Augusta, he was a pillar of support and a great asset; he was a good teacher, an inspiring personality, and technically a splendid surgeon.

During the early days after the war, some tension developed between "town and gown." Certain surgeons and physicians in Salt Lake City felt that the tax-supported Medical School faculty should not compete with their private practices. Some felt that Utah had too small a financial and population base for a medical school; other doctors had no enthusiasm for the new school. Yet over the years most of these factors of dissension dissipated, and at present a greater understanding and cooperation between the University and privately practicing surgeons and physicians generally prevails.

When Dr. Price became dean of the Medical School in 1956, he was succeeded by Dr. Walter Burdette in 1957, a PhD and MD from Yale who was interested in cancer genetics, emphasizing research and fostering publication of departmental results. The VA Hospital was brought into the residency program in surgery during his tenure, and he was present when the new University Hospital was opened in 1965, leaving for a position in Houston, Texas, shortly afterward. Considerable dissatisfaction accompanied his tenure because of his poor results with open-heart surgery. Displaced from the University by Burdette's desire to do cardiothoracic surgery himself, Dr. Russell Nelson — whose fine reputation and skill had established a leading cardiovascular department at the LDS Hospital — contributed much

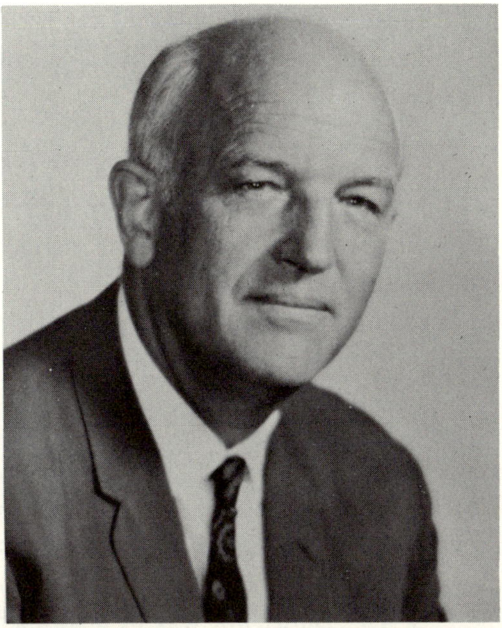

William H. Moretz, MD, came to the Department of Surgery in 1947 with three years of Army experience as well as surgical training at the University of Rochester. In 1955 he left to become professor and chair of surgery at the Medical College of Georgia, serving as president of that medical school from 1972 to 1983.

to the University's later cooperative program.

Dr. Keith Reemtsma came to Utah in 1966 from Tulane University School of Medicine in New Orleans. He was instrumental in broadening the base of the clinical material for the surgical residency program by involving community hospitals in the teaching program. In 1968 he signed a formal agreement with Holy Cross Hospital in Salt Lake City and McKay-Dee Hospital in Ogden. At that time, he appointed Dr. Dominic Albo, Jr., as chief of the University service at Holy Cross and Dr. John Dixon as chief of surgery at McKay-Dee. This was the catalyst for what was to become the University of Utah Affiliated Hospital System, which later included LDS Hospital, Primary Children's Medical Center, and the VA Hospital in Salt Lake City. This affiliated hospital group now has students, residents, and fellows in all specialties represented within each hospital. LDS relinquished its independent surgical residency program, and Dr. Charles Smart was appointed chief of the University service at LDS, completing the involvement of community hospitals and the teaching program at the University.

During Reemtsma's professorship (through 1971), formal divisions were created in the Department of Surgery, including orthopedics, urology, neurosurgery, plastic surgery, ENT, cardiothoracic, and pediatric surgery. This organizational structure led to better relationships among the specialties, and advances in each field were more appreciated. The Renal Transplant Program blossomed, and work with Dr. Willem J. Kolff's dialysis became important. The residency program was strengthened, but it was under Dr. Frank Moody that the surgical residency moved from regional to national prominence.

From 1972 to 1983, Dr. Frank Moody enhanced gastrointestinal research, and three of his residents, Drs. Larry Chung, Bing Rikkers, and James Becker, moved to chairs or important positions in surgery elsewhere in the U.S. The Burn Unit was formed under Drs. Glen Warden and Jeff Saffle. Dr. John Dixon developed the Laser Institute, a division of the Department of Surgery, and the preliminary work with lasers for opening obstruction for nonoperative cancer of the esophagus, coagulation of GI bleeders, and many other uses was introduced.

Dr. William A. Gay, Jr., a cardiovascular surgeon and chair from 1984 to 1990, has been interested in the mechanism and prevention of myocardial injuries. His "Cardiac Transplant Cooperative Program" with the LDS Hospital surgeons is exciting, successful, and nationally recognized. He is a strong force in strengthening the residency program and in unifying the surgical department. In 1990 he served as Vice President for Health Sciences, returning to head the department again in 1991.

Veterans Administration Hospital

Opened in 1932, the VA Hospital on Twelfth Avenue developed a close association with all the Medical School departments in 1946, under the direction of the Dean's Committee. Under Drs. Dean W. Tanner and Jay Gubler, a cooperative residency program educated many of Salt Lake City and Utah's general surgeons. The present larger VA Hospital at Fort Douglas was opened in 1952, and in 1958 an additional formal agreement of affiliation was signed under Dr. Walter Burdette as chair of the Department of Surgery.

In recent years, as in all the major hospitals of Utah, many sophisticated technical advances affecting surgical practice have been instituted. These include vascular surgery laboratories with modern ultrasound, nuclear medicine diagnostic labs, CT scanning, and NMR equipment.

Drs. Knox Fitzpatrick, Clynn Ford, Clifford Snyder, Mark Wolcott, and Peter Lawrence are among the important surgeons operating and supervising surgical training and operations at the VA Hospital.

Advances in the Practice of General Surgery

Since World War II, general surgery has seen many important changes. New or modified operations have been devised in addition to the transplant procedures. These include radical extirpation such as pancreaticoduodenectomy with common duct reconstruction for cancer of the pancreas, hepatectomy, total colectomy with various anal pull-through or "reservoir pouches," combined thoracicoabdominal operations, and many others in the cancer field. Breast surgery has moved away from the more radical mastectomy to preservation of the chest wall muscles. Segmental breast removal, combined with x-radiation, hormonal manipulation, and chemotherapy, is gaining increasing acceptance with patients and surgeons, as have various types of breast reconstruction performed post-mastectomy. Adhesive intestinal obstruction is now often alleviated with release of adhesions and use of splinting tubes. Ileal bladders are constructed to replace the urinary bladder, a necessity in some cancer operations. These examples are typical of the many changes.

Newer instruments such as intestinal stapling devices have supplanted many hand-sewn anastomoses. Endoscopic instruments, beautifully designed to extract stones of the common duct and to inject dyes for diagnosis, are now used extensively. Most recently, laparoscopic cholecystectomy has been introduced and is currently being used at the University and elsewhere. Gastroscopic and colonoscopic instruments have virtually eliminated many open-surgery procedures, as have laser and electro-fulguration devices used in gastrointestinal disease.

Advances in pre- and postoperative care, with early ambulation, short-stay surgery, parenteral nutrition, and intensive care units in hospitals, also demonstrate major attitude changes which have improved safety and contributed to better surgical results.

Much improvement in structural ancillary procedures and hospital monitoring in the recent decades includes professional review organizations, hospital credential committees to screen qualifications of prospective surgeons, and other committees which grant or limit hospital privileges. Required monthly result-oriented morbidity and mortality conferences improve education and supervision of surgical care, as do tumor conferences and weekly surgical departmental meetings.

Because knowledge of antibiotics is universal, these comments are addressed primarily to their use in surgery of the intestine. Colon and stomach surgery have been made safer as cephalosporin, penicillin derivatives, and synthetic analogues have replaced the pioneer sulfa drugs. Postoperative treatment of pneumonias and wound infections demonstrates much better results with use of these agents which supplement the more advanced knowledge of surgical pathology, physiology, and all related basic sciences.

County and state medical societies are more active in surgical programs than in the past. Grievance committees, as well as legal committees, have been instituted to review the real or potential malpractice suits which have changed medicine practice with much economic impact since World War II.

In Utah, hospitals with residency programs have provided well-trained young surgeons as operators, assistants, and pre- and post-operative attendants, making surgery safer and better. The University of Utah and affiliated hospital programs have led to much-improved balance and scope of clinical training for the physicians and surgeons of the future.

The Salt Lake Surgical Society, founded in 1937, has been an excellent organization for continuing education of regional general surgeons. This body, meeting monthly at the Alta Club, includes most of the state's diplomates of the American Board of Surgery and those seeking qualification, as well as hospital residents. The Society and the Utah committees of the American College of Surgeons have been strong forces in encouraging high surgical ethics and standards.

General Surgery in the Private Hospitals

To list all the state's surgeons of importance is impossible because of space limitations. Many surgeons in private practice with large volumes and wide experience have maintained an interest in teaching and have been current in rapidly advancing changes. However, some deserve special consideration when discussed in relationship to their primary hospitals.

Founded in 1875, the Holy Cross Hospital became (with St. Mark's, 1872) one of only two hospitals of importance in Salt Lake City until 1905, when Dr. W. H. Groves' Latter-day Saints' Hospital was dedicated and opened. From the 1940s and beyond, Holy Cross has played an important part in clinical surgery in Utah, with major new buildings and facilities. The staff and the residency program, associated with the University of Utah, have created a sound and successful community hospital.

Drs. Kenneth Castleton, later dean of the Medical School, and Wallace Brooke, both now retired but active in Medical School activities, had significant private practices. The late Dr. Phillip Howard was a dedicated and effective teacher. Drs. Dominic Albo, Knox Fitzpatrick, Hallard Harmon, and others of fine reputation and career success have made the general surgical division at Holy Cross an important addition to Utah's surgical history.

From the early 1940s until their deaths, Drs. Ralph T. Richards, Floyd Hatch, and Eliot Snow were notable for their surgical dedication and success at LDS Hospital, as was Dr. Frederick Hicken, now retired. In 1968 Dr. Walter Gaisford was appointed as the first full-time surgical director at LDS, and the general surgical program, with other surgical specialties, was completely integrated with the University of Utah programs. He was followed by Drs. Charles Smart (1974–84) and Larry Stevens (since 1984). Drs. Vincent Rees, Adolph Nielsen, Talmage Nielsen, Mark Muir, and other well-trained surgeons were and are notable. Many and constant improvements have been made in ancillary services at LDS, such as x-ray, intensive care, laboratory, radiation, and medical oncology. By 1989 the hospital had nineteen operating rooms and did approximately 18,000 operations annually, of which about 20% were general surgical procedures. Under the present leadership of Dr. Larry Stevens, an outstanding transplant program has been developed, including kidney, liver, and pancreas replacements.

St. Mark's, Salt Lake's first hospital of note, has moved three times since its establishment in 1872, and in its present Thirty-ninth South location was purchased in 1988 by the Hospital Corporation of America. Under the auspices of the Episcopal Church from its founding, St. Mark's was most active in industrial medicine and surgery, but in recent years, with its new 300-bed facility, has acquired a broadly based staff and a completely certified group of American Board of Surgery specialists. Its operating room supply management methods have been notable.

Dr. Martin Lindem, a member of the founding group of the American Board of Surgery, started a large practice in 1927. He was an outstanding Utah surgeon and a stalwart in improving St. Mark's standards, as was Dr. John H. Clark, for many years chief of surgery and staff representative on the board of directors.

Drs. Harold Lamb and Gilbert Wright in a somewhat later period had an impact on surgical practice in Salt Lake City, as did the pioneer anesthesiologist Dr. Hugh Brown. Drs. Tony Lindem, Brian Rasmussen, Barry Robb, and other surgeons of recent date have carried on a fine tradition.

The McKay-Dee Hospital in Ogden and its precursor, the Thomas D. Dee Memorial Hospital, were associated with major and important surgeons such as Drs. Ezekial Dumke, Dean W. Tanner, Rulon Howe, John Dixon (who later served as dean of the Medical School), Dan Hunter, and others of note.

In the early years of the century, Drs. Ezra and Edward Rich, brothers from a large polygamous family, were the leading surgeons in the Ogden area. Ezra's son Clark and Edward's son Edward, Jr., followed their fathers into regional prominence.

Dr. A. Z. Tanner graduated from Rush Medical School in Chicago and returned to LDS Hospital, starting a practice in Farmington in about 1910. His sons Noall Z. and Joseph organized the A. Z. Tanner Memorial Clinic in Layton, which Joe later left for the Stanford Medical School faculty. Their brother Dean brought further distinction to the family name in practice in Ogden and Salt Lake City following World War II.

Dr. Ezekial Dumke, who took extra surgical training in New Orleans, held the lead in surgical volume at the Dee Hospital. He and his medical colleagues had little time for further training outside the region, so they organized the Ogden Surgical Society, which first met in the spring of 1946. Drs. Dumke, Ezra Rich, George Fister, Dean Tanner, and others had excellent contacts with outstanding and sometimes famous surgeons from their own medical school days and used them to create a successful educational forum which won wide recognition and community backing.

The Budge Hospital group in Logan and the Utah Valley Hospital in Provo are important in Utah surgery. The latter institution has had remarkable and dedicated surgeons, among whom were Drs. William Dixon and Donald Poppen.

The Pioneer Valley Hospital in the Salt Lake Valley should be noted for Dr. Wallace Chambers and others in general and thoracic surgery.

Altogether, Utah has been fortunate in its general surgery history and care, with outstanding success in this field over the years.

CHAPTER TWENTY

Pediatric Surgery

DALE G. JOHNSON, MD

THE FIRST FULLY TRAINED SURGEON in Utah with a practice limited to infants and children, Dr. Dale G. Johnson, was recruited from Philadelphia in 1971 and appointed chief of surgery at the Primary Children's Hospital. Children's surgery had been performed in Utah, of course, but 1971 was the first time that any Utah surgeon with specialty training had felt it practical to limit his practice to the pediatric age group.

Pediatric surgery really had its North American beginnings with the career change in 1917 of Dr. William E. Ladd, a Boston surgeon. A ship had been torpedoed in Halifax harbor in Nova Scotia, and scores of children looking out on the harbor were injured as the blast exploded the windows. Dr. Ladd volunteered to help, and his experience resulted in a lifelong commitment to the surgical problems of infants and children. His subsequent leadership in surgery at the Boston Children's Hospital and his classic writings on the surgery of infants and children earned him a reputation as the father of pediatric surgery in North America.

Evolution of Children's Surgery in Utah

The first Utah surgeon with any significant special training in pediatric surgery had been, remarkably enough, Dr. Ladd's chief resident at the Boston Children's Hospital for eighteen months in 1939 and 1940. Dean Tanner was from Ogden, Utah, and he had general

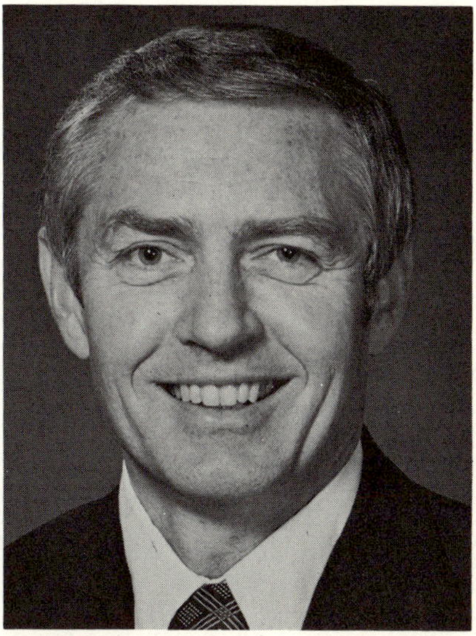

Dale G. Johnson.

surgical training at the Peter Bent Brigham Hospital as well as Boston Children's. He returned to Utah in 1946, after serving in the war with the Peter Bent Brigham Hospital surgical unit.

Dr. Tanner moved to Salt Lake City with a one-half-time academic appointment as chief of surgery at the Salt Lake Veterans Administration Hospital. With the rest of his time he attempted to establish a practice in pediatric surgery based mostly at St. Mark's Hospital. His practice was, therefore, a mixture of adults and children, and he was not clearly identified as a pediatric surgical specialist by other general surgeons in the community, who were also competing for patients. No one else had experience with the more complex reconstructive procedures, however, so from 1946 into the 1960s he was referred the diaphragmatic hernias, omphaloceles, and anorectal reconstructions, and he performed the first operations in Utah for esophageal atresia, biliary atresia, and Hirschsprung's disease.

Dean Tanner was one of those unusual individuals who doesn't seem to require regular sleep. It was his habit to work into the night, and his colleagues in Boston still remember him as the chief resident who made routine ward rounds every morning at one or two A.M. He was also very broadly based in his clinical practice, both by virtue of his training in Boston and the war, and because he was filling a void in specialized clinical experience in those early years in Utah. His practice included repair of meningomyelocele as well as a fairly large volume of cleft lip and palate surgery. He also did the patent ductus and Blalock shunt surgery he had learned from Robert E. Gross, who had preceded him as Dr. Ladd's chief resident. After a year or so in Salt Lake City, Dr. Tanner moved his practice to Layton, Utah, near his family home, and he continues to practice there to the present.

A second Utah surgeon with formal training in pediatric surgery was Dr. Adolph M. Nielsen, who spent an extra six months at the Chicago Children's Memorial Hospital with Willis Potts before coming to Salt Lake City in 1949. After graduating from the University of Utah in 1936, Nielson attended Rush School of Medicine in Chicago. He had an eighteen-month internship in surgery at the Salt Lake General Hospital before spending three years in the U.S. Army Medical Corps, from 1942 to 1945. He continued general surgical training at Wesley Memorial Hospital in Chicago, followed by the six months at Children's Memorial. Although Nielsen had extra training and a major interest in children's surgery, he too felt he could not limit his practice to pediatric surgery exclusively. The time wasn't right and the specialty was still struggling for recognition.

A third individual who focused on children's surgery in Utah during the fifties and sixties had partial training in both pediatrics and surgery. He practiced general pediatrics but felt strongly about managing the surgical problems in his own patient population. He was not well accepted by either the pediatric or surgical communities, and he received referrals from neither. He is now deceased, and it is difficult at this point to evaluate the nature of his surgical practice.

Utah's Hospital for Children

The Primary Children's Hospital began as a chronic care nursing home for children in 1922. A new building was constructed in 1952, but the function was still chronic care. Dr. Alfred M. Okelberry, a

Harvard-educated orthopedic surgeon, was a major force in the surgical activities of the hospital during the fifties and even earlier, and he made a significant commitment to children's orthopedic surgery in those early days. Expansion projects in 1961 and again in 1966 increased the bed capacity and support facilities, making possible the hospital's conversion to acute care for general medical and surgical problems in children. In 1964 two anesthesiologists, a radiologist, a pathologist, and a neurologist were on board as the first specialists in Utah based in a children's hospital. Dr. L. George Veasy was appointed physician-in-chief in 1967, and under his direction the hospital continued to thrive in its new role as an acute care center.

In 1968, a short distance away at the University Hospital, Dr. August L. (Larry) Jung was developing what would become the Intermountain Newborn Intensive Care Unit while newborn intensive care and the specialty of neonatology were still in their own infancy on a national level. A satellite NBICU was subsequently developed at Primary Children's Hospital, renamed Primary Children's Medical Center (PCMC) in 1968. These developments were essential to the creation of a program in pediatric surgery.

Exploratory discussions were carried on for at least two years before Dale G. Johnson was finally appointed as chief of surgery at PCMC in July of 1971. His background included five years at the Massachusetts General Hospital and certification in general surgery. He then spent two years in experimental surgery at the Walter Reed Army Institute of Research and a third at the Harrison Department of Surgical Research, University of Pennsylvania. Two years of training in pediatric surgery at the Children's Hospital of Philadelphia followed, and Johnson remained five years on the faculty of the University of Pennsylvania, with appointments as assistant professor of pediatric surgery at Penn and senior surgeon at the Children's Hospital. Recruitment to PCMC was a joint effort with the University of Utah, and the initial appointment included the academic titles of associate professor of surgery and pediatrics and head of pediatric surgery. This appointment also initiated the affiliation of the University and PCMC in a resident teaching program in general surgery.

There was considerable anxiety on the part of surgeons in private practice, particularly those in urology and general surgery, over the appointment of a hospital-based pediatric surgeon. The concern was naturally over the possible loss of patient referrals because of the built-in advantage for referral to a hospital-based surgeon. In fact, two years earlier the job description had involved teaching, program development, and charity patients without the privilege of private practice. Dr. Johnson argued that a surgeon who did no surgery would soon be neither a teacher nor a surgeon. After two years of negotiation, the point was conceded, but it is fair to say that there are still those in the private practice community who feel that the original decision to recruit a hospital-based surgeon, whatever his specialty, was a mistake.

A key figure in the negotiations was Keith Reemtsma, chair of the Department of Surgery at the University of Utah since 1966. Though not formally trained in pediatric surgery, Dr. Reemtsma had a genuine interest in the specialty. He had been corresponding and meeting with Dr. Johnson, one of the founding members of the American Pediatric Surgical Association, for at least a year. By chance, in March of 1971 Reemtsma had been appointed by the American Board of Surgery to chair a subcommittee instructed to evaluate the final petition for specialty certification of pediatric surgeons. Reemtsma left Utah to assume the chair at Columbia in the spring of 1971, before Dr. Johnson arrived, and the American Board of Surgery unanimously approved certification in pediatric surgery in June of 1972.

Toward Specialty Recognition

As a specialty, pediatric surgery has had a long struggle with identity problems. In its beginnings, it represented general surgery of the infant and child in the broadest sense. The early pediatric surgeons did not limit their focus to traditional general surgical problems of the chest and abdomen, because their whole field was filled with problems crying for solution. The early pioneers for many problems in pediatric orthopedics (Sir Dennis Browne, London), pediatric neurosurgery (Robert Zachary, Sheffield), pediatric cardiovascular surgery

(Robert E. Gross, Boston), and pediatric urology (Durham Smith, Melbourne, and W. H. Hendren, Boston) were all general pediatric surgeons who recognized the need for development of these areas for children, even though specialties for corresponding organ systems in adults were already well established.

It has been inevitable, however, that as general pediatric surgeons have initiated development of surgical subspecialty interests, subsequent trainees have devoted full time to specific organ system problems in order to push progress further. Thus new pediatric surgical subspecialists have evolved and are still evolving oriented to the traditional organ system categories rather than to the pediatric surgical patient as a whole. Subspecialty division (some would say fragmentation) of pediatric surgery in the near future will look very much like the subspecialty divisions in adult surgery. This is not a bad trend; it is the natural outgrowth of increasing knowledge and the demand for the best that is available. As with adult surgery, however, there will remain an important role for the surgeon trained to evaluate and manage surgical problems of the whole pediatric patient who can also integrate these skills with those of the organ system specialist.

The first organization for pediatric surgeons in North America was founded in 1948 with the birth of the Surgical Section of the American Academy of Pediatrics. Key members of that organizing group included Alexander Bill, Robert E. Gross, C. Everett Koop, William E. Ladd, W. T. Mustard, Willis Potts, and Orvar Swenson, all of whom were major contributors to the development of pediatric surgery. They felt a need to communicate about common professional and scientific problems, and they needed support from one another because they were challenging the territory of established specialties. Moreover, they wanted recognition for the new standards they felt they were developing for the surgery of infants and children.

By 1948, at the time organized pediatric surgery was making an appearance, eighteen specialty boards had been approved. Dr. Ladd had insisted from the beginning that certification by the American Board of Surgery be required for membership in the Surgical Section of the American Academy of Pediatrics. The natural course, therefore, seemed to favor a subsidiary board under the American Board of Surgery, and that was the relationship that finally took form.

In April 1973 a "Certification of Special Qualifications in Pediatric Surgery" was approved by the American Board of Medical Specialists. The American Board of Surgery was designated the primary board to issue this certificate, and the first examination was given in 1975. The certificate was time-limited for ten years, and with this examination pediatric surgery became the first surgical subspecialty to require mandatory recertification.

Development of the Program in Utah

In 1971 it was not difficult to develop a busy clinical pediatric surgery service in Utah because the time was right and all the pieces were in place. Primary Children's Medical Center was the only acute care children's facility in a five-state referral area. The staff now included first-rate pediatric radiology, pathology, neonatology, and cardiology. Most of the pediatric subspecialties not available in-house at PCMC were easily accessible through the University's Department of Pediatrics. Dr. Johnson brought experience from eight years of academic practice at the Children's Hospital in Philadelphia, and, consistent with the specialty of pediatric surgery, he limited his practice to infants and children.

The pediatricians in the huge referral area were marvelously supportive. Many of the general surgeons felt threatened for a while, but most came to realize that the majority of the referral problems were not those they felt comfortable dealing with anyway. Some of the common herniorrhaphies, pyloromyotomies, and appendectomies were also referred to the service, but these were spread across the whole community, and the losses from any one individual's practice, with the possible exception of Adolph Nielsen's, were not enough to cause real pain. Because Dr. Nielsen had a long-established interest in pediatric surgery, he was most likely to lose from a hospital-based program. His personal practice was affected by changing referral patterns, but he has continued to support the developing program at PCMC.

Dr. Johnson saw his responsibilities in program development as four-fold. First, no teaching or clinical research was possible without the development of an adequate volume of clinical cases. Second, the brief rotation times for the general surgical residents required that they not only learn well the common procedures appropriate for future practice in general surgery, but also be able to recognize the complex problems they should not touch without further specialized training. Third, any program, however well initiated, will eventually stagnate without ongoing exploration of new ideas, techniques, and challenges. Fourth, national and international recognition was important for program development and for the prestige of the institution.

Some of these goals have been realized more completely than others. The clinical volume has grown to an appropriate level for the size of the institution. Dr. David Stewart was on the pediatric surgery faculty in 1974 and 1975. Dr. Michael E. Matlak (pediatric surgical fellowship, National Children's Hospital in Washington, D.C.) joined Dr. Johnson in 1977, and Dr. Richard E. Black (pediatric surgical fellowship, Cincinnati Children's Hospital) joined the group in 1981. Volume has been fairly steady at around 1,200 cases per year, with approximately 200 newborns and a large majority under the age of two years.

General surgery resident feedback concerning the training and teaching on the service has been uniformly positive. The rotation has been consistently among the most popular in the program, the only complaint being a lack of free time for reading and family.

While research output has suffered because of heavy clinical demands, the division has nevertheless published extensively on surgical aspects of gastroesophageal reflux in children, with some important original contributions relating to twenty-four-hour pH monitoring in this age group. Publications on the surgical management of acquired obstructions of the airway and the management of Wilms' tumor have built a national reputation, and through numerous oral presentations the service has also attained wide recognition for expertise in esophageal reconstruction and in newer approaches to management of complex anorectal malformations.

Utah's pediatric surgeons have been both visible and internationally recognized. Among his many professional assignments, Dr. Johnson has served on numerous programs and administrative committees for the American College of Surgeons, the Society of University Surgeons, the American Surgical Association, and as examiner for the American Board of Surgery. He has also served as a member of the board of governors, as a member of the education, publications, cancer, and nominating committees (four times), as secretary, and as president (1986) of the American Pediatric Surgical Association. Beginning in 1985 he served a three-year term as secretary of the Pacific Association of Pediatric Surgeons (PAPS — Australia, Western Canada, Indonesia, Japan, New Zealand, Taiwan, Western U.S.), and he was president of PAPS in 1990. Visiting professorships have included the Mayo Clinic, Cook County Hospital, Indiana University, Stanford University, the Universities of Michigan, Alabama, Iowa, and Nebraska, and Yale University in this country, plus children's hospitals and numerous universities in Mexico, Chile, Brazil, Australia, South Africa, Singapore, Japan, and Poland. Dr. Johnson's bibliography includes 85 papers, 6 major reviews, 21 chapters in significant textbooks, and 2 technical films. His abstracts and presentations fill nine pages.

Dr. Matlak has achieved national visibility in the area of pediatric trauma management education, and he has developed pediatric trauma education programs for both professional and lay participants nationally as well as in Utah.

Growth of Pediatric Surgery Outside PCMC

Dr. Dennis Vitale established a practice in pediatric surgery at the Utah Valley Hospital in 1979, after a move from Sacramento. Dr. Vitale remains busy in solo private practice, and so far he has not established ties, except for occasional referrals, with the service at PCMC.

Expansion of Children's Specialty Surgical Services

During the eighteen years that specialized general pediatric surgery has been developing at PCMC, surgical subspecialists — some full-time faculty and some in private practice — have focused their interests and training on the surgery of children. Dr. Sherman S. Coleman actually predates this period, since he joined the PCMC staff in 1963. As chair of orthopedics at the University of Utah for many years, and as chief of surgery at the Shriners' Hospital, Dr. Coleman developed a national reputation through his interest in and writings on pediatric orthopedics and pediatric bone tumors.

Drs. T. Ray Broadbent and Robert Woolf had established high standards for pediatric plastic surgery even before general pediatric surgery came on the scene. Their work with cleft lip and palate was unsurpassed, and Dr. Broadbent brought national recognition to the institution and to the training program which he established. Craniofacial reconstructive surgery and microsurgery were later developments, however, introduced at PCMC with the recruitment in 1983 of Dr. Louis Morales. Morales had trained in plastic surgery in Georgia, and his subsequent pediatric craniofacial fellowship was at the Children's Hospital in Philadelphia. He was originally appointed as a full-time faculty member at the University of Utah, but he is currently in private practice. Dr. David Thomas also brought a background of training in craniofacial reconstruction, and he joined Dr. Broadbent in private practice in 1986.

In 1987 Dr. Graham Lister was recruited from Louisville, Kentucky, as chief of plastic surgery at the University. Dr. Lister is renowned internationally for his work in reconstruction of congenital malformations of the hand and forearm.

Dr. Marion L. Walker joined the faculty and the hospital-based surgical staff at PCMC in 1976, following his fellowship in pediatric neurosurgery. He was joined from 1981 to 1986 by Dr. Bruce Storrs and is currently associated with Dr. David Moss. Dr. Walker's work with lasers in pediatric neurosurgery and with dorsal rhizotomy for spasticity has brought wide renown to his service and to the institution.

Dr. Tom Williams joined the staff as a private practice pediatric ophthalmologist in 1977, and Dr. Jane Kivlin joined as a full-time University faculty member in the same subspecialty in 1981.

Dr. Peter Stevens completed an Australian fellowship in pediatric orthopedics and joined the PCMC staff from private practice in 1978.

Dr. Steven Scott focused on bone tumors during his pediatric orthopedic fellowship, and he complements the division as a University faculty member. Dr. Tom Hawke became the third orthopedic surgeon with a pediatric fellowship to join the staff, also from private practice, in 1987.

Pediatric heart surgery at PCMC was developed by Drs. W. Ray Rumel, Russell M. Nelson, J D Mortensen, and Conrad B. Jenson. Dr. Jenson handled most of the cases in the early years until Dr. Edwin C. McGough, with tenacious determination, focused his interests and his energies on the pediatric cases. Eventually Dr. McGough won the clinical referrals through both his growing expertise and his incredible dedication to the details of clinical care.

Dr. William A. Gay, a cardiovascular surgeon, became chair of surgery at the University in 1984; he came from Cornell with wide experience in pediatric heart surgery. His responsibilities at the University and his development of the heart transplant program have so far limited his involvement with children.

Dr. Don Doty moved from the University of Iowa with a national reputation and large experience as a pediatric cardiovascular surgeon. The circumstances of his private practice have currently directed his focus more toward adult problems, however.

Dr. Richard Middleton at the University and Drs. Hal Bourne and Anthony W. Middleton, Jr., in private practice all had extra training and significant interest in pediatric urology. Dr. Tony Middleton was the most recently trained of the three, and his pediatric caseload was large for many years even though he maintained a major stake in adult urology. In 1984 Dr. Richard Middleton, as chair of urology at the University, recruited Dr. Brent Snow, just out of his pediatric urology fellowship at the Children's Hospital of Philadelphia, as a full-time pediatric urologist. Dr. Snow has since developed the largest individual practice in pediatric urology, although a variety of urologists in private practice still do a significant number of pediatric cases.

For many years tonsillectomies and myringotomies in children were the mainstay of the surgical schedule at PCMC. This has changed over the years, partly through changing indications, but also because outpatient surgical units have sometimes made these procedures more convenient for patient and surgeon outside of the Medical Center. Many of the large number of ENT surgeons who have loyally supported the children's hospital for years are approaching retirement age, and the changing socioeconomic environment suggests that their surgical schedules may not be replaced by younger trainees. However, pediatric otolaryngology has also developed as a subspecialty allowing a practice limited to infants and children, and Dr. Steven Gray joined the University faculty and the PCMC staff as a pediatric ENT surgeon on July 1, 1990.

Summary

The development of pediatric surgery in Utah has paralleled, with some time lag, the development of children's surgery throughout the country. The justification for a specialist in pediatric surgery versus adult general surgery is the same as the justification for a pediatrician versus an adult specialist in internal medicine. The physiology is different, the disease entities are different, and the management is different. Just as general pediatrics has spawned a variety of pediatric medical subspecialists, so the field of general pediatric surgery, which seemed to be all-encompassing in its early years, has stimulated the development of pediatric surgical subspecialists with a finer focus. In each case there is some danger of overspecialization, but we do not yet see the time when either the pediatrician or the general pediatric surgeon will become obsolete.

The new Primary Children's Medical Center on the University of Utah campus has opened with a magnificent physical plant, state-of-the-art equipment, and a vastly expanded and highly specialized faculty and staff in both surgery and medicine. Significantly, this has been accomplished by blending the resources of both the private practice and academic communities. The surgical care of children has come a long way in Utah, and the next decade should keep PCMC among the top-ranking pediatric centers in the country.

CHAPTER TWENTY-ONE

Thoracic Surgery

HAROLD V. LIDDLE, MD

THE SPECIALTY OF THORACIC AND CARDIOVASCULAR surgery was first introduced in Utah by Dr. William Ray Rumel when he established a practice in Ogden in 1940. One year later he moved to Salt Lake City permanently. Dr. Rumel started his medical education with the two-year course available at the University of Utah and received a doctorate of medicine from Northwestern University in 1935, where he ranked third in his class of 120 students. He interned at St. Luke's Hospital in Chicago and then spent two and one-half years in surgical training at the St. Luke's and Cook County hospitals.

In 1938 Rumel went to the Lahey Clinic in Boston, where he met Dr. Richard Overholt and was so captivated by thoracic surgery that he became Overholt's second fellow and trained with him from 1938 to 1940. Dr. Overholt kindled a fire that was to burn brightly for the next thirty-seven years. Dr. Rumel was certified by the Board of Thoracic Surgery as a founding member in 1948. He was unique in the Intermountain West in that he entered practice as a specialist in thoracic surgery, as distinct from general surgery, and thereafter he remained fiercely devoted to the principle that thoracic surgery was an independent specialty. He was dedicated to teaching students, residents, and nurses the principles of thoracic surgery and stressed the need for qualified research in the specialty. He pioneered the development of these principles in Utah and during his illustrious career was their most devoted disciple. The enduring characteristics of this remarkable man were his devotion to thoughtful and caring attention to patients and his imaginative drive to pioneer new ways to address the existing host of chest diseases.

In 1941 Rumel performed the first successful lobectomy, in a patient with bronchiectasis, and the first division of a patent ductus arteriosus in the Intermountain area. The following year he performed a successful pneumonectomy for carcinoma in a patient who survived for nineteen years, when he died of causes unrelated to the original diagnosis. Dr. Rumel created a Blalock shunt for cyanotic heart disease in 1947, did a pericardectomy for constrictive pericarditis in 1948, and in 1949 was the first Utahn to repair a coarctation of the aorta.

It is important to understand that during this first ten-year period of his practice, thoracic radiographic services were limited to simple chest x-rays and to fluoroscopy with none of the sophisticated options now available. Cardiac catheterization was not introduced anywhere until 1945 and was not available in Utah until about 1947; therefore, the diagnoses of the various forms of heart disease upon which he operated were established only by artful historic and physical examination.

In 1951 Dr. Rumel performed the first mitral commissurotomy, a surgical treatment which became the springboard for his most enduring contribution to cardiac surgery. The operation he designed and performed in hundreds of patients with mitral valve deformities remains, perhaps, the best reconstructive procedure available. The lack of commercially available thoracic surgical instruments stimulated Dr. Rumel's inventiveness, and he designed and manufactured many that bear his name.

Dr. Louis E. Viko, a superb clinical cardiologist at the Intermountain Clinic, was also a pioneer in his field and a major supporter of Dr. Rumel's early ventures in this area. Dr. Alan Lindsay, who succeeded Dr. Viko, also made major contributions to clinical cardiology and to teaching students, residents, and fellow staff physicians the art and science of electrocardiology. He espoused a healthy and welcome sense of conservatism in the management of heart disease.

Dr. Edwin Lawrence came from Yale University in 1946 to be associated with Dr. Rumel and remained in Salt Lake City, practicing

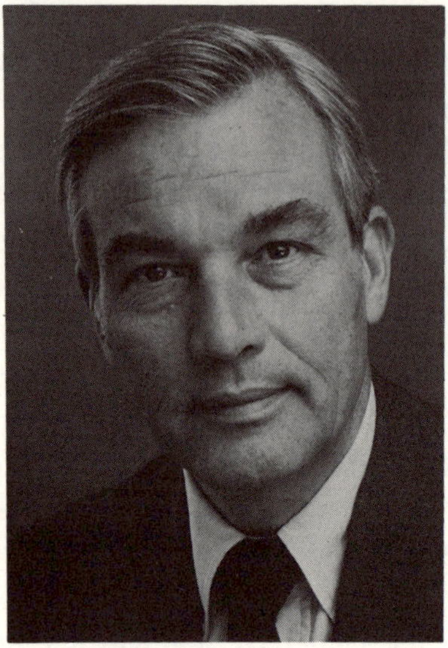

Harold V. Liddle.

largely at SLGH, where he also became the first cancer coordinator before returning to Indianapolis after one or two years.

Dr. Preston R. Cutler had graduated from Temple University Medical College in 1942 and, after six years of training, first in general and then in thoracic surgery at the Baltimore City Hospital, returned to Salt Lake City to join Dr. Rumel in September 1948. For the next several years these two men provided the thoracic surgical services for the LDS, Primary Children's, Veterans, Holy Cross, St. Mark's, and Salt Lake General hospitals and for the State Tuberculosis Sanatorium in Roy, near Ogden, Utah.

Dr. Ralph Rigby, who trained in endoscopy with the famous Dr. Hollinger at St. Luke's Hospital in Chicago, had established a very highly respected endoscopy practice at St. Mark's Hospital. In that early period he was courageous indeed to limit himself to such a narrow field of specialty.

Dr. Elmer Kilpatrick was established at Holy Cross Hospital in the practice of pulmonary diseases, also contributing importantly to the care of tuberculosis patients at the State Sanatorium. In 1953 Dr.

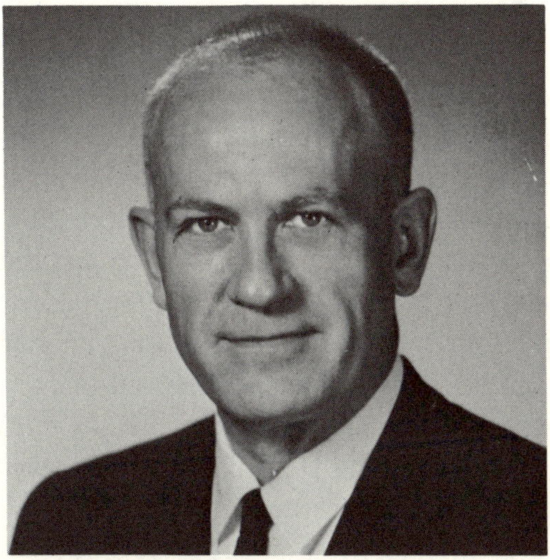

William Ray Rumel.

Thomas Keyes joined the Holy Cross staff as a thoracic surgeon, and in 1955 Dr. Wallace Chambers established a practice in thoracic and general surgery at St. Mark's.

Although Drs. Rumel and Cutler continued to provide consultative services at the State Sanatorium, Dr. Keith Farr had come to Ogden to do needed surgery on tuberculosis patients. By this time, resectional surgery had largely replaced the historic collapse treatment of tuberculosis, but in the early 1960s drug treatment virtually eliminated the need for surgical intervention in this disease. Not very many years elapsed before antibiotic therapy dramatically reduced the need for resection for lung abscess and bronchiectasis. As a result of these rapid pharmacologic advances, the original clinical basis of thoracic surgery became permanently altered. The equally rapid development of cardiac and vascular surgery more than filled the void, however, and the growth in the numbers of physicians devoted to cardiac surgery was explosive from the mid-1950s on.

The LDS Hospital had forged a preeminent position in the specialty of thoracic surgery in Utah by the mid-1950s, in large part because of Dr. Rumel's dedication to the independence of the specialty and his teaching. In 1954 Dr. William Dixon established a practice in general and thoracic surgery in Provo and pioneered thoracic and cardiac surgery in that area.

Dr. Homer R. Warner returned from the Mayo Clinic in 1953 and spent one year with Dr. Hans H. Hecht at the University Hospital. Dr. Hecht was an outstanding clinical and research cardiologist who, notwithstanding substantial reluctance from his peers, had established a catheterization laboratory at SLGH in 1947. In 1954 Dr. Warner went to LDS Hospital, where he began a pioneering program in computer sciences which has remained at the forefront of medical computer applications since that time. He also established a clinical laboratory for cardiac catheterization at LDS which was subsequently directed by Dr. Alan F. Toronto and more recently by Dr. Hiram W. Marshall.

In 1964, this laboratory was among three or four in the country to use a digital computer program for data management. Dr. Warner developed a program to display pressure tracings and to manage the physiologic data necessary for clinical diagnosis, an application which was the first step in the development of the HELP system, a computer program unique in this country. After twenty-five years of development, it is now applied to on-line physiologic monitoring of patients in the various intensive care areas, including calculation of cardiac indices; to assimilation and presentation of laboratory and radiographic data; to the presentation of data from the respiratory laboratory; and more recently to nursing notes. Drs. Warner and J D Mortensen established a cardiovascular research laboratory in which many significant projects were undertaken.

By the early 1950s the volume of thoracic surgery had grown so rapidly that Drs. Rumel and Cutler became convinced that the thoracic service would be an appropriate training opportunity for young physicians. Initially Dr. Rumel approached the University of Utah to solicit its involvement in such a program, but because of philosophical differences concerning the role of thoracic surgery as an independent specialty, the Department of Surgery at the University declined to become involved. With the support of the administration of the LDS Hospital, Dr. Rumel applied successfully to the Board of Thoracic

Surgery for a thoracic surgical residency program in 1953 which he directed until 1967. He was also chair of the Division of Thoracic Surgery from 1956 to 1967.

During his thirty-two years of practice, Dr. Cutler increasingly limited himself to general thoracic surgery and developed a large volume of both pulmonary and esophageal surgery. In this period, the volume of cardiac surgery grew so rapidly nationwide that decreased emphasis on the non-cardiac variety made it difficult for thoracic residency programs all over the country to train young doctors adequately in general thoracic surgery. Dr. Cutler was a vital contributor throughout his career, and the program suffered when he retired in 1980.

Dr. J D Mortensen came from the Mayo Clinic to join Drs. Rumel and Cutler in 1955, and they formed the Rumel Chest Clinic. In 1958 Dr. L. George Veasy joined the Clinic as a pediatric cardiologist and remained until January 1, 1968, when he became physician-in-charge of the Primary Children's Hospital, a position he has held for more than twenty years.

Dr. Mortensen performed the first successful open-heart surgery on a child at the LDS Hospital in 1956; the operation was performed there because at that time Primary Children's could not offer the complex services required. During the next five years Mortensen performed a wide variety of adult and pediatric cardiac operations (including the first Senning operation for transposition of the great vessels) and introduced many peripheral vascular operations to this area. These endeavors contributed heavily to the preeminence of the LDS Hospital in the late 1950s.

In the early 1960s Mortensen undertook visualization of the coronary arteries by the flush technique and on the basis of that demonstration of coronary anatomy was the first to do direct surgical coronary endarterectomy. It was at this time that he realized that selective coronary arteriography, which Dr. Mason Sones had developed at the Cleveland Clinic in 1962, was an indispensable minimum if direct coronary surgery was to succeed. It is important to recognize that in 1964 surgery for coronary artery disease was considered an unacceptable treatment modality by a great many physicians. Dr.

Mortensen retired from clinical practice in 1976 but has continued to pursue a very active program of research at the Utah Biomedical Test Laboratory (UBTL), where he developed the first intravascular oxygenator, a forerunner of an implantable artificial lung.

During this period, cardiac surgery was being performed simultaneously in Utah by external hypothermia induced in a tub of ice slush, by a modification of the well technique first described by Dr. Gross and later by Dr. Kirklin, and, finally, with extracorporeal circulation.

Dr. Rumel had established daily teaching rounds for the thoracic nurses in 1952, and in 1958, with the participation of his associates, he was instrumental in the founding of a master's degree program for thoracic nurse specialists through the College of Nursing at the University of Utah. The Rumel Chest Clinic physicians then established Utah's first intensive care unit for thoracic surgical patients at LDS Hospital at a time when there were very few surgical intensive care units anywhere in this country. The first class of these new nurse specialists staffed the new ICU and made such an important contribution to the success of the thoracic program that they deserve individual recognition. They were: Alma Burgess, Marian Drury, Genevieve Lemon, Lynn May, Glenna Birkenshaw, Barbara Smith, Frances Funk, Sandra Noal, and Vera Snell.

Dr. Russell M. Nelson also returned to Salt Lake City in 1955 and was initially on the academic staff of the College of Medicine, where in November of that year he performed the first cardiac operation in Utah utilizing cardiopulmonary bypass. That operation was performed at the SLGH on an adult with an atrial septal defect. In March 1956 Nelson performed the first successful pediatric cardiac operation at the SLGH, a total repair of tetralogy of Fallot in a four-year-old girl. In 1959 he joined the staff of the Salt Lake Clinic, became associated with the LDS Hospital, and continued to make major contributions to the development of the thoracic specialty both in the clinical sciences and as the second director of the residency program. Nelson's surgical volume was sufficiently large that it was a critical component of the residents' experience. He was an innovative and facile surgeon responsible for many improvements in cardiac operations. He also established a research laboratory at LDS Hospital.

The first artificial heart valve had been described and implanted by Dr. Albert Starr in Portland, Oregon, in 1962. Utah's thoracic surgeons utilized this valve, as well as an assortment of other artificial valves, almost immediately. By the late 1960s, Dr. Nelson's experience with artificial aortic valve implantation was such that he was able to report a large series of patients with an exceptionally low operative mortality. He became involved with the administrative aspects of medicine and was elected president of the Utah State Medical Association. He was chair of the Division of Thoracic Surgery at LDS Hospital from 1967 to 1974 and director of the University of Utah Affiliated Hospital residency program in thoracic surgery from 1967 to 1984. He was honored nationally by being elected president of the Society for Vascular Surgery and a director of the American Board of Thoracic Surgery. In 1984 Dr. Nelson left private practice to serve The Church of Jesus Christ of Latter-day Saints as a member of The Council of The Twelve Apostles.

No history of thoracic surgery would be complete without recognition of the vital contributions made by Dr. Scott Smith, who was attracted from St. Louis by Dr. Rumel specifically to develop a program of anesthesia for cardiac and thoracic surgery in this area. With a federal grant Smith established a training program in anesthesiology at the University of Utah and affiliated hospitals (including LDS) in which an outstanding group of anesthesiologists, including Drs. Jack D. Stringham, Leland O. Learned, and Edward Hruska were trained. Drs. William Dillon and Betty Dillon trained in anesthesiology at the Cleveland Clinic and came to Salt Lake City to practice. Dr. Smith was joined initially by Dr. Hruska and later by Dr. Harry C. Wong and, in concert with Drs. Stringham and Betty Dillon, these physicians made possible a safe and enlightened anesthesia environment for the conduct of thoracic surgery at LDS Hospital. Dr. William Dillon was subsequently a principal contributor to the cardiac surgical program at the Primary Children's Hospital.

Throughout this period, Dr. Philip B. Price, the first chair of the Department of Surgery at the University of Utah, had conducted a program that included chest surgery under the aegis of the general surgery department. Dr. Price, like many other prominent surgeons of that day, felt it inappropriate to separate thoracic surgery from the specialty of surgery as a whole. However, the momentum of the specialty of thoracic surgery would prove overwhelming, and in 1970 the American Board of Thoracic Surgery became a primary board and thoracic surgery a totally independent entity. When Dr. Price vacated the chair of surgery at the University after a long and illustrious career, he became dean of the College of Medicine, and Dr. Walter Burdette, whose principle contributions lay in basic research in genetics, was appointed the new chair.

In 1956 Drs. Mark W. Muir and Robert J. Beveridge entered practice at the LDS Hospital. Dr. Muir, a general surgeon trained at the University of Pennsylvania, had a strong interest in vascular and general thoracic surgery and participated in the activities of the thoracic division for many years. Dr. Beveridge was the second resident to complete the thoracic training program at LDS Hospital and entered practice there. During his career the residents appreciated Dr. Beveridge because he gave them the opportunity for independent decision making in patient management and provided them an important volume of general thoracic surgical experience. Dr. Beveridge was chair of the Division of Thoracic Surgery at the LDS Hospital from 1980 to 1986, when he retired from active practice.

In 1957 Dr. C. Maxfield Parrish returned to Salt Lake City and established an enduring thoracic surgical practice at the Holy Cross and St. Mark's hospitals, as well as a reputation in peripheral arteriography and vascular surgery. In 1958 Dr. W. Gerald Rainer joined the Intermountain Clinic in thoracic surgery for only one year before relocating to Denver, Colorado.

Dr. Clynn Ford returned to Salt Lake City from his training at the Cincinnati General Hospital in January 1960 and for five years was associated with the University and VA hospitals. He then filled the thoracic surgical position at the Intermountain Clinic and in 1965 became associated with LDS, where later he established the peripheral vascular laboratory. In late 1975 he was the first surgeon at

LDS to use a dilute solution containing potassium to induce elective cardiac arrest. He was also the first among his peers to re-introduce *in-situ* vein grafting in peripheral arterial disease. Throughout his career Dr. Ford has provided important contributions to the thoracic surgical teaching meetings.

Dr. Conrad B. Jenson trained at the University of Minnesota and, after an additional period in general thoracic surgery in Los Angeles, he returned to Salt Lake in 1961 to practice with Dr. Russell Nelson at the Salt Lake Clinic. After a few years Drs. Nelson and Jenson left the Clinic and established their own group practice at LDS Hospital, where they had long and productive careers. In 1969 Dr. Jenson undertook the challenge of pediatric cardiac surgery and broadened the spectrum of procedures being performed successfully at Primary Children's Hospital, where he was chief of cardiac surgery for ten years. In 1970 Dr. Jenson was the first surgeon to employ the mammary artery as a coronary graft conduit. He retired from practice in 1987.

In the summer of 1964, Dr. L. Stephen Richards, Jr., returned to Salt Lake City from the University of Minnesota to join the Salt Lake Clinic as the thoracic surgeon. Over the succeeding quarter century, he made an important contribution to the residency program because he, too, had a large general thoracic surgical volume in addition to his cardiac surgical practice. Dr. Richards was chair of the Division of Thoracic Surgery at LDS Hospital from 1974 to 1980.

Dr. Harold V. Liddle, who had practiced in Pennsylvania for four years, was recruited by the Rumel Chest Clinic in 1964, in part to introduce the technique of selective coronary arteriography to the Intermountain West. As might be expected, several years elapsed before this diagnostic test achieved wide acceptance by either the community of internists or the thoracic surgeons; during this time the procedure was performed by the Sones technique, which did not lend itself to universal application. In the late 1960s the Judkin method of selective coronary arteriography gained increasing acceptance among internists and thoracic surgeons at the LDS and Holy Cross hospitals. It was a unique circumstance in this country that the surgeons rather than the cardiologists were the invasive diagnosticians for coronary disease, a circumstance that persisted for many years.

Dr. Liddle introduced the method of trans-venous insertion of pacemaker leads in 1964 and in that same year began to perform the Vineberg operation (mammary artery implant) for coronary artery disease. That operation was not destined to have enduring success and was abandoned in 1970. In 1968 he performed the first direct vein graft for coronary artery disease in the Intermountain West. In January 1976, in concert with Mr. Richard Berryessa, the cardiopulmonary perfusionist for the Rumel Clinic, he introduced the use of cold potassium cardioplegia at the LDS Hospital after determining the safe limits of the technique by the intraoperative use of a mass spectrometer to measure myocardial gas tensions and by measuring coronary sinus lactate levels during and following periods of cardiac arrest.

Administratively, Dr. Liddle served as the Speaker of The House of Delegates of the Utah State Medical Association from 1974 to 1977 and in 1978 was elected president of the Society of Thoracic Surgeons and, the following year, president of the Western Thoracic Surgical Association. He was a director of the American Board of Thoracic Surgery for six years and then served as president of the Council of Medical Specialty Societies. He retired from practice in 1988.

Notwithstanding the original reluctant acceptance of coronary arteriography and direct coronary artery surgery, these two procedures are now among those most frequently performed in every major hospital in Utah and the rest of the country.

Dr. Keith Reemtsma had become chair of the Department of Surgery at the University of Utah College of Medicine in 1966. Very quickly his enlightened leadership brought about the affiliation of the thoracic surgical services at the University with the Division of Thoracic Surgery at the LDS Hospital. He invited Dr. Nelson to direct the residency program, which was then expanded to provide training at the University and VA hospitals as well as at LDS and Primary Children's. Dr. Reemtsma's tenure from 1966 through 1971 was a period of very effective reinforcement of the specialty of thoracic surgery and the beginning of national recognition of the training program. He brought Dr. Richard K. Hughes to the University to direct the thoracic program at that hospital from 1968 through 1977.

The combined University of Utah Affiliated Hospitals residency program then was strengthened in the number of available positions (three each year) and in the educational opportunities available to the residents. Since that time, this residency has become one of the most sought-after in the country.

Although Dr. Rumel and the other members of the faculty had always had a strong commitment to teaching, the residency program was the principle catalyst for the creation of regular weekly teaching meetings designed both for resident education and for the continuing medical education of the faculty. Since the meetings involved the faculty from the University and the community hospitals, they became the formal educational arm of the Affiliated residency program.

By 1985 it was apparent that more residents were being trained and certified in this country than existed job opportunities. The faculty agreed that all residency programs should be cut back, and beginning in 1986, the resident rotation in the Utah program was staggered and the residents reduced to two each year. The program's directors included Dr. William Ray Rumel, 1954–67; Dr. Russell M. Nelson, 1967–84; and Dr. William A. Gay, 1984–present.

Dr. James W. Webster completed training at the Texas Heart Institute in 1968 and then joined Dr. Beveridge in practice at the LDS Hospital. A superb surgeon with an engaging sense of humor and a modesty that was most becoming, he soon became very active on hospital committees. Dr. Webster had a parallel profession in the Army National Guard in which he excelled even when in competition with men many years his junior. While he was engaged in Guard activities a tragic accident cost him his life in August 1982.

In 1969 Dr. Reed Gardner of the LDS Hospital biophysics department designed a device which has become known as the Intraflow. Providing for a continuous flow of a dilute solution of heparin through the indwelling catheter, the Intraflow was critically important to clinicians because it guaranteed that arterial pressure lines in patients would remain open as long as they were needed.

In 1969 Dr. Ralph McFarlane established a cardiothoracic surgical practice in Ogden at the McKay-Dee Hospital, where he practiced for almost twenty years. Dr. Richard Rees was associated with Dr. McFarlane for a period of time and Dr. Noel Nellis practiced independently in Ogden for several years after completing his training at the University of Utah Affiliated Hospitals in 1970.

In 1973 Dr. J D Mortensen and his associates at the Utah Biomedical Test Laboratory (UBTL) enlisted the participation of Dr. Alan H. Morris at the LDS Hospital in a project to develop a program of extracorporeal membrane oxygenation (ECMO) for patients with pulmonary failure. Initially conducted at the UBTL, the project was brought to the LDS Hospital and the first successful application of the technique performed in 1974. A remarkable number of new developments arose from this project. The HELP system, originally developed by Dr. Homer Warner, was expanded to provide computer interface with the new pulmonary intensive care unit where the ECMO project was conducted. A rapid transit capability for patient transportation which ECMO required was the forerunner of the Life Flight program. As a result of the computer application in the pulmonary ICU, an experimental program was developed which is unique in the world, in which ventilator management of patients is controlled by the computer. The computer determines the necessary changes in ventilator settings and the timing of those changes, which the ICU personnel implement. The same program has also been successful in managing patients who are on extracorporeal circulation for pulmonary failure.

Dr. Rumel's illustrious career was interrupted in 1976 when he developed an idiopathic cardiomyopathy. He succumbed to this illness on September 22, 1977, at the age of sixty-six. His driving determination and great imagination were sorely missed by his family, the thoracic community, and his host of friends.

Following the departure of Dr. Hughes from the University Hospital in 1977, Dr. Kent W. Jones returned to Salt Lake City from his training at Duke University. Under the chairmanship of Dr. Frank Moody, Dr. Jones continued the thoracic program at the University, although he was affiliated with Drs. Nelson and Jenson at the LDS Hospital. After a year, he was joined at the University by Dr. William DeVries, who had been a co-resident with Dr. Jones at Duke.

In 1980 Dr. Jones left the University for full-time practice with Drs. Nelson and Jenson at LDS Hospital. By the mid-1980s his practice was the backbone of the training program. He is responsible for the organization of the transplant program at LDS. He has become known nationally as a speaker at scientific meetings and is involved with the educational activities of the Society of Thoracic Surgeons and the Western Thoracic Surgical Association. After Dr. Jones left the University, Dr. DeVries headed the Division of Thoracic Surgery, which undertook the clinical application of the first artificial heart implant. In 1984 he performed the celebrated operation on Dr. Barney Clark. Dr. Lyle Joyce, who had just completed training in the University's Affiliated Hospitals program, joined Dr. DeVries at the University and was an important member of the team which performed that historic operation.

This was an important year in thoracic surgery in Salt Lake City for another reason. Dr. William A. Gay, a thoracic surgeon, was recruited by the University to chair the Department of Surgery. He initiated the program of cardiac transplantation and performed the first successful cardiac transplant operation in Utah in March 1985. Dr. Gay, with Dr. Paul Ebert, pioneered the application of cold potassium cardioplegia which was to revolutionize open heart surgery and to reduce to a minimum the remaining major risks of that surgical technique. After instituting the transplant program at the University, Drs. Gay, Jones, and Doty and their medical colleagues formed the Utah Transplant Affiliated Hospitals (UTAH) program which, from the outset, has been among the most successful in the country. This team of surgeons works together to assist each other in procurement and management of transplant patients. The program is clarion testimony to the effectiveness of a combined community effort for which all three surgeons are responsible. It is a continuation of the cooperative spirit initiated by Drs. Reemtsma, Rumel, and Nelson. The team of cardiologists consisting of Drs. Michael Bristow, Dale Renlund, and John O'Connell have played a critical role in the success of the program by testing and applying new chemotherapeutic agents during and following the surgery.

When Dr. Gay came to Salt Lake City, he brought with him a long-time associate, Dr. S. V. Karwande. They were joined in 1985 by Dr. Nelson Burton, who left for private practice in 1988. In 1986 the University team attracted a very able thoracic surgeon, Dr. Wayne Rickenbacher, to complement the department. Dr. Karwande assumed responsibility for the thoracic surgical service at the VA and has successfully established a very rich program in cardiac as well as general thoracic surgery. He has largely filled the void in the training program in general thoracic surgery resulting from Dr. Cutler's retirement.

This chronology of Utah's thoracic surgeons now returns to 1972, when two young surgeons, Drs. Maunsel Pearce and Edwin C. McGough, completed the thoracic residency in the University of Utah Affiliated Hospitals program and began very productive careers in Salt Lake City. Dr. Pearce established a practice at Holy Cross Hospital, where he was later to become president of the staff and a member of the Board of Directors. Dr. McGough had worked at the VA Hospital before forming a partnership with Dr. Pearce. Although Dr. McGough had also worked at St. Mark's Hospital, his principle contribution was in pediatric cardiac surgery at Primary Children's.

Dr. Clifford Kwan-Gett came to this country to work at the Cleveland Clinic in 1966. An Australian who completed an engineering degree before going to medical school at the University of Sydney, where he also had two years of postgraduate training, Kwan-Gett came to Utah with Dr. Willem Kolff in 1967 and in the next two years designed and built the first artificial heart, initially of silicone rubber. Later, with the help of Donald Lyman, a variation of polyurethane was developed for the manufacture of the heart. Originally the pumping chamber was made in two halves, but because of clotting problems along the seam, it was later made as a single unit. In order to make the chamber pliable but inelastic, he then used several layers of polyurethane in its construction. Dr. Kwan-Gett also designed and built the driving system for the heart and, remarkably, he did all of this at his home. The "Kwan-Gett heart," since called the "Jarvik heart," and the driving system remain today very much as originally designed by Dr. Kwan-Gett. In 1971 he entered training in thoracic surgery which he completed in 1973, but because the American Board of Thoracic Surgery would not accept his credentials for certification without his having completed a general surgery residency, he did so, finishing in 1977. He then practiced with Dr. Parrish for ten years before joining Drs. Pearce and McGough.

Dr. Rudolfo Morales joined the Rumel Chest Clinic in 1976 upon completing his residency at the University of Utah Affiliated Hospitals and spending six months at Boston Children's Hospital with Dr. Aldo Castenada. He was an excellent surgeon with a gift of gentleness that was appreciated by patients and nurses alike. After a year he left Salt Lake City to go to San Jose, California.

In 1977 a team of investigators at the University and LDS Hospital successfully applied total left heart bypass in a patient with profound left heart failure and maintained the patient's circulation for six days. It was several years before ventricular support devices were in use in the rest of the country.

Dr. Donald B. Doty, who had established a national reputation in pediatric and adult cardiac surgery at the University of Iowa before coming to Utah in 1983, became associated with Drs. Nelson, Jenson, and Jones in practice at the LDS and Primary Children's hospitals. Doty has written many articles and a major text on thoracic surgical technique. He became chair of the Division of Thoracic Surgery at LDS Hospital in 1986 and has been an important contributor to the success of the transplant program.

Dr. Roger Millar had a long association with cardiac surgery at LDS Hospital, beginning with undergraduate research activities with Dr. J D Mortensen. He graduated from the University of Utah College of Medicine and then trained with Drs. Kent Jones and William DeVries at Duke University before starting a practice in Oregon. In 1987 he returned to Salt Lake City to practice with Drs. Jones and Doty.

In the decade of the eighties, nine highly qualified young men completed training in cardiovascular and thoracic surgery and entered private practice in Utah. Three of these were trained outside the state and include Dr. Klint Stander, who opened a cardiac surgery program at the Utah Valley Hospital in Provo, and Drs. Steven Cain and Michael Coleman, who have established a cardiac surgical practice at the McKay-Dee Hospital in Ogden.

The remaining six surgeons completed the thoracic surgical residency program in the University of Utah Affiliated Residency and have remained in practice in Utah. Dr. Glade Smith joined Dr. Stander in Provo and Drs. Robert Place and Kent Thorne entered practice with Drs. Pearce and McGough at Holy Cross. Drs. Michael Collins and George Robinson established a private practice at the LDS Hospital, and when Dr. Ronald Quinton completed an obligation to the military, he joined them. Dr. Quinton was the twelfth graduate of the University of Utah Affiliated Thoracic Surgical Residency to practice in the communities of the Wasatch Front.

In the forty-eight years after Dr. Rumel's first cardiac operation in Utah, every major pulmonary and cardiac illness which lent itself to surgical correction was successfully treated in this state. Physicians in Utah were at the forefront of the application of new techniques in both physiology and surgery, and in many instances they pioneered and established those techniques. It is a proud heritage for successive generations of thoracic surgeons in the state.

Acknowledgments

The author wishes to express his great appreciation to Dr. J D Mortensen, Dr. Preston R. Cutler, Dr. Russell M. Nelson, and Dr. Robert J. Beveridge for the materials they so painstakingly assembled which have been the basis for this document. Mrs. Margene Withers provided important historic information concerning nursing. Dr. Harry C. Wong provided information concerning the history of anesthesia. Dr. Alan H. Morris and Dr. Reed Gardner were very helpful concerning research developments. Drs. Harry C. Wong, Russell M. Nelson, L. George Veasy, and J D Mortensen very kindly provided thoughtful editing of the manuscript.

CHAPTER TWENTY-TWO • 1

Plastic and Reconstructive Surgery: LDS Hospital and Primary Children's Medical Center

THOMAS RAY BROADBENT, MD

DR. T. RAY BROADBENT completed four years of general and thoracic surgery at Duke University in 1950 and became interested in taking two additional years of training in plastic surgery under Dr. Kenneth L. Pickerell at Duke. Clarence Wannacott, administrator at LDS Hospital, and Dr. Paul Richards, surgeon, suggested Salt Lake City to him as a place to practice. Except for having been a student at BYU, he had no roots in the area.

When Broadbent arrived in Salt Lake City in 1952, four physicians were doing plastic surgery: Robert R. Robinson, B. F. Robbins, A. C. Callister, and Oscar Billeter. Dr. Billeter, who had completed a partial preceptorship in Detroit with Dr. Clair Straith at the Straith Clinic, practiced at St. Mark's Hospital. He was not very active because of his cardiac status, a concern that had caused the early termination of his preceptorship.

Dr. Robbins was a generalist in family practice and surgery, a fine gentleman with an interest in cleft lip and cleft palate patients, who served the Primary Children's Hospital admirably for many years. His welcome to Salt Lake City was instrumental in Broadbent's staying in the Valley. He said, "I have cared for these children as well as I could, but knowing your training is more up-to-date, I think you should now take care of them." After the first visit it was a rare baby with a cleft that he didn't refer.

Dr. A. C. Callister was something different. When the Board of Plastic Surgery was created in 1937, self-appointed plastic surgeons were invited to join on a geographic basis, so Dr. Callister had become a founding member. The newcomer's courtesy call was upsetting, for he told Broadbent that too many plastic surgeons were in town already and he wasn't wanted. Later Callister would try, unsuccessfully, to block Broadbent's application to take the Board examinations.

Mr. Wannacott at LDS and his successor Mr. Brent Goates were always, by contrast, very supportive and helpful in those formative years. Dr. Callister had an interest in cleft lip surgery, and much of the work on the new plastic surgery service would be secondary corrections of his work.

Dr. Robert R. Robinson was the only fully trained plastic surgeon in Salt Lake City. He had wartime experience and had been trained by the St. Louis group, led by Drs. Vilray P. Blair, Louis Byars, James Barrett Brown, Frank McDowell, and Minot Fryor. Dr. Robinson was as fine a physician and gentleman as one could find. His work was technically superb, but even more, he was a patient's full physician, any hour, night or day. Dr. Robinson practiced at Holy Cross Hospital and clearly contributed as much to high-quality care as anyone on the staff. He invited young Broadbent to share an office with him in the newly constructed Doxey-Layton Medical Building at 508 E. South Temple, which he did for a few months. They agreed that since Billeter was at St. Mark's and Robinson himself was at Holy Cross, an association with LDS Hospital would offer Broadbent more opportunity. Discouraged by a colleague's suit against him, Dr. Robinson retired prematurely and moved back to his native Missouri in the sixties. He had done much to establish high standards in plastic surgery in the Intermountain West.

It was soon realized that the drawing area for patients extended from Kansas City, Missouri, to California and from Canada to Mexico. Preceptorships were offered in two training centers in California and one each in Kansas City and Portland. A residency with graduated responsibility and a balanced didactic program, like that at Duke, did not exist in the Intermountain region.

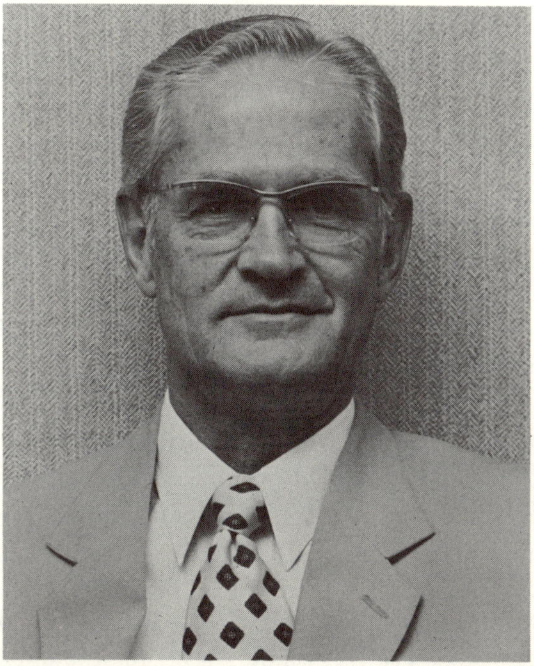

Thomas Ray Broadbent.

The practice and scope of plastic surgery in Salt Lake City and at LDS and Primary Children's grew steadily, extending to trauma, including burns, head and neck cancer resection and reconstruction, congenital deformities, and elective surgery, each claiming about 25% of a doctor's time. A good bit of elective surgery was hand surgery following the poliomyelitis epidemic of the fifties.

The broad scope and variety of patients available offered an opportunity for training residents. Arrangements were made at LDS Hospital for general surgery residents to take a three-month rotation on plastic surgery. The experience was of considerable value to surgeons in general, for their view of surgery was broadened. Further, they began to see surgery for its reconstructive value and not merely as an ablative type of endeavor. Several residents rotating through plastic surgery changed course and went on to become some of the community's fine plastic surgeons.

In 1955 and 1956 the plastic surgery service was given division status within the Department of General Surgery at LDS. Interns began to rotate on service for a month at a time, principally to be instructed on proper wound closure and care. A natural corollary was for them then to supervise the emergency room and the trauma work in that area.

In 1956 discussion was initiated with the American Board of Plastic Surgeons and the National Residency Review Training Committee toward establishing a plastic surgery training program at LDS Hospital. Hospital, department, and division data were collated and submitted for review. At that time the division staff consisted only of Dr. Broadbent as senior staff, with rotating interns and general surgery residents. LDS Hospital and its church service clientele, Primary Children's Hospital, and Salt Lake General Hospital provided most of the teaching material, with consultative service at the Shriners' Hospital as well as the Utah State Prison Infirmary. Outreach clinics were held in Provo and Logan once a month in addition, with lectures to hospital and society staffs throughout the Intermountain area once or twice a month.

In the fifties, training programs were awarded to individuals, not institutions, and Dr. Broadbent applied for a formally approved two-year program with one resident appointment per year. Drs. Douglas McComber and Gus Garcia of Denver and Albert Davis of Southern California were sent to evaluate the proposed program and found the work load and resident opportunities adequate and the didactic programs satisfactory. The latter consisted basically of patient rounds at 6:30 each morning and late in the evening, anatomy dissection course, art drawing or sculpting course, pathology conference with pathologists on current surgical pathology and scheduled material, physiology lectures, participation in general surgery conferences, and dermatopathology conferences with the dermatologists and pathologists.

The first resident, Dr. Albert Hochstrasser, was accepted in July of 1957. Board-certified in general surgery, Dr. Hochstrasser came to the area from Washington, D.C. Since finishing the program, he has practiced in his native city of Lucerne, Switzerland.

With Dr. Hochstrasser and those to follow, the training philosophy was to resist having a resident service of charity patients. Instead, all patients were mixed on the same ward. Graduated responsibility and case assignment depended solely on the resident's ability to handle the problem in preoperative planning, operating, and follow-up care, regardless of the patient's ability or inability to pay.

During this period, Dr. Robert M. Woolf, a well-trained general surgeon, had left Salt Lake City to train in plastic surgery at Duke University. It was their mutual intention that Woolf would return to join Dr. Broadbent in practice and in conducting the training program. He arrived in 1958 for a twenty-eight-year association before his retirement in January of 1986. Together Broadbent and Woolf enlarged and expanded the residency program to involve a weekly operating session at the state prison hospital — a great experience for the residents — and eventually the University of Utah and VA hospitals. They shared the work load in head and neck cancer, burns, and supervision of the emergency trauma service. Before short-stay and Surgicenter care evolved, the overall in-patient load commonly ran twenty-five to thirty patients.

Because of the obvious need for cost containment and patient convenience, the short-stay service at LDS was initiated in the late 1960s. Very few utilized that service for the first two or three years. Now it is the wave of the present and future. The concept grew out of Dr. Stewart Gordon's study in Toronto. He wanted to see what he could do on an out-patient basis where all patients had formerly been treated as in-patients. He found that within a two-year period he was treating 50% of his former in-patients as out-patients. He concluded that this required three things: better hemostasis, better bandaging, and better and less anesthetic. This concept, with economic pressures, has shortened the length of stay as well; for example, rhinoplasties from two to three days as in-patients to an out-patient basis, and reduction mammoplasties and breast reconstructions after mastectomy from five to seven days in the hospital to a zero- to one-day stay.

The residency grew to be more than two staff men could cover with two plastic surgery residents (one first-year and one second-year), a general surgery resident, and an intern. In cooperation with Dr. Keith Reemtsma, chief of general surgery at the University of Utah Hospital, a full-time chief in plastic surgery was recruited, and Dr. Clifford C. Snyder arrived in 1967. Broadbent and Woolf withdrew from the University and VA hospitals. Thereafter the residents were to spend half their time at those two hospitals, including laboratory research experience, and half at the LDS/Primary Children's rotation. From that time to 1985, the program was known as the University of Utah and Affiliated Hospitals Plastic Surgery Residency Program.

In 1985 all services at LDS were requested to cut costs and to be discontinued if they were available elsewhere in the community. National studies on human resources production and distribution suggested overproduction of residents, and Salt Lake City had more plastic surgeons per capita than any other city in the United States or Canada. Gradually the volume of work suffered, and the government's Title XIX rule put restrictive pressure on the autonomy of a resident in the operating arena. The plastic surgery residency program at LDS was terminated in 1985.

The future of education and training of plastic surgeons rests now with new minds and imaginative financing. The scope and opportunities are endless, limited only by a lack of imagination. As with any endeavor, those who follow should ascend higher than their predecessors. Nearly all of the students trained in the residency program have been certified by the American Board of Plastic Surgery. They are great people with their patients, continuing to learn, and some have become teachers, innovators, artists, and authors.

CHAPTER TWENTY-TWO • 2

Plastic and Reconstructive Surgery: University of Utah

CLIFFORD C. SNYDER, BS, MD

AT THE REQUEST OF DR. KENNETH B. CASTLETON, Dean of the Medical School, and Dr. Keith Reemtsma, chair of the Department of Surgery, Dr. Clifford C. Snyder was appointed August 25, 1967, to organize and chair a Division of Plastic Surgery and, as chief, to reorganize the entire surgical service at the Salt Lake City Veterans Administration Medical Center. He requested that Dr. Reemtsma entice Dr. Mark Wolcott, a long-time colleague from the Veterans Administration in Washington, D.C., to join him a year later. With Wolcott's expertise, the final VA transition was uneventful.

Drs. Thomas Ray Broadbent and Robert M. Woolf had been supervising trainees in an approved residency program in plastic surgery which involved the LDS and Primary Children's hospitals and included the Utah State Prison Infirmary. This program was later coordinated with the University–VA program to become the University of Utah and Affiliated Hospitals Plastic Surgery Residency Program. Dr. Grant Hickman was the senior consultant in plastic surgery at the VA Hospital at the time, and he concurred with this arrangement. When Dr. Robert (Robbie) Robinson, pioneer plastic surgeon in Salt Lake City and chief of plastic surgery at the Intermountain Shriners' Hospital for Crippled Children, decided to move to the Midwest, he requested that Dr. Snyder fill his position. After confirmation by Dr. Sherman Coleman of the Shriners' Hospital, Dr. Reemtsma, and Dean Castleton, this doctor-hospital relationship became continuous for twenty gratifying years. The plastic surgery residents rotated through the Shriners' Hospital program, alternating on-call emergency services with the orthopedic residents.

An established federal regulation at all VA hospitals that veteran patients could not be exposed to medical students for examinations was abolished, and the Salt Lake City VA Hospital became the first institution to become part of a university's teaching program.

Before accepting the University–VA appointments, Dr. Snyder was to be permitted to organize and develop a surgical research laboratory at the VA complex. A building on the VA grounds was restructured to satisfy his needs, and through research grants, six operating tables, ceiling operating lights, surgical instruments, bovies, and other necessities were installed. This animal-care facility was soon used by all services or individuals under VA auspices. Having pioneered microsurgery in the Salt Lake Valley, Snyder inaugurated and taught formal courses in micro-techniques to surgical staffs from other VA hospitals. An annual research teaching course for the University of Utah Honors Program was initiated in the VA research lab in 1971 and has been taught without interruption for twenty years.

The residents and staff have been privileged to do research in these original facilities. Research models were set up for plastic surgical procedures for correction of exstrophy of the bladder, paraplegia, nerve growth factor, replantation of limbs, renal transplantation, temporomandibular joint reconstruction, vascular and neural microsurgery, snake venom research, and training in surgical techniques for veterinary surgery staff members from universities across the nation.

During Snyder's thirteen-year tour of duty at the VA Medical Center, the number of admissions to the surgical service increased 33%. The hospital was designated one of the system's few plastic surgery centers and received problem patients from Idaho, Wyoming, Montana, and Northern California. Allocated resident-training positions in surgery for VA service-connected residents were filled by the Dean's Committee at the University.

The University of Utah and Affiliated Hospitals Plastic Surgery Residency Program became a well-rounded complex with teaching

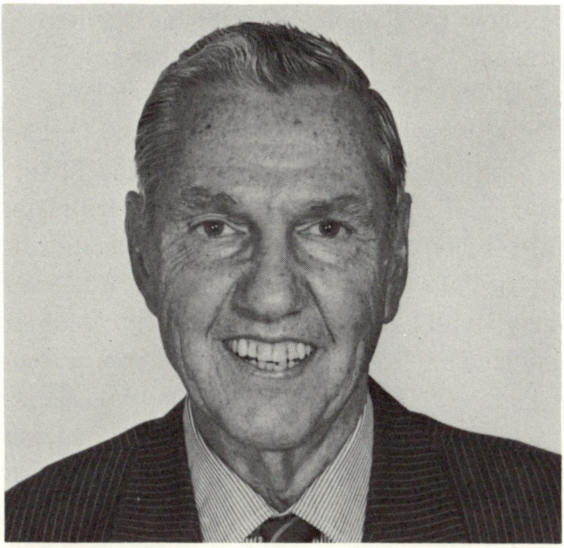

Clifford C. Snyder.

and learning facilities in congenital anomalies, burns, head and neck tumors, aesthetic surgery, hand problems, research, cranio-maxillo-facial abnormalities, trauma, and reconstructive procedures. The teaching staff included both full-time and clinical professors. The resident staff remains four in number, two junior and two senior trainees, with July as the starting month. An ample supply of qualified resident-applicants who meet the required years of pre-plastic surgery training has been available; two senior residents have graduated in each of the past twenty years. Sponsored by the program, some trainees have enjoyed interim visits to other programs at Los Angeles, Newport Beach, San Mateo, Atlanta, Boston, Honolulu, Dallas, Mexico City, and Taipei. Dr. Snyder has trained ninety-one residents who have established offices throughout the nation as well as in foreign countries.

Residents sharpened their surgical and research skills by participating in various projects. A few of interest follow: "Blood Brain Barrier" with Arthur Benson; "Peripheral Neurogenesis" with Larry Ruth; "Total Jaw Prosthesis" with David Dingman; "Neurovasculomuscular Pedicle for Paraplegia" with Earl Browne; "Epineural Cuff Neurorrhaphy" with James Clayton; "Irradiated Nerve Homografts" with Don Teal; "Cobra Venom for Keloids" with Craig Davis; "Frostbite Therapy" with Gene Sullivan; "Free Osteo-myoneurovascular Rib Graft for Pollicization" with Philip Metz; "Artificial Nerve" with Ted Saeih; "Rib Graft Hernioplasty" with James Pickens; "Silicone Tube Tenorrhaphy" with William Seare; "Microsurgical Neurorrhaphy" with Larry Patton; "Bovine Pericardium Augments in Human Surgery" with Larry Ruth; "Elastic Sutures for Tenorrhaphies" with Gary Hunter; "Mono Versus Polysutures in Neurorrhaphy" with James Pickens; "Traumatic Neuroma" with James Pickens; "Dupuytren's Contracture" with James Fowler; "Mammary Prostheses" with Kathleen Tucker; "Snake Bites" with Gary Hunter; "Sterno-clavicular Joint Transfer for T-M Joint Substitute" with George Levine; "Craniopagus Conjoined Twins" with Robert Wilson and Dee Allred; and "Laser Anastomoses" with James Kilgore.

Full-time faculty staff members of the Division of Plastic Surgery at the University included Dr. Paul V. Slater, who now enjoys a generalized plastic and reconstructive surgical practice in Cheyenne, Wyoming. Dr. Earl Z. Browne, Jr., a former resident in the program, was also an assistant dean in the Medical School and is currently chief of plastic surgery at the Cleveland Clinic. Dr. Michael A. Teague is practicing in Baton Rouge, Louisiana, with another former resident, Dr. Charles Greenwald. The two were the first in that region to replant an amputated hand successfully. Dr. Larry G. Leonard was acting chief of plastic surgery at the University and currently is deeply involved in surgery of the hand, in which he excels. His wife, Dr. Claire Leonard, is on the pediatric staff of the University Medical School. Dr. Louis Morales, Jr., whose major interest is craniofacial surgery, was intimately involved in the separation of craniopagus conjoined twins and is a busy surgeon today in the Salt Lake Valley.

Over time, Dr. Snyder's interest in clinical surgery has waned but has increased in the direction of research surgery and the teaching of medical history, which culminated in a year's sabbatical and the publication of several research papers and a text on teaching medical history. Appointments as Professor Emeritus of Surgery and Associate Dean of the Medical School provide time for him to be of further benefit to the University. Teaching Honors Program courses for twenty years has been an education in itself, but being made the University of Utah Distinguished Honors Professor for 1988 was his greatest thrill.

Dr. Leonard fulfilled the position most satisfactorily during Snyder's sabbatical; and following Snyder's retirement as chair of the division, Dr. Morales was appointed as interim head. The University's plastic surgery program is now under the direction of a superb upper-extremity surgeon and able leader, Dr. Graham Lister, who has demonstrated his concern for both academics and patient care. The high standards of plastic surgery in the state of Utah established by the practicing specialists, staff members of the affiliate hospitals, and members of the Utah Plastic Surgery Society are worthy of note. It takes many bees to make a hive.

CHAPTER TWENTY-THREE

Neurological Surgery

CHESTER B. POWELL, MD, FACS
J. LOUIS SCHRICKER, JR., MD, FACS

SURGERY OF THE NERVOUS SYSTEM is perhaps the oldest surgical discipline after mankind began emergency suturing of wounds and amputation of limbs. Archaeologic discoveries show that almost all cultures worldwide have left evidence of trepanation. Surgical progress was severely handicapped until the discovery of effective anesthetic agents by Morton in the 1840s, Pasteur's discovery of the role of microorganisms in infections, and Lister's demonstration in 1867 that it was possible to prevent surgical infections. It is not surprising that with these fundamental discoveries medicine and all forms of surgery made revolutionary progress in the second half of the nineteenth century. In the 1880s, reports of primary operations for brain tumor and abscess appeared in England (Godlee, Horsley) and Scotland (Macewen).

In 1864 in the United States, W. W. Keen coauthored with Weir Mitchell a treatise on gunshot wounds and other injuries of nerves based on his Civil War experience. In 1887 he performed the first resection for a benign brain tumor in the Western Hemisphere. He also performed and described procedures for sciatica, trigeminal neuralgia, hydrocephalus, brain tumor, craniosynostosis, and spasmodic torticollis, and in 1898 he introduced the Gigli saw in this country. He was also an active general surgeon. Harvey Cushing, on the other hand,

Note: Dedicated to Augustus C. Behle, MD, who, I have reason to believe, would find this both fascinating and gratifying. C.B.P.

was the first to confine his surgery and published research to the nervous system, thereby defining the specialty of neurological surgery.

Nineteenth-century Surgery in Utah

After the completion of the railroad in 1869, twenty-two years following the arrival of the Mormon pioneers, large-scale mining became profitable. Mines proliferated, worked by a new wave of European immigrants, and, not surprisingly, trauma became more prevalent. An epidemic of plumbism (lead poisoning) — a frequent side-effect of the mining operations — was a major factor in the founding of St. Mark's Hospital in 1872 and Holy Cross Hospital in 1875. At St. Mark's between 1872 and 1903, 2,900 cases of lead poisonings were seen, and many of the 667 injuries treated were industrially related back and head injuries.

In the last three decades of the nineteenth century, in response to the growing population and the needs of the two hospitals, a number of better-trained physicians arrived, practicing both medicine and surgery. Almost no documentation of their practices exists, with the exception of Dr. Samuel H. Pinkerton. A younger physician, Dr. Franklin Meacham, worked with Dr. Pinkerton through 1892 and wrote a detailed report of the surgery for that year. Of 692 operations, 91 were on the head, face, and neck. Among the latter were two operations for compound depressed skull fractures. The first case was that of a twelve-year-old boy who sustained a fall resulting in a left hemiplegia and recovered after the doctor placed a burr hole and elevated the depression. The second was a thirty-five-year-old man who also sustained a fall, was operated upon four hours after the injury, and recovered completely.

Five cases of "inveterate sciatica" were successfully treated by bloodless stretching of the sciatic nerve. Dr. Pinkerton's "rare surgical" treatment of facial neuralgia was reported in detail in the newspaper; several months later the patient reported no recurrence of pain.

While Dr. Pinkerton practiced as a general surgeon in the true sense of the word, there is no indication that he had a special interest

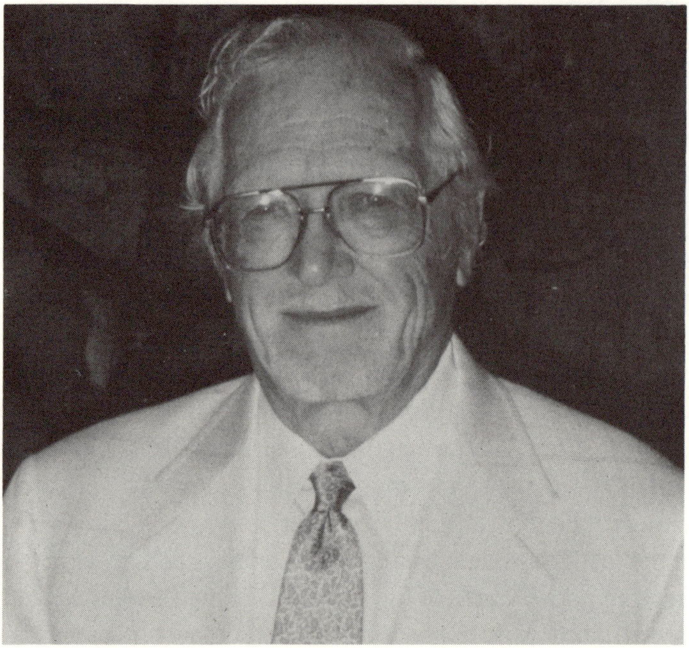

Chester B. Powell.

in any type of surgery. With a younger physician who became his protege, it is a different story.

A Trend Toward Neurosurgical Specialization

Dr. Augustus C. Behle, born January 24, 1871, was a physician's son. After studying on his own in his father's Blackfoot pharmacy, he became a registered pharmacist in Idaho at the age of nineteen. He graduated from Rush Medical College in Chicago in 1894, returned to Salt Lake City, and simultaneously interned at St. Mark's Hospital and practiced medicine for a three-year period. In 1897–98 he visited eastern clinics and did postgraduate work at Johns Hopkins, with special interest in bacteriology and pathology, under the guidance of Osler, Kelly, Welch, Flexner, and Halstead, but apparently had no contact with Cushing. At Dr. Pinkerton's behest, Dr. Behle revised St. Mark's operating room techniques of antisepsis, including steriliza-

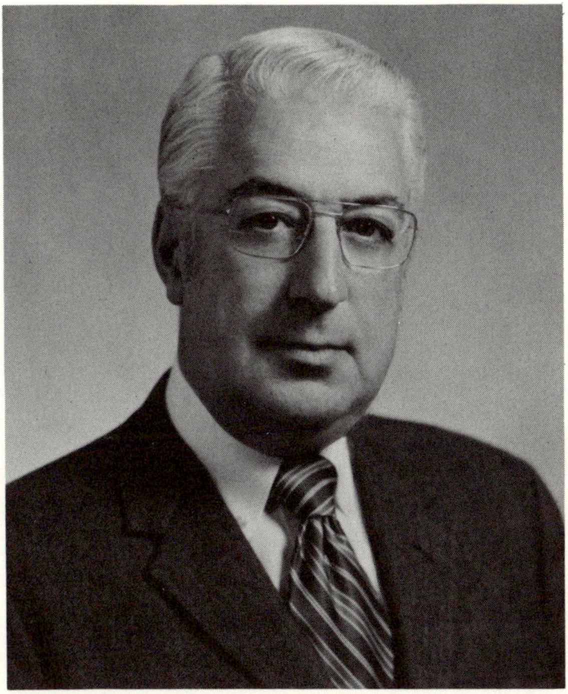

J. Louis Schricker.

tion of hands, cleansing of fingernails, introduction of rubber gloves and face masks, and sterilization of sutures. The result in the control of infection was (to quote Professor William H. Behle's biography of his father, here and below) "revolutionary." Behle also introduced the microscopic study of surgical specimens. He spent 1903 in Europe visiting prominent surgeons, including Theodore Kocher. As a result of a visit with Conrad Roentgen, he brought x-ray to St. Mark's.

Dr. Behle's interest focused in three areas, thyroid, cleft palate, and brain surgery, including "removal of tumors, draining of cysts, repairing compound fractures," and treating hematomas. He used the "Elliott trephine originally, then later used a Hudson or Ajax burr followed by a Gigli saw. He always used fine silk sutures in brain surgery." In cases of sciatica he would "expose the nerve surgically and stretch it." He operated upon the spine. "A man from Malad

[Idaho] was brought in with a fractured neck and quadriplegia. [Behle] felt the cord was not severed but only compressed and performed an emergency operation decompressing the cord, with the patient's recovery." Five weeks later he had a second "identical" case, which he operated upon successfully. In 1912 Behle published an article in *Northwest Medicine* on the pituitary gland and its importance to the surgeon.

Other surgeons in the first decade of the twentieth century performed occasional neurosurgical operations. According to Dr. Eliot Snow, Drs. Samuel Baldwin and Joseph Tyree, general surgeons with primary interest in orthopedics, performed trephines for subdural hematoma and elevated depressed fractures. However, by virtue of his lifelong interest in surgery of the nervous system, his efforts in obtaining advanced training, and the amount of actual neurosurgery he performed, Dr. Behle must be considered Utah's first neurosurgeon.

Neurosurgery as a Specialty —Reed Harrow, MD

The first neurosurgeon trained as such arrived in Utah in 1932, several years before the American Board of Neurological Surgery was incorporated in 1940. Reed Harrow had graduated from the University of Pennsylvania Medical School, where his interest in neurosurgery was aroused by Drs. Charles Frazier and Frances Grant, under whom he completed his residency. Dr. J. Louis Schricker, who was closely associated with Dr. Harrow in later years, stated that Harrow's reception by the surgical community was less than warm and his early years difficult, but that his keen diagnostic acumen and meticulous surgical skills soon established a niche for him in the community and laid the foundation for the neurosurgical service at LDS Hospital.

At that time neurosurgery, although an acknowledged specialty, was primitive by current standards. Diagnostic procedures were largely limited to spinal puncture, x-rays, and air studies (introduced by Dandy in 1918). Myelography (visualization of the spinal canal by opaque contrast media) was rarely used until Mixter and Barr's clarification of the herniated disc syndrome in 1934 popularized it as a localizing diagnostic tool. Infection was still a major surgical problem, the sulfa drugs just appearing. Bone flaps easily became infected, especially in secondary procedures, and were either steamed-sterilized or replaced with metal plates. Surgical lighting of the intracranial cavity was a problem only partially solved by flexible lighted retractors. With no blood banks, blood was replaced post-operatively from cross-matched donors, and intravenous fluid and electrolyte management was in its infancy. Cerebral edema was controlled largely through dehydration or subtemporal decompressive surgery.

Dr. Harrow had other problems locally. He had no trained operating room personnel and had to utilize other surgeons as assistants. Dr. Cyril Vance, an obstetrician, was a frequent assistant and became a close personal friend. He interested Dr. Harrow in neurosurgery of birth defects, and they became the state's pioneer pediatric neurosurgical team. Dr. Eliot Snow also assisted Dr. Harrow in the early years. He remembers Dr. Harrow giving a talk on subdural hematomas at the pathology conference shortly after his arrival. Only a week later Dr. Snow had a patient who presented these very features of a chronic subdural hematoma; he referred the patient to Dr. Harrow and assisted him at surgery.

Dr. Harrow was physically of small stature, slim, and restlessly hyperactive. Dr. Schricker says, "He was fiercely independent, a private person who presented an outer facade but who had no close relations with colleagues or family. He was a musician and an outstanding pianist. He did like to fish with Cyril Vance. At surgery he was demanding and very meticulous in his technique, expecting the same of his assistants, and was not at all shy at expressing his displeasure at clumsiness or poor techniques." He tended to be curt with patients and was noted for his disdain for medical records. Dr. J. Floyd Cannon, who had known him from medical school days, recalled that Dr. Harrow accumulated a vast pile of incomplete charts in the record room. Finally the record librarian cornered him in the hall one day and led him into the record room, showing him several large cartons. Dr. Harrow smiled and asked if he could take them home. Delighted at his cooperation, the record librarian agreed, whereupon — and Dr. Cannon swore this was true — Dr. Harrow took the records home and spent the evening feeding them to his furnace.

Dr. Paul Bucy in Chicago commented on Harrow's independence: "With his training and experience, we invited him to become a charter diplomate of the Board of Neurological Surgery. We didn't get a response and when I later chanced to meet him, he said, 'I'm getting along all right. I don't need *that.*' "

Dr. Harrow's neurosurgical practice was typical for those years and reflected his training. He performed craniotomies for tumors, abscesses, and hematomas with diagnoses based on sharp neurologic assessment and air studies. He treated trigeminal neuralgia with alcohol injections and operated when injections were ineffective or unsuitable. Cranial surgery included orbital decompression for malignant exophthalmus. He operated upon several superficial arterial venous malformations but no aneurysms. Spinal surgery was performed for intraspinal tumors, and from the mid-forties on he performed disc surgery although he had no special training with these lesions. Thoracolumbar sympathectomies were in his repertoire. He repaired myelomeningoceles and treated hydrocephalus with choroid plexus cauterization. His fine surgical results reflected his excellent surgical technique. Among Dr. Harrow's assistants, two, Drs. Donald C. Bernson and Steward A. Wright (the latter with an additional year of observation under Dr. Naffziger) continued their own practices at LDS and St. Mark's hospitals, respectively, in neurosurgery. Dr. Bernson left Salt Lake City in 1974.

Dr. Chester B. Powell has two vivid recollections of Dr. Harrow. Visiting before he came to Salt Lake, he found Dr. Harrow most cordial and encouraging. In the early years of his practice as a young and very young-looking neurosurgeon — needing on several occasions the help and support of an older neurosurgeon — he found Harrow a willing, gracious, and strongly supportive consultant, for which he was very grateful.

Contemporary Neurosurgery in Utah

Chester B. Powell was the second trained neurosurgeon to practice in Utah. In medical school at the outbreak of World War II, he was deferred by the registration laws until he had completed his training. As a student he met and was strongly influenced by Drs. Percival Bailey and Paul Bucy, and in internship at St. Luke's Hospital he came under the influence of Dr. Eric Oldberg, one of Cushing's last residents. Powell continued his neurosurgical residency under Oldberg at the University of Illinois.

During active duty in the Army, Dr. Powell was assigned to Bushnell General Hospital in Brigham City, Utah. The Intermountain scene and climate were a "revelation" after Chicago, and the Powells resolved to consider Utah seriously. Then Dr. Phil Howard asked Dr. Oldberg if he had any residents interested in coming West to join the post-war expansion of the staff of Holy Cross Hospital. At Howard's invitation, the Powells returned to Utah briefly, and it was an easy decision once they were back in the mountains.

Powell brought with him diagnostic expertise in electroencephalography and cerebral angiography and was the first to use them in Utah. These techniques, with new contrast agents for myelography, enormously increased diagnostic capabilities over air studies and led to the expansion of neurosurgical treatment: defining and localizing early intracranial lesions, aneurysms, and other vascular lesions; differentiating between gliomas and benign tumors; and localizing with precision lumbar and cervical discs and intraspinal tumors.

At that time angiography was performed by percutaneous needling of the carotid artery. An injection was made for each exposure, necessitating multiple injections for antero-posterior (AP) and lateral projections and for arterial and venous phases. There were reports of rapid film changers, but none were available. Dr. Ralph Meyer, who had come through the University of Chicago radiology residency and was as much a neuroradiologist as existed at that time, suggested that he and Powell build one. His elegantly simple, efficient hand-operated changer took six cassettes pushed through by a hand lever, exactly sufficient to visualize the entire arterial-capillary-venous phases. The changer permitted complete angiography in AP and lateral projections with only two injections. The results were outstanding.

Angiography proved invaluable for aneurysms, which now became an important part of the neurosurgical repertoire, as well as the definition of intracranial neoplasms.

EEG played an important role in the diagnosis and localization of brain tumors. It was also used in a number of patients with intractable epilepsy, taking records off the cortex exposed under local anesthesia to define epileptogenic foci which were then excised, for the most part with favorable results and clinical improvement.

Infants with early hydrocephalus, referred in surprising numbers, were treated with choroid plexectomy by cauterization with a ventriculoscope, a cystoscope adaptation. This was not very effective generally, and a procedure coming into vogue was a shunt from the lumbar subarachnoid space into the ureter following a nephrectomy. Powell began working with urologists who performed the necessary nephrectomies. These children were stabilized for a while but did not do well in the long run, most often because of dehydration (since there were no partial pressure valves in the shunts) and electrolyte depletion.

This short-lived effort was succinctly characterized by St. Mark's urologist Jimmy Palmer, who was accustomed to greet Powell with, "Hey, Chet! How are your pee-brains doing these days!"

An interesting aspect of the neurosurgical scene in 1948 was the total lack of any neurosurgeons in Nevada, Idaho, Montana, or Wyoming and the prevailing concern over the transportation of back- and head-injured patients. As a result, many calls for distant consultations were received necessitating emergency out-of-town surgery. It was soon apparent that this was not compatible with a busy local practice without chartered flights. Returning from a call to Moab and passing over the shoulder of Mount Timpanogos, its late spring crown of snow reflecting the colors of the setting sun, Powell was forcibly struck with the realization that he could do this himself! With a pilot's license and a Bonanza, and later a twin Cessna, he continued for many years to fly not only to attend out-of-town calls, but also to a monthly clinic in Elko, Nevada, and to medical meetings across the U.S., Mexico, and Canada.

From the fifties through the seventies, great advances occurred in neurological surgery: the development of anterior surgery for cervical intervertebral discs; the development of shunts for hydrocephalus and precision instrumentation for stereotactic procedures; great advances in the understanding of electrolytes and body fluid management; the development of advanced dehydrating agents; great strides in neurosurgical anesthesia, the advent of the surgical microscope and the associated clarification of microsurgical anatomy; development of microsurgical instrumentation; and finally the appearance of the revolutionary diagnostic aid the CT scanner, followed shortly by magnetic resonance imaging. With these advances the evolution of neuroradiology was a natural consequence, to the specialists' mutual benefit. Simultaneously, older and obsolete procedures were discarded and laser surgery and advanced mechanical resection instruments have replaced older and cruder techniques. The fifties and sixties also saw the arrival of well-trained neurosurgeons, in Utah and the adjacent states, beginning with Dr. Schricker's return from the Armed Forces to join Dr. Harrow in 1957.

Dr. J. Louis Schricker first returned home to Salt Lake City in 1944 after medical studies at Washington University in St. Louis. During his internship at LDS Hospital he became interested in neurosurgery through his contacts with Dr. Harrow. He entered military service in 1946, took a residency in neurosurgery under Dr. Henry Schwartz, and was sent to Denver's Fitzsimmons Hospital to establish a neurosurgery service. He remained its chief until his resignation and return to civilian life in 1957. He joined Dr. Harrow in the office and went on LDS staff on June 17, 1957. A month later Dr. Harrow slipped and fell in his home, hit his head on the floor, and was unconscious for a brief period. He tried to return to his practice but was unable to operate because of increasing neurologic symptoms. He retired in the spring of 1958 and died in 1975.

A neurosurgical unit was established at LDS in 1958. A neurosurgical intensive care unit followed in 1963.

In 1962 Dr. Laverne S. Erickson joined Dr. Schricker, followed by Drs. William Stoops and Howard Reichman in 1964 to make a staff of five. After one year Dr. Reichman chose academia and became professor at Loyola Medical School in Chicago. Dr. Stoops pioneered in surgery for Parkinsonism but unfortunately succumbed to acute leukemia in 1971.

In 1969 Dr. Bruce Sorensen returned to Salt Lake City after completing a neurosurgery residency in Cleveland, Ohio, and was joined by Charles Rich in 1970, after the latter had completed training in Boston, to form a lasting partnership. Dr. Erickson went into solo practice in 1967, joined Dr. Reichman in Chicago for three years, then went on staff at the University and VA hospitals on his return to Salt Lake City in 1981.

University of Utah Medical School and Neurosurgery Residency

In 1955 Dr. Petter Lindstrom was appointed the first full-time professor of neurosurgery at the University Medical School, where he remained ten years, enlisting, in 1961, Dr. Theodore Roberts as the second full-time staff neurosurgeon.

With the growth of the University of Utah Medical School and its importance and prestige in the Intermountain West, the development of a modern neurosurgical department became a paramount goal, achieved largely through the foresight and efforts of Dr. Roberts. To supply an adequate patient basis, Dr. Roberts and Dr. Powell (as clinical professor of neurosurgery since 1948) added the neurosurgical service at Holy Cross and had the good fortune to enlist Dr. Peter Heilbrun in their group. The residency became a reality when the program was accepted in 1972, with Drs. Pedro Arlant of Sao Paulo, Brazil, and Robert Hood as first residents. To date, twenty residents including two women have completed the program and are practicing neurosurgery.

Dr. Roberts' other accomplishments were considerable as well. He introduced retrograde angiography by femoral catheterization. He began microsurgery in the laboratory in the sixties and then took it into the operating room, probably the first in the area to operate on aneurysms under the microscope. He also pioneered transphenoidal pituitary surgery regionally, accumulating finally a series of more than 150 cases. He spearheaded the development of the Brown-Roberts-Wells stereotactic instrument for use with the CT scanner, achieving an accuracy of 1 mm in reaching any intracranial lesion. The instrument was probably the first and is certainly the most widely used such device.

Dr. Roberts moved to Seattle in 1985 and was succeeded by Dr. Heilbrun, who has expanded the department with an active research program. Heilbrun has established the pediatric neurosurgical program with Dr. Jack Walker through the Primary Children's Medical Center and has enlarged the staff, including Dr. Ronald Apfelbaum, of international stature.

The Richard Lende Winter Neurosurgical Conference

In 1970 Dr. Richard Lende, a brilliant young New York neurosurgeon, enlisted a group of colleagues, including Dr. Shelley Chou, formerly of Salt Lake and St. Mark's and now professor and head at the University of Minnesota, for an informal skiing and discussion group. With Alta's incomparable slopes, success was assured. After Dr. Lende's unfortunate death due to anesthesia complications, the group, spearheaded by Drs. Roberts, Heilbrun, and Powell, has grown to a membership of more than 100. Roberts' and Heilbrun's consecutive chairmanship was inherited by Dr. Robert Hood, and the meeting, now based at Snowbird, has become, with its outstanding scientific programs and international attendance, a major annual neurosurgical event.

Utah's Neurosurgical Future

To date thirty-nine neurological surgeons, excluding residents, have practiced in Utah. Of these four are dead, twelve have moved out of state, two are enjoying retirement, and twenty-one continue in active and ever-busier practice. Magnetic resonance imaging is now in many respects superseding computer tomography, revealing even more and earlier lesions. With current advanced surgical techniques, modern instrumentation, with CT and MRI stereotactic guidance, these lesions are being treated earlier, more effectively and with gratifyingly reduced morbidity and mortality. Neurosurgeons no longer are considered optimists treating incurable disease, and with the phenomenal growth of the specialty in Utah, it would seem that Dr. Wright's gloomy prediction to Powell in 1948 that in Utah "there is no room for another neurosurgeon" was an incredible understatement.

The future directions of neurosurgery both generally and in Utah are clearly indicated: continuing advances in neurophysiology and oncology, an ever-expanding diagnostic armamentarium, more exquisite and finely tuned surgical and parasurgical techniques, and remarkable advances in anesthesia. Despite the problem-ridden economics of medicine, the incursion of third-party carriers, the clear trend to ultimate socialization of medical practice, and the pressures of an increasingly litigious society, it is an exhilarating and exciting prospect.

CHAPTER TWENTY-FOUR

Surgical Oncology

LELAND B. COWAN, MD • R. DIRK NOYES, MD

DR. LELAND R. COWAN IS GENERALLY regarded as the first real oncologist in Utah. In the 1920s there was no recognized specialty of oncology; chemotherapy was nonexistent and radiation therapy was in its early development. Most cancer was treated surgically either by general surgeons or general practitioners, few of whom had any specialized training in cancer. Leland R. Cowan opened his Salt Lake City practice in the Medical Arts Building on South Temple Street in 1926, after what for those days was considered an extraordinarily long period of training — five years of postgraduate medical education, including a full cancer residency at the institution now known as Sloan-Kettering Memorial Hospital in New York City. Initially Dr. Cowan did some general surgery and general practice, but by the early 1930s he restricted his practice entirely to cancer and allied diseases. The original training program at Memorial Hospital qualified a physician in both cancer surgery and radiation therapy, so Dr. Cowan could be considered a surgical and a radiation oncologist.

As the pioneering oncologist in the Intermountain area, Dr. Cowan gradually developed an enormous referral base, attracting patients from nearly all the Western states. Although earlier in his career he worked in several hospitals in the area, including St. Mark's and Holy Cross, Cowan's primary hospital was LDS, and in later years he worked exclusively in that institution.

Cowan was known and remembered by all his colleagues for his

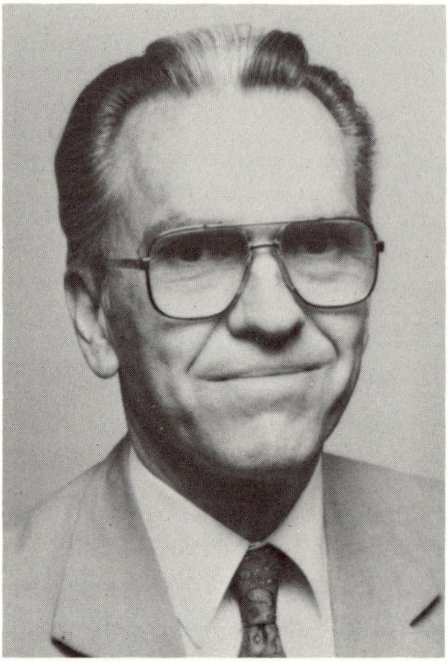
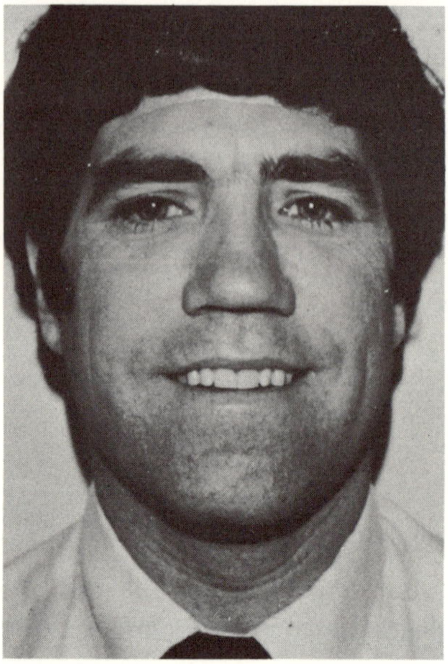

Leland B. Cowan, left, R. Dirk Noyes, right.

prodigious work schedule and long hours. He routinely started his hospital rounds before 5:30 A.M. and was seeing patients in his office from shortly after 6:00 A.M. to 7:00 P.M. or later each day. Throughout his nearly fifty-year practice (until 1976), Dr. Cowan always kept up with medical advances by frequently attending medical meetings, seminars, and postgraduate courses.

In 1964 Dr. Leland B. Cowan joined his father in practice after a residency in surgical oncology at Memorial Hospital which included six months of radiation oncology. A small cobalt unit was installed in their office, and the younger Cowan practiced both surgery and radiation therapy.

Dr. Charles R. Smart, born in Ogden in 1926, graduated from Temple University with an MD degree in 1955. He trained in general surgery until 1961, then completed a cancer fellowship at UCLA in 1961–62 and remained on the faculty there until 1966, when he became the first surgical oncologist at the University of Utah. He established the Intermountain Tumor Registry, a central recording

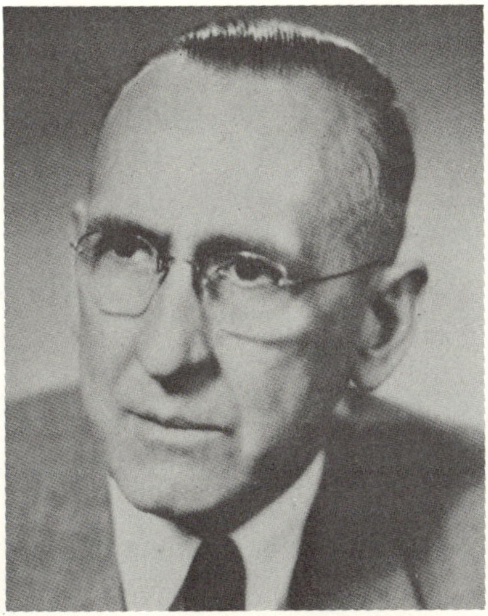

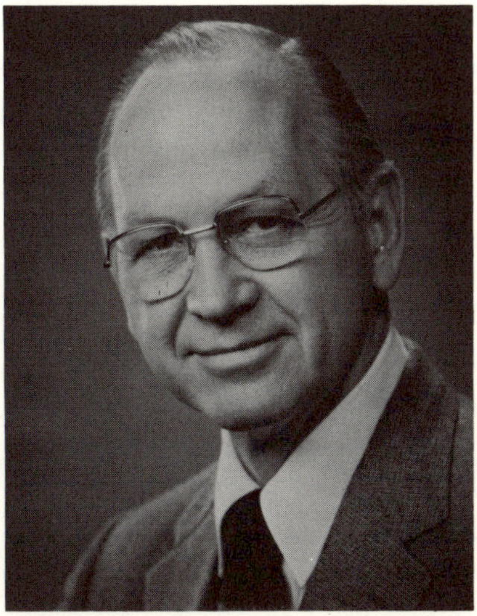

Leland R. Cowan, MD, left, the first "oncologist" in Utah qualified in both surgical oncology and radiation therapy, practiced at LDS Hospital from 1926 to 1976. Charles R. Smart, MD, right, was the pioneer surgical oncologist at the University of Utah Hospital, 1966–69. He moved to LDS Hospital in 1969 and was Chief of Surgery there, 1974–83. Dr. Smart was chief of the early cancer detection branch at the National Cancer Institute, 1983–91.

repository for all cancer cases in the region. The Registry was later expanded into many other states and served as a national model. After the Radiation Center moved to LDS, Smart joined the staff at LDS Hospital in 1969, doing cancer surgery, chemotherapy, and immunotherapy. He was the local pioneer of the isolation and perfusion techniques for the treatment of advanced melanoma. He was promoted to clinical professor of surgery at the University of Utah in 1974 and full-time chief of surgery at LDS Hospital, leaving the clinic.

Dr. Smart and Dr. Merrill L. Wilson, who had a two-and-a-half-year cancer surgery fellowship at Memorial Hospital, formed the Smart-Wilson Cancer Clinic and were joined in 1971 by Dr. Charles B. Edwards, who spent one year at Memorial Hospital and two years at M. D. Anderson Hospital in Houston, Texas, from 1969 to 1971.

In 1973 Smart, Wilson, and Edwards formed with the two Cowans what later became the Leland R. Cowan Cancer Clinic. They were joined by William McCaa as medical oncologist from 1975 to 1979, and in 1977 by Dr. Clyde D. Ford in the same capacity.

From the beginning, Dr. Smart's expertise in chemotherapy added a new dimension to the practice. Shortly after the new clinic was formed, Dr. Cowan, Jr., took a two-and-one-half-year leave of absence to pursue additional training in radiation therapy, after which he took his specialty boards in radiation oncology. Upon his return in 1976, the clinic moved to the Doxey-Hatch Medical Center.

After seven years in the Doxey-Hatch Medical Center on Thirty-ninth South, the clinic moved in 1983 to the Medical Tower adjacent to Cottonwood Hospital. Cowan used a rotational cobalt unit until his retirement in 1990. In 1978 Smart accepted a part-time position as assistant director and later director of the cancer department in the office of the American College of Surgeons in Chicago. He resigned both this appointment and his position as chief of surgery at LDS Hospital in 1983 to become the chief of the Early Cancer Detection Branch of the National Cancer Institute in Washington, D.C.

Dr. H. M. Jackson was another trained general surgeon who did a fellowship at Sloan-Kettering Memorial in New York in 1948, following his Army service, and established a practice at the Intermountain Clinic. As were most early surgically trained oncologists, Jackson was also very comfortable in giving both adjuvant (supplemental) and therapeutic chemotherapy, and he built a very large referral practice of oncologic patients. He also practiced at the LDS Hospital for his surgical procedures and remained an associate of the Intermountain Clinic until his retirement in 1983.

In 1980 Jackson was joined in practice by Dr. R. Dirk Noyes, who had completed a fellowship in surgical oncology and spent one year on staff at M. D. Anderson Hospital, University of Texas in Houston. With the firm establishment of medical oncology as a subspecialty in Utah, Dr. Noyes did not administer chemotherapy in practice with Dr. Jackson, but instead concentrated his efforts in national clinical cancer trials. Through the leadership of Drs. Henry Plenk and Bill Sause, Noyes became active in the Radiation Therapy Oncology Group (RTOG), eventually becoming chair in 1988 of both the GI

Surgery and the Intraoperative Radiation Therapy (IORT) committees of this national cooperative group. Through the efforts of Drs. Sause and Noyes, LDS Hospital became the leading institution in the country for the accrual of patients to the national IORT trials from 1985 to 1989. The many national and international presentations and publications in the field of IORT firmly established LDS Hospital as one of the leaders in clinical research in this evolving, technically challenging, innovative treatment of advanced cancer.

Other physicians noted in the field of surgical oncology in Utah include Dr. William Rees, who did a surgical oncology research year with Dr. Morton at UCLA during his residency. He has contributed significantly to the state oncology program as cancer liaison for the American College of Surgeons since 1985. Dr. Phillip Schneider, who was trained at the National Cancer Institute and recruited to the University in 1985 from the University of California at Davis, had a research interest in surgical approaches to hepatomas. He was lured back to U. C. Davis in 1988 and was replaced in 1990 by Dr. Ben Kim. Dr. Kim, who currently works at the University and whose primary research interest is tumor immunotherapy, came to Utah from Case Western Reserve.

While more and more complicated cancer problems are now referred to surgical oncologists, most cancers are still handled by general surgeons.

CHAPTER TWENTY-FIVE

Orthopedic Surgery

TRUDY McMURRIN • BASED ON CONTRIBUTIONS BY ALFRED M. OKELBERRY, MD • SHERMAN S. COLEMAN, MD • WALLACE E. HESS, MD

WHILE ORTHOPEDICS FACED MANY FAMILIAR challenges as it was differentiated from the general body of medical practice, few of the newer disciplines have had such a significant or immediate impact on so many lives.

The first orthopedic surgeon in Utah was Dr. Samuel C. Baldwin, who joined the staff of the brand-new Dr. William H. Groves' Latter-day Saints' Hospital in 1905 and was able to restrict his practice exclusively to orthopedic surgery by 1914. Born in Louisville, Kentucky, in 1855, Baldwin graduated from Louisville Medical College in 1884 and practiced in Kentucky until 1887, when he moved to Helena, Montana.

Baldwin traveled to observe the work of the outstanding world authorities of the time and was a disciple of Dr. Louis A. Sayre of New York. Sayre, considered the father of orthopedic surgery in the U.S., introduced the practice of prolonged plaster fixation for diseases of the bones and joints. During Dr. Baldwin's medical school days, strips of heavy manila paper impregnated with glue were applied to a patient in successive layers to make a light and effective rigid dressing. When plaster of Paris was introduced, Baldwin became expert in its use. If a body cast was to be worn for a few years, he would sometimes make a celluloid cast. When completed on the mold, the jacket was then cut down the front and hooks applied for lacing so that the cast could be removed for skin care.

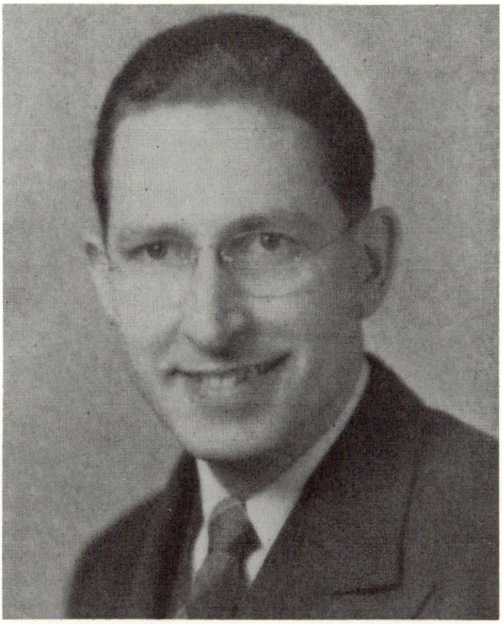

Alfred M. Okelberry.

While Baldwin made it look easy, Dr. Wallace E. Hess well remembers having to sit over a big box of this early powdered plaster, trying to work it into crinoline while rolling the fabric and finding that most of the plaster fell into the water bucket as the roll was dipped.

Dr. Baldwin introduced locally the Bradford Frame, a device for treating deformities of the spine. The frame was rectangular, constructed from water pipe with canvas tightly stretched between the sides and end. Traction on the legs or neck was added in cases of spinal compression. Special attention was given to the patient's general health. When the deformity had been corrected or had become static, a body cast was applied so the patient could be rolled from side to side to improve mobility.

Baldwin had a special interest in the management of tuberculosis of the spine and was skillful in treating chronic osteomyelitis by the Orr method, the most advanced procedure of the day. He had been elected a member of the American Orthopaedic Association in 1903,

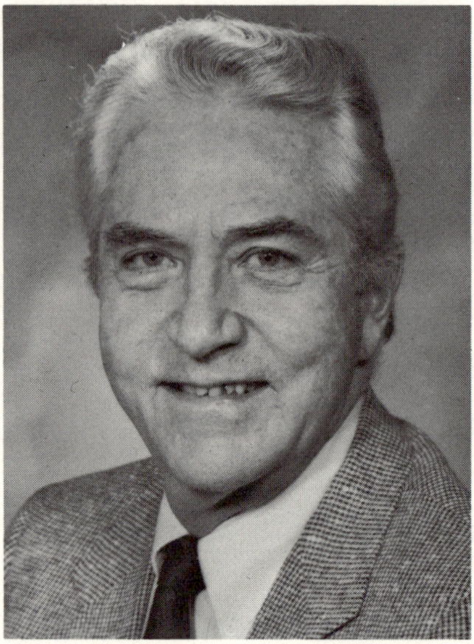

Sherman S. Coleman.

when that group had a limited membership of 100, and Dr. Alfred M. Okelberry remembers his generosity in sharing his national contacts for the benefit of Utah's young surgeons.

Baldwin's work with the young patients at Primary Children's Hospital is considered his most important, followed by his ten-year study of progressive muscular dystrophy, during which he located more than 400 cases in the Intermountain region, the largest number documented in the nation to that time. Dr. Okelberry recalls Baldwin's unselfish devotion to the children and their delight at receiving jelly beans from the distinguished doctor's vest pockets. After his death at eighty-nine in 1944, Dr. Baldwin's studies of muscular dystrophy were continued at the University of Utah School of Medicine.

Dr. Joseph Edgar Tyree, born in Virginia in 1880, had a peripatetic education before his graduation with an MD from Rush Medical College in Chicago in 1906. He spent a year studying pathology under Dr. Gideon Wells, one of the nation's leading pathologists, and later interned under Dr. John B. Murphy, a surgeon of international renown. In 1910 he went west to practice at the Miners' Hospital in Park City,

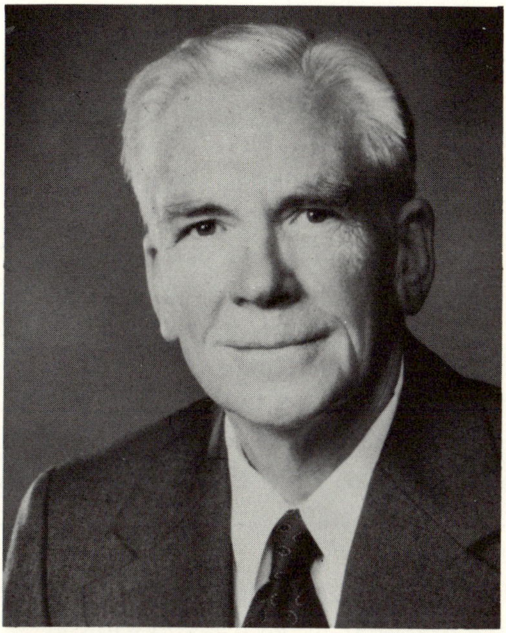

Wallace E. Hess.

Utah. In January of 1915 he was one of six founding members of the Salt Lake Clinic and joined the staff of LDS Hospital.

Patients from throughout the Intermountain region were referred to Dr. Tyree, whose excellent techniques and sound judgment allowed him to specialize more and more. He introduced modern orthopedic surgical methods to Utah — including operative arthrodesis of hip, knee, and spine conditions associated with tuberculosis — and gave the new specialty a boost. Dr. Okelberry remembers Tyree as an outstanding teacher and a fine gentleman as well.

Dr. Alfred M. Okelberry, who received his MD from Harvard in 1934, began general practice in 1935. He took a preceptorship with Dr. G. Gill Richards in internal medicine and with Drs. Baldwin and J. E. Tyree in orthopedic surgery and limited himself to orthopedic surgery from 1941. He was one of the few orthopedists who stayed in Salt Lake City during World War II, and he remained a guiding light in the field until his retirement in 1971. In 1952 he was instrumental in the planning and development of Primary Children's Hospital as a unique medical facility for children. Dr. Okelberry did pioneering work on open reduction of acetabular fractures, and his early experiences were reported at the meeting of the Western Orthopedic Association in 1956. He was well known also for his generous mentoring of the younger physicians entering the orthopedic specialty.

Infections were exceedingly difficult for the orthopedist to treat before the availability of chemotherapeutic and antibiotic agents. Prontosil, neo-Prontosil, sulfanilamide, and sulfathiazole were introduced in the late 1930s, but infections still sometimes lasted for years despite the most careful and imaginative treatment. The first penicillin given in the LDS Hospital was administered in 1943 for a troublesome staphylococcal infection. A thirty-eight-year-old man had suffered a fracture of his upper right femur when a horse fell with him. After other remedies had failed to eradicate the infection that developed around the pins inserted to hold the bones in place, Dr. Okelberry decided to try to obtain the new drug, which was still undergoing clinical trials managed by a committee. The penicillin, paid for by the Sugar House Lions' Club, caused a rapid reduction of the patient's pain and fever, and his overall condition improved quickly.

It was fortuitous that the "wonder drugs" were developed, because these years saw not only the wounds of war but also great increases in industrial activity and motor vehicle traffic. Orthopedic surgery as a specialty was booming. During a five-year period in the early forties, Tyree and Okelberry treated about 750 fractures at LDS Hospital. At night the overworked LDS staff could look across the valley from the top floor and see tracer bullets on the firing range at the Remington Arms ammunition plant.

The shortage of physicians, residents, and interns during the war is legendary. According to Okelberry, some of the secretaries and nurses were drafted to write medical histories and became so skillful that "After reading one of those histories, one could almost arrive at a diagnosis."

When Dr. Paul A. Pemberton arrived in Salt Lake City in 1945, seeking a "kinder climate" for the arthritis he had developed in England during the war, he was the area's only board-certified orthopedist. He had received his MD degree from the University of Oregon in 1929 and completed an orthopedic residency at Cleveland Clinic. Dr. Philip Price, chief of surgery at the University of Utah, saw the chance to institute an orthopedic surgery residency and asked Pemberton to submit a plan. Pemberton developed what he thought was "a dandy" of a proposed residency, but Price declared that there weren't enough hours in the day for such a program. They agreed on a residency that would comprise one year at Salt Lake General Hospital (SLGH), one year at St. Mark's (which included the Shriners' unit), and one year at the old VA Hospital on 12th Avenue. According to Dr. Pemberton, the program was soon approved by the American Board of Orthopaedic Surgery.

Through extensive experience with the Navajo Indians and other patients, Pemberton developed an operative procedure for congenital dislocation of the hip that bears his name. In 1957 he reduced his practice and was succeeded at the Shriners' Hospital and the Medical School by Sherman Coleman, while Dr. Robert Lamb continued with some of the Indian clinics and congenital hip repair at St. Mark's.

Before the development of the Salk and Sabin vaccines in the mid-fifties, summer was known as "polio season," a time of dread for the region's parents. Although more than 200 polio cases occurred in Utah during each of the next five years, it is the epidemic of 1951 that is remembered most. All of the acutely ill were hospitalized at SLGH on Dr. Pemberton's service, with the overflow sent to LDS. Dr. Reed Clegg, who had started practicing at LDS in 1946, treated the young patients there, as well as stricken adults. By his retirement in 1971, Dr. Clegg had served many years as the physician for the University of Utah athletic teams, pioneering in the new area of sports medicine.

An orthopedic residency was begun at the Primary Children's Hospital in 1954, and Dr. Paul R. Milligan was the driving force behind the residency established at LDS Hospital in 1956. Milligan had graduated from the University of Kansas Medical School in 1939 and, following a stint in the military, completed his residency in Chicago in 1948. He and an eight-member staff won approval for their two-year program in 1958, and Dr. Hess recalls that the first resident was Heng Chi Ho, a Taiwanese who later became a four-star general in the Nationalist Chinese air force.

Dr. Wallace E. Hess graduated from Temple University Medical School in Philadelphia in 1943. After serving as battalion surgeon under General George Patton, he completed a hard-to-get residency in orthopedic surgery in Memphis, Tennessee, and New York City in 1950. Hess was director of the orthopedic residency program at LDS Hospital from the early sixties until his retirement in 1983. As the orthopedic service continued to expand rapidly during these years, one of the most important additions, according to Dr. Okelberry, was a clean air room in surgery where hip replacements could be done with greater safety from infection — a facility for which "Dr. Hess worked long and hard."

In 1961 LDS Hospital led the community in its concern for preparedness, establishing a disaster planning committee chaired by Dr. Okelberry. LDS had a full complement of interns and had been reaccredited, but a shortage of nurses and beds was a continuing problem. Dr. Madison H. Thomas arranged for members of the 328th Army Reserve Hospital to participate in a December 5 disaster drill, and the committee further improved the emergency strategy.

The disaster plan proved itself on November 11, 1965, when a jet airliner crashed at Salt Lake International Airport. Dr. Okelberry and other staff members assembled quickly, and the nineteen patients taken to LDS were treated promptly and efficiently. Other patients were admitted to the University, Holy Cross, and St. Mark's. Smoke inhalation injuries required the most care, and all involved were grateful for the specially trained nurses as well as the emergency oxygen equipment. The Disaster Committee continued its drills, updating emergency communications and expanding treatment capabilities.

Another milestone was the creation of a medical-surgical intensive care trauma unit at LDS Hospital in 1976 with the appointment of Dr. Terry Clemmer. An air ambulance service was also initiated, reducing the time from injury to definitive treatment. Life Flight helicopters made 174 flights between July 17 and December 31, 1978, and this number had increased to 575 by 1979, while 140 patients were transported that year by fixed-wing aircraft.

Wartime medical students were frustrated and concerned over whether they belonged in medical school or on the front lines with their friends and relatives. For Sherman S. Coleman, a young Utahn studying at Northwestern Medical School, the problem was solved when the war ended during his junior year. He proceeded to an internship at the Los Angeles County General Hospital and returned to Chicago in 1948 to complete a master's degree in surgical anatomy. His mentor, Dr. Barry J. Anson, helped to shape Coleman's future when the next year he asked him to give the anatomical portion of the American Board of Orthopaedic Surgery's certifying examination as his surrogate. "What a stroke of fate!" says Coleman, who had planned a career in general surgery.

The surgical residency programs were reserved for newly discharged medical officers, so Coleman accepted an appointment to teach the surgical basic science program at Northwestern, where he was tutored and inspired by great orthopedists Clinton L. and Edward L. Compere and Sam W. Banks. In 1951 Coleman eagerly volunteered to serve on a "surgical team" in Korea, but while he was stationed at Camp LeJeune in North Carolina, at home in Chicago his oldest son fell victim to the nation's last great polio epidemic, and the young orthopedist experienced the psychological ravages and uncertainty of acute poliomyelitis and lengthy recovery firsthand.

The Navy stationed Coleman in Indianapolis, where he pursued his anatomical studies. After the war, he took a residency at Northwestern in orthopedic surgery, the last year of which he spent in Salt Lake City at Primary Children's Hospital. Prompted by the inspiration of Dr. Okelberry, he began his sustained interest in the early diagnosis of congenital dysplasia and dislocation of the hip.

When Dr. Coleman was offered the position of chief of staff of the Shriners' Hospital and the chair of the University's orthopedic surgery division in 1957, he willingly returned home after fourteen years away. Soon he was offered the American British Canadian Traveling Fellowship, and with several colleagues toured Scotland

and England, where his interest in leg lengthening was kindled. A Mr. W. A. Anderson had devised the technique of performing essentially a closed osteoclasis of the tibia utilizing a "karate" blow to a midtibia weakened by multiple drilling. Coleman practiced this technique for several years, reporting that "in later efforts my fifth metacarpal informed me that in some instances too few drill holes had been made in the tibia prior to the osteoclasis!"

The move to Utah had offered a chance for Coleman to develop his interest in pediatric orthopedics, and beginning in 1960 he made a two-day visit every month for three years to the Navajo Reservation in the Four Corners area, where ultimately he examined more than 2,000 newborn infants. The incidence of abnormal hips was about 5%, so he evaluated and treated a great number of children with dysplasia.

By the late sixties, despite expansion of the hospitals' orthopedic staffs, "the writing was on the wall," in Dr. Hess's words, that residencies without University affiliation would not survive. Coleman was chair of the Educational Committee, and under his leadership the residency became "The University of Utah, LDS Hospital and Affiliated Hospitals Orthopedic Residency." The directors of orthopedic training were Drs. Coleman for the University and Shriners', Hess for LDS, William S. Allred for Primary Children's, John N. Henrie for Holy Cross, Albert C. Martin for St. Mark's, and Andrew C. Ruoff for the VA.

By 1970 the residency was fully integrated. The efforts of many skilled and dedicated people were involved, but Coleman's colleagues give him the lion's share of credit for developing the affiliated residency into one of the most sought-after in the country. This tradition has been continued and enlarged upon since 1981 by Coleman's successor, Dr. Harold K. Dunn.

Utah orthopedists also have established a tradition of involvement with and recognition by major professional organizations. In 1976 Coleman was elected president of the American Orthopaedic Association (AOA). He was a founding member of the Pediatric Orthopaedic Society, a Trustee of the Orthopaedic Research and Education Foundation (OREF), a member of the American Board of Orthopedic Surgeons, and the A. R. Shands lecturer for the AOA in 1985. Hess served two terms on the Board of Councilors of the American Academy of Orthopedic Surgeons (AAOS) and capped a distinguished career as president of the Western Orthopedic Association in 1983.

Orthopedics has benefited from significant technological improvements through the years. Between 1977 and 1983, the average stay for orthopedic procedures dropped from 8 to 5.2 days, a trend which continues.

Recently, much excitement has been generated by the arthroscopic techniques developed by Provo surgeon Dr. Robert W. Metcalf. His seminars on the subject have been in great demand nationally. Metcalf was the athletic team physician for Brigham Young University for many years before joining the staff of the University of Utah, where he has taught arthroscopy to many residents. The method for introducing a small fiberoptic scope into the knee joint through minimal incisions, taking photographs or movies, and repairing cartilage and ligaments has been just one of the recent revolutionary changes in surgical techniques, matched only by the total replacement of hips and even more recently of knee joints.

One of Metcalf's colleagues, Dr. Thomas D. Rosenberg, developed an x-ray technique for recognizing early degenerative changes in the knee. Dr. Lonnie Paulos and others of the younger generation are making orthopedic history in sports medicine and keeping the spotlight on developments in Utah.

Mark H. Greene, Jr. was the pioneer hand surgeon in Utah. After completing his training in orthopedic and hand surgery at Los Angeles County Hospital–USC, he joined Doctors Pemberton and Lamb at St. Mark's Hospital in 1956. From 1957 to 1990 he staffed a hand clinic at Shriners' Hospital, where orthopedic residents rotated for three months. Since 1982 he limited his practice to hand surgery. When he joined the Society for Hand Surgeons in 1962 it had only 40 members.

In 1989 the total number of orthopedic surgeons practicing in the state was 110. As this number grows, so do the contributions and accomplishments of the practitioners of this highly visible and gratifying medical discipline.

CHAPTER TWENTY-SIX

Otolaryngology — Head and Neck Surgery

JAMES L. PARKIN, MD, MS

THE PRACTICE OF OTOLARYNGOLOGY HAS CHANGED dramatically during the past century, and especially in the past twenty-five years, because of research with new drugs, equipment, and surgical procedures. Review of the otolaryngology literature of the early twentieth century reveals an emphasis on infectious diseases of the head and neck. The complications of otitis media such as mastoiditis, meningitis, brain abscess or lateral sinus thrombosis, rarely encountered now, were then significant factors in pediatric and adult morbidity and mortality. Anatomical and surgical research reported on the fascial planes of the neck and the treatment of abscesses of the head and neck.

With the development of effective antimicrobial agents such as penicillin and sulfa, many thought that the need for otolaryngologists would diminish, and indeed training positions decreased in the late forties and early fifties. The development of microsurgery, head and neck oncology, and advances in nasal and sinus surgery rejuvenated the specialty, however.

Before World War II, most otolaryngologists trained as EENT (Eye, Ear, Nose and Throat) specialists. The formal training often consisted of one year of post-medical school experience with six months each in ophthalmology and otolaryngology. Many specialists went to Europe for training at leading institutions for one or more years.

The American Board of Otolaryngology was the second Board established for the certification of specialists. The training period

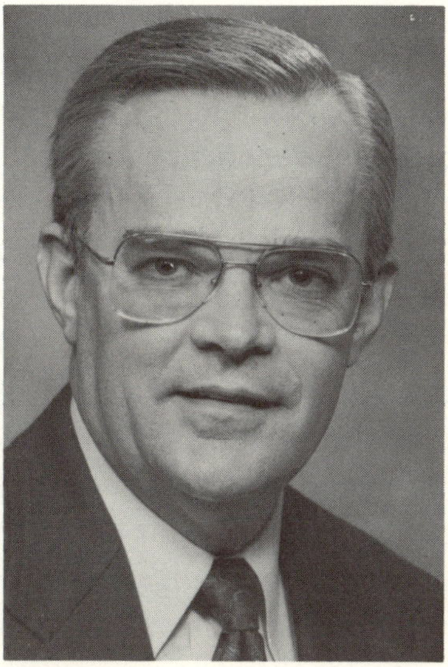

James L. Parkin.

required for eligibility for Board examination increased slowly and has fluctuated through the years. Five years of postgraduate training are now required to qualify for examination, one year of which must be in general surgery and three years in otolaryngology. The additional year is left to the discretion of the department chair.

National and state specialty societies were usually joint ophthalmology-otolaryngology groups. In 1978 the American Academy of Otolaryngology was established after separating from the American Academy of Ophthalmology and Otolaryngology. The Utah Oto-Ophthalmological Society followed the national example shortly thereafter, with separate ophthalmological and otolaryngological societies.

The specialty underwent many internal debates regarding its name. Confusion is reflected in the variety of names attached to academic departments and divisions throughout the country: otolaryngology, otorhinolaryngology, otolaryngology and maxillofacial surgery, head and neck surgery, otolaryngology and communicative disorders, and many more. In 1982, after much debate within the Academy, the membership voted to change the name to otolaryngology — head and neck surgery. The division in the Department of Surgery at the University of Utah followed this example, and the name was formally changed to Otolaryngology–Head and Neck Surgery.

Many patients recall the experience, especially in rural areas, of otolaryngology procedures performed in doctors' offices and even on kitchen tables. With the development of new anesthesia techniques, increasing awareness of safety during surgical procedures, and the development of better facilities, otolaryngologic procedures were shifted from the home and office to the hospital and now, to some extent, to the outpatient surgical center. The development of non-flammable anesthetic agents which replaced ether, cyclopropane, chloroform, and other flammable agents allowed for the safe use of electrocautery techniques during surgery which have diminished postsurgical bleeding problems in common procedures such as adeno-tonsillectomy.

Before the development of antibiotics, mastoidectomy was a much more commonly performed procedure. From the 1920s to the 1940s, mastoidectomies were usually performed with a hammer and chisel. The procedure consisted of removing the mastoid cortex and establishing drainage to a coalescent mastoid infection. Use of the operating microscope in otolaryngology was pioneered in Sweden and subsequently by prominent ear surgeons in the United States, including Lempert, Shambaugh, and House. High-powered electric drills and air drills were developed which enhanced the speed and completeness of mastoid surgery when performed under the microscope. The development and refinement of better anesthetics and improved microscopes, drills, and other microsurgical instruments has greatly increased the complexity of otologic and neuro-otologic procedures undertaken by the modern otolaryngologist.

Newer techniques for evaluating the hearing mechanism have improved the otolaryngologist's diagnostic abilities. Audiological equipment has progressed from the tuning fork to pure tone audiometers, speech audiometers, brain stem–evoked response audiometry, electrocochleography, and tympanometry, to name a few instruments and techniques. Improved radiological imaging from plain films to tomography, contrast studies, computerized axial tomography, and magnetic resonance imaging has also enhanced the otolaryngologist's diagnostic accuracy.

As otolaryngologists have become more involved in the treatment of malignant lesions of the head and neck region, they are dependent upon developments in other fields, including pathology, anesthesiology, diagnostic and therapeutic radiology, and medical oncology. The application of laser technology in the head and neck region has been pioneered at the University of Utah under the leadership of John A. Dixon. Roy Kim Davis and James L. Parkin continue research in this important scientific area.

Probably the greatest change in operative technology in the past five years is in surgery of the paranasal sinuses. Development of special fiberoptic endoscopes has led to new techniques with reduced morbidity.

Surgery of the larynx has also changed dramatically in the past twenty-five years. With the development of suspension laryngoscopy instrumentation and microscope applications in laryngeal surgery, microsurgery of the larynx can now be performed safely. Marriage of the laser to this technology has further enhanced laryngeal surgery.

Otolaryngologists have long been involved in the care of maxillofacial trauma, with nasal fractures still one of the most common traumas seen in emergency rooms. The development of facial plating systems has improved precision and resulted in the treatment of more complex maxillary and mandibular fractures.

With an affluent, aging American population, more patients are interested in cosmetic surgery. The otolaryngologist — head and neck surgeon has been influential in the development of cosmetic surgical procedures. Many otolaryngologists take post-residency fellowships in head and neck plastic and reconstructive surgery to refine their skills. The American Academy of Facial Plastic and Reconstructive Surgery has been formed to promote education, foster research, and assist residents and surgeons interested in this aspect of the specialty. Some have also chosen to subspecialize in pediatric otolaryngology, and post-residency fellowships are available.

Utah in the Early Days

Early Utah physicians did little or no specializing. Dr. Samuel L. Brick opened an office in Ogden in 1886 and practiced EENT for the next thirty years. At about the same time, Dr. Ira A. E. Lyons was listed in the Salt Lake directory as an oculist and aurist from 1911 to 1931. These men did eye surgery for cataracts, strabismus, and external eye infections, but the extent of their ENT surgery is not known.

In Salt Lake City and Ogden, the beginning of the twentieth century saw the first specialists who really did anything comparable to modern otolaryngology. Most of the physicians who limited themselves to this specialty were general practitioners who had gone to Vienna or Berlin to take additional training.

In 1898 Dr. Leslie W. Snow opened his office in Salt Lake City as an EENT man and continued practicing until his death in 1936. In 1903 Dr. Fred Stauffer started his Salt Lake City EENT practice and was joined by his son, Dr. F. Leaver Stauffer, in 1925. Dr. Leaver Stauffer was highly respected for his ear, nose and throat and bronchoscopy work. William Donoher began an EENT practice in 1906 and continued until he moved to California a year before his death in 1936. During most of that time he limited himself to ENT and thus probably was the first pure otolaryngologist in the state.

At about the time Dr. Donoher came to Salt Lake City, Dr. Robert R. Hampton opened a practice limited to EENT and confined himself to both specialties until 1921, when Dr. E. M. Neher returned from Europe and took over the ophthalmology that was done in their office. Dr. Hampton did a fine grade of otolaryngology until his death at sixty-five in 1940. Following Dr. Hampton's death, Dr. James A. Cleary came from Nebraska and practiced ENT at Holy Cross Hospital until his death in 1964.

The Specialty Comes of Age

The separation of ENT from EENT began in Salt Lake City when two general practitioners, A. Ray Irvine and A. J. Ridges, went to Europe for special training. Dr. Irvine returned in 1910 and did EENT work. Dr. Ridges returned from Berlin, where he had received exceptionally good training with Gustav E. Killian, and from 1915 until he retired in 1949 he did ENT exclusively.

Meanwhile, in Provo, Eldon D. Clark and Stanley M. Clark practiced EENT from 1921 until about 1964. In the 1970s and 1980s the availability of otolaryngology specialty services expanded throughout central and southern Utah. Dr. Jerry Marsden began practice in St. George, Utah. Dr. David Hilding, a prominent academician from Yale and the University of Illinois, established a practice in Price, Utah. Drs. Robert Arbon, Randal Gibb, William Nelson, Robert Peterson, Steven Rowley, and others established practices in the Provo area.

In northern Utah, the early otolaryngologists included Drs. Charles Coulson, Rich Pugmire, Clinton Leroy Pugmire, Ralph W. Pugmire, J. Dwight Harding, Glen F. Harding, Clarence Charles Hetzel, Sr., and Clarence Charles Hetzel II. Dr. Hetzel, Sr., was typical of Utah's early EENT specialists; although he had a demanding practice, he found the time and energy to serve his family and his community and was active in local and national specialty and medical societies.

Like many other early physicians and otolaryngologists, Clarence Charles Hetzel II, Dr. Hetzel's son, followed in his father's footsteps, pursuing a medical education and specialty training in EENT. Dr. Hetzel, with many other Utah physicians, served in the Armed Forces during World War II. He returned to Ogden to resume practice with his father.

D. Wilson Hales came to Ogden in 1952 and did the first otologic microsurgery in 1950. Cache Valley depended upon Ogden and Salt Lake City specialists for otolaryngology care until Douglas B. Hart located his practice in Logan.

Early in 1943 Dr. Samuel Crowe, chair of the Department of Otolaryngology at Johns Hopkins Medical School, was asked to recommend a candidate for academic otolaryngology at the University of Utah. Dr. David A. Dolowitz, who was completing his training at Johns Hopkins in 1943, was offered a part-time clinical teaching position and a private practice opportunity by Dr. Philip Price. In

September Dr. Dolowitz came to Salt Lake City and purchased a home. Three days after he started work, the Army asked him to take the place of an incapacitated otolaryngologist in one of the Johns Hopkins field units. Dolowitz obtained leave of absence from Dean Callister and went overseas to serve in the South Pacific, returning to Salt Lake City in 1946.

Many Utah otolaryngologists who served during the war returned to practice in Utah at about the same time, and office space was very difficult to find. Dr. Robert G. Snow found space in a remodeled automobile showroom, where he stayed until a medical building was constructed on Fifth East and South Temple. He joined the Salt Lake Clinic in 1959. Dr. Dolowitz opened an office in the basement of his home on Gilmer Drive and practiced there until an office was built on the corner of First South and Ninth East.

At first Dr. Dolowitz had difficulty being accepted by the otolaryngology community. In those days a meeting of the Salt Lake Medical Society was held every month; a scientific session was followed by a business meeting. When Dr. Dolowitz attended his first meeting, Dr. Ridges presented the case of a woman in her eighties, a Mrs. Day from Idaho. She was presented as a case of osteomyelitis of the frontal bone with cardiac fibrillation. Because of her cardiac problems she was considered inoperable. Dr. Dolowitz was asked to review the case to see if the new University professor had anything to add. The x-rays showed not only osteomyelitis but a carcinoma in the middle of the frontal bone, and he recommended frontal sinus surgery. Dr. Hans Hecht, a cardiologist at the University, agreed to try to get the patient in sufficient cardiac status to withstand surgery. Dr. Dolowitz subsequently removed a thick portion of the frontal bone and made a primary closure; pathology confirmed the carcinoma. The patient had a successful recovery with eradication of her tumor. The case became well known in the community and helped to establish Dolowitz's reputation.

Limited at first to providing lectures to third-year students and outpatient clinical instruction to fourth-year students, the University's Division of Otolaryngology grew slowly. Specialists in the community provided excellent support for the otolaryngology clinics held at the old Salt Lake General Hospital (SLGH) at Twenty-first South and State streets, and many assisted in lecturing the medical students as well. Dr. Robert Snow aided Dr. Dolowitz in setting up guidelines for both the clinics and the lectures. Dr. Ralph Rigby established an endoscopy clinic and was available on an emergency basis to remove foreign bodies. Drs. Leon Saunders, James Cleary, Earl Phillips, Whitney Haight, Mowatt Muirhead, and William Beck all gave unselfishly of their time and effort.

Membership in national societies was not always available to Western and particularly Intermountain otolaryngologists. When Dr. Dolowitz applied for membership to the Triological Society (Laryngological, Rhinological and Otological), his application was tabled for three consecutive years. Finally, he was permitted to meet with the Society's executive council and was told that because Salt Lake City was merely an oasis in the desert, they did not think they should take a member from that area. Dr. Dolowitz persuaded them to allow him to discuss research papers presented at the annual meeting. He discussed two in detail, which apparently impressed the executive council, and his membership application was accepted. He went on to serve as a vice president of the National Triological Society and president of its Western section. Other Utah practitioners who have been accepted into this society include Drs. Roy Kim Davis, Wilson Hales, David Hilding, James L. Parkin, Michael Stevens, Gary Thomas, and Dean Zobell. An additional honor awarded Dr. Dolowitz was his selection as an active member of the American Otological Society; other Utah members include David Hilding and James Parkin.

Dr. Dolowitz established a residency training program at the University in 1963, and the first to complete it was Glen Lund, who finished in 1967. The program has trained many Utah otolaryngologists, including Drs. Craig W. Anderson, Richard Aoki, Marsden Blanch, Boyd Cole, Paul Doxey, Keith Finlayson, Ronald Gordon, Arlen Heiny, Leland Johnson, Garner Meads, Jr., William Nelson, Barry Nielsen, Richard Nielsen, and Michael Stevens. Other graduates have established their practices elsewhere.

In the mid-1960s Dr. Dolowitz recruited Gary K. Thomas from Temple University in Philadelphia to join him on the full-time faculty at the University. When Dr. Dolowitz resigned in 1967, Dr. Thomas became chair of the division. Dr. Gary McCandless was recruited as head of audiology. In 1972 Dr. James Parkin was recruited from the University of Washington to join the division faculty. When Dr. Thomas decided to return to his native Idaho to practice in 1974, Dr. Parkin was named chair of otolaryngology. He received his medical school education at the University of Utah, with internship, residency, and fellowship in auditory neurophysiology at the University of Washington.

More faculty members were recruited to meet the increasing needs of the otolaryngology division. Dr. Michael Stevens completed his otolaryngology training at the University of Utah and became a full-time faculty member. Dr. Leland Johnson obtained his medical education at Cornell University in New York and his otolaryngology training at the University of Utah, where he too joined the full-time faculty.

In 1985 Roy Kim Davis was running the Head and Neck Service at Walter Reed Army Hospital in Washington, D.C. A graduate of the University of Utah Medical School, he had received his residency training at Madigan Army Hospital and his head and neck oncology fellowship in Boston under Dr. Stuart Strong. Dr. Davis was recruited by Utah because of his special expertise in head and neck oncology. Dr. Steven Gray, son of Salt Lake otolaryngologist Dean Gray, completed his residency training at the University of Iowa. He did a pediatric otolaryngology fellowship under Dr. Robin Cotton in Cincinnati, Ohio, and returned to the faculty of the University of Iowa. Dr. Gray was recruited as a full-time pediatric otolaryngologist in 1990.

Through generous contributions of former patients, colleagues, and Dr. Dolowitz himself, the Dolowitz Lectureship in Otolaryngology was established at the University of Utah in 1987 to bring a prominent otologist or neurotologist to Utah each year for continued education.

The Division of Otolaryngology has been active in many research areas. Dr. Dolowitz is a recognized pioneer in understanding vestibular physiology, utilizing corticosteroids in otolaryngology, and identifying hereditary factors in sensorineural hearing loss. Evidence for the University's eminence in laser research, pioneered by Dr. John Dixon, was given when the Smithsonian Institution asked the University to prepare a public exhibit in Washington, D.C., for the twenty-fifth anniversary of laser technology.

Dr. Kim Davis has been recognized through a clinical investigator development award from the National Institutes of Health. His research has centered around head and neck oncology topics, and in cooperation with the Rocky Mountain Tumor Registry, he has published series dealing with various types of head and neck cancer.

A frontier of otolaryngology research in the last twenty years has been the area of cochlear implantation — technology designed to restore meaningful hearing to profoundly deaf individuals. The cochlear implant project at the University of Utah was established in 1972 as a joint project with Dr. Derald Brackmann of the House Otologic Medical Group of Los Angeles. A multichannel cochlear implant device was developed by the University of Utah's artificial organs division and implanted in the first patient by Dr. Brackmann in 1975. After the project was separated from the Otologic Medical Group, research continued at the University, where the Ineraid cochlear implant was developed. Otologic surgeons from many countries have been trained in the implantation of this device, which is recognized as one of the most successful multichannel cochlear implant systems in the world.

The town-and-gown relationship in Utah remains strong. Many practicing otolaryngologists continue to play important roles in the educational activities of the Division of Otolaryngology at the University. Dr. Robert Ferguson served for many years as director of education for otolaryngology at Holy Cross Hospital. He has been succeeded in this effort by Dr. Richard Nielsen. Dr. Glen Lund was instrumental in developing an otolaryngology residency position at the Primary Children's Medical Center. Many of the community otolaryngologists have provided time and effort in supervising the residents in surgery and the clinics at the Veterans Administration Hospital.

Space does not permit recognition of many other individuals who have played crucial roles in the development of otolaryngology in the state of Utah.

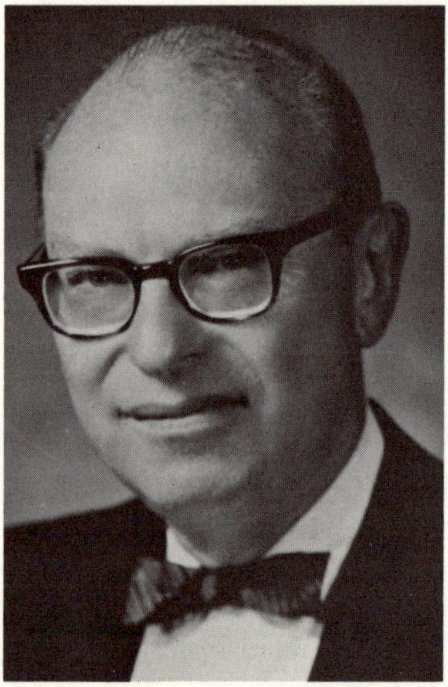

David A. Dolowitz, MD, pioneer otolaryngologist at the University of Utah Medical School. Recruited in 1943, he took a leave to serve in a Johns Hopkins Hospital unit in World War II. Returning in 1946, he became the first professor and head of the division until his resignation in 1967. A Dolowitz Lectureship was initiated in 1987.

Acknowledgments

This chapter would not have been possible without the significant assistance of Drs. Robert G. Snow, D. Wilson Hales, and David A. Dolowitz. These individuals not only were significant players in the history of otolaryngology in Utah, they also took the time to record for review and use their thoughts and remembrances, which have been incorporated in this chapter. I express my deepest appreciation to them.

CHAPTER TWENTY-SEVEN

Ophthalmology

DEAN SPEAR, MD

THE FIRST MEDICINE IN UTAH was practiced by the Indians. Their armamentarium consisted principally of herbs, roots, leaves, bark, and berries, from which they brewed tea and tonics, salves, and poultices. These were supplemented by rituals and dances.

Dr. Robert M. Christiansen writes in the *Utah Medical Bulletin* of July 1968: "As the pioneers began to settle in Utah, the mid-wife's cure for eyewater began to replace the Indian's cures." Quacks soon appeared, claiming "particular attention at all times, paid to surgery, and diseases of the eyes."

"After the appearance of the railroad, cinders from locomotives became a problem," writes Christiansen. "At least one frontier physician criticized train crews who carried cocaine and used a sharpened match or the point of a knife to remove cinders."

The first trained ophthalmologist in Utah was a woman — Dr. Romania Bunnell Pratt. Born in Indiana in 1839, she emigrated to Utah with her mother in 1855. She married the son of Mormon Church leader Parley P. Pratt in 1859 and had a number of children. While the youngest was still an infant, upon the advice of Brigham Young she went east to study medicine.

Financial difficulties interrupted her studies, but, with Young's aid, Pratt graduated from the Women's Medical College in Philadel-

Note: This essay is based on extensive research by Dr. Robert Hales, whose premature death prevented him from completing his assignment.

phia in 1877. Four years later she went to New York City to take courses in diseases of the eye and ear under Dr. Benjamin B. Noyes. She returned to Salt Lake City and did general practice with a special interest in eye, ear, nose and throat. She was undoubtedly the first doctor in Utah to remove a cataract.

Many of the pioneer specialists practiced both ear, nose and throat (ENT) and Eye (EENT). Dr. A. Ray Irvine went to Vienna in 1910 for a course in EENT, followed by training in Eye at the Wills Eye Hospital in Philadelphia. He joined the newly formed Salt Lake Clinic in 1915 and can be considered the state's first true ophthalmologist. He moved to Los Angeles in 1921, becoming the "Dean of Ophthalmology" there and the founder of a family of nationally known ophthalmologists. The next pure "eye man" was Dr. E. M. Neher, who was the first Utahn to be certified by the American Board of Ophthalmology and the first and only one elected to the prestigious American Ophthalmologic Society, which requires publication of one's scientific experiments.Dr. Neher kept a number of rattlesnakes caged in his basement and proved that a membrane, now known as the eye cap, extends over the cornea and is shed when the snake sheds its skin.

Dr. Horace Merrill was the first to limit himself to Eye in Provo but moved to San Diego in 1935. Dr. L. Weston Oaks took the reins in Provo, limiting his practice to Eye after taking courses in Vienna and Berlin in 1935. In 1967 his nephew Merrill Oaks took over his surgical practice.

Most of those doing ophthalmology in Utah were physicians who had tired of the rigors of general practice or were dissatisfied with their proficiency. The vast majority of those who converted to ophthalmological practice also did ear, nose and throat, and this was the rule throughout the United States, the strict ophthalmologists being located in the large cities until about World War II. As an illustration, the 1939 financial report of the Utah Oto-Ophthalmological Society indicates approximately thirty members practicing in the state, of whom only two were doing ENT and four doing Eye exclusively. All the rest did both.

Bascom Palmer was raised in South Carolina, trained under Dr.

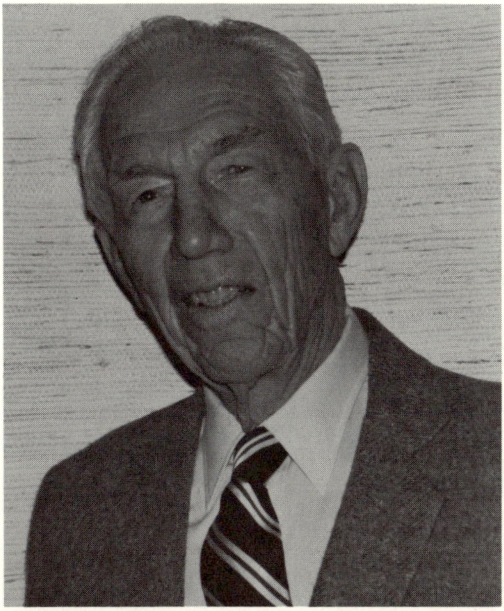

Dean Spear.

Frank Birch in Minneapolis–St. Paul, and entered the office of Dr. Robert R. Hampton in Salt Lake City about 1933. Dr. Palmer was board-certified and practiced ophthalmology exclusively. He was ambitious, cocky, and enjoyed a good time. Early in his practice he traveled to Nevada, examined patients, and arranged for their surgery in Salt Lake City. With his outgoing personality and competence, he soon established a large surgical practice. Even after the war, when many well-trained ophthalmologists were practicing in Salt Lake City, he continued to perform most of the cataract extractions in the city until he retired in 1961 at the age of fifty-nine. His secretary of many years says that he retired because he disliked the intrusions of government into the practice of medicine. He was chief of the ophthalmology division at the University of Utah College of Medicine from the early forties to about 1955.

After doing general practice in Nevada for nine years, Dr. Everett Muir spent three years in an ophthalmology residency and joined Dr.

E. M. Neher in 1939. Shortly thereafter, he joined the U.S. Army. By the time of Muir's return to civilian life, Dr. Neher had died and his office had been taken over by Dr. Charles Ruggeri. Dr. Muir then joined Dr. Palmer.

In Ogden no one dominated the field of ophthalmology as Bascom Palmer did in Salt Lake City and Weston Oaks in Provo. Glen Harding had three years of training in ophthalmology and started practicing in Ogden in 1940. He was called to active duty in 1942 and gained considerable experience in the U.S. Army, returning to Ogden in 1946.

Dr. Ralph Pugmire began an eye practice in Ogden in 1942. Oliver Richards began his practice in 1959 and did a great deal of surgery. In 1942–43 Dee Hospital recorded sixty surgical eye cases, compared with six in 1927.

In 1960 Dr. Louis Snider moved from Salt Lake City to Ogden and continues to practice there.

Winn Richards, who served a term in the Utah Legislature, Robert Brodstein, and Phillip Hale formed a partnership and in the latter half of the seventies performed a large number of cataract extractions with the insertion of intra-ocular lenses. At first extra-capsular extractions with iris-supported lenses were performed. At a scientific meeting a different type of lens was advocated, and the three partners began to use it with drastic results. The implants, all from the same manufacturer, were used in twenty-four cases, of which thirteen developed what came to be known as the UGH syndrome — uveal erosion, glaucoma, and hyphema. Six or seven of these patients had to have the implants removed. Microscopic examination of the lenses removed revealed extreme roughness. The symptoms gradually cleared in most of the patients, and all of the removed lenses were eventually replaced with lenses from a different supplier.

Robert H. Hales finished a three-year residency at the University of California in San Francisco and returned home to Provo in 1963. He staffed the Low Vision Clinic in Salt Lake City under the Division of the Visually Handicapped, whose chairman was Fred Whitney. He gave lectures to sophomore medical students on physical diagnosis of the eye and conducted the Wednesday afternoon clinic for several years after the Division of Ophthalmology was established under Dr. Henry VanDyk. He also published a textbook on contact lenses.

Dr. Hales became active in Medical Society affairs, serving on various committees and as president of the Utah State Medical Association, the Cordes Medical Society (an association of former University of California residents), and the Utah Ophthalmological Society.

Hales and Merrill Oaks performed the first two lens implants in Utah in 1975 and assisted each other with more. During the latter half of the seventies, Hales and Oaks in Provo and Winn Richards and Robert Brodstein in Ogden did a large number of lens implants, seeming to promote the procedure more aggressively than the ophthalmologists in Salt Lake City.

At the end of World War II, four eye men practiced in Salt Lake City: Bascom Palmer, Rowland Merrill, and Charles Ruggeri had arrived before the war, and Dean Spear came from Northwestern early in 1945. Alan Crandall, Sr., soon arrived, following his training at the University of Pennsylvania. In addition to his private practice, he contracted for eye care for the employees of the Utah Copper Company.

In 1947 Homer Smith began an illustrious career. He has been president of the Salt Lake County and Utah State Medical Associations, executive secretary and president of the Pacific Coast Oto-Ophthalmological Society, a member of numerous committees and ultimate Guest of Honor of the American Academy of Ophthalmology, secretary of the Board of Governors of the American College of Surgeons, and a member of the Joint Commission on Accreditation of Hospitals. These assignments and more were carried out while Dr. Smith conducted a busy private practice.

Dr. Richard Sonntag began practice in Salt Lake City in 1950 after a year of general practice and four years of eye training at Temple University Medical School. One of his early cataract patients was David O. McKay — the president of the Mormon Church. Thereafter cataract patients flocked to Sonntag, many wanting to be operated on by the same surgeon who had successfully operated on President

McKay. Dr. Sonntag served a term as president of the Salt Lake County Medical Association and a year as president of the LDS Hospital staff. He worked long hours with little time off and is still conducting a limited practice after thirty-nine years.

Orson White has been curious all his life. When he was a resident at the University of California in San Francisco, the etiology of retrolental fibroplasia, the greatest cause of childhood blindness, was still unknown. White, interested in deep sea diving, was aware of the toxic effects of oxygen. He presented a paper at a Cordes Society Meeting. Three and a half years later White's theory was confirmed. He wrote the chapter on optics and refraction in the standard textbook of Vaughn and Ashbury, where he offers mathematical proof that the cornea is not a structure of refraction, as has long been held, but merely forms the anterior surface of the aqueous, which then becomes a major source of refraction. He has conducted studies on the penetration of a missile passing from one medium into another, during which he shot a bullet into an artificial vitreous of Karo syrup.

Dr. White performed the first corneal transplant in Utah in 1955. After combatting unwarranted political stumbling blocks, he founded the first eye bank in 1972 with funds contributed by the Salt Lake Exchange Club and later by the Utah Lions Club. In 1974 the Eye Bank received twenty-two eyes. In 1986 it received 452 eyes, supplying corneas for 372 transplants. Those not used for transplants were used for research and teaching.

Andrew W. Lyle graduated from the Baylor University College of Medicine in Baltimore and in 1970 served a third year as senior resident at the University of Utah. As the only resident in the new program under Dr. VanDyk, Lyle was able to do a lot of surgery. After a short, unhappy affiliation with Drs. Quinn and Tanner, he set out on his own. His self-confidence, ambition, and deft technique soon won him a large surgical practice. He operated upon retinal pathology, glaucoma, and cataracts. He founded the Eye Institute of Utah and advertised it extensively on television. Though many questioned his judgment, no one questioned his surgical ability. His van met patients at the Salt Lake airport who had flown in from all over the Intermountain region to be operated on in his own operative suite. He incurred the animosity of the ophthalmic surgeons in the Salt Lake area, who accused him of unethical conduct, including returning surgical patients to the referring optometrists for postoperative care.

Dr. Keith Gates received an MD from the University of Utah in 1947. After serving in the Air Force he did general practice in Logan for two years, went to the University of Michigan for an eye residency, and returned to Logan as the only eye man there until Russell Warren joined him in 1976. Dr. Gates served one term in the Utah State Legislature, during which he incurred the wrath of the Medical School officials by introducing a bill (which was defeated) to reduce the number of medical students.

Russell Warren, after serving a three-year residency at the University of Iowa, began practicing in Logan in 1975.

Utah Ophthalmologic Society

The date of the first recorded Utah Ophthalmologic Society meeting was 1931, and the meeting format remained unchanged for many years. Interested physicians gathered at a Salt Lake City hotel or private club dining area, enjoying a congenial, relaxing time before having dinner. A discussion of business problems was followed by a scientific meeting where members or guests presented papers.

At the November 1941 meeting, the Department of Public Welfare submitted a fee schedule listing $5.00 for a refraction and $100.00 for a cataract extraction. The most spirited discussion concerned the practice of an optical company giving rebates to physicians who wrote prescriptions for their glasses. This common, but shady, practice prevailed for many years. One of the members supported the idea because it "pays my rent." A motion condemning rebates as unethical carried unanimously. In about 1974 the ophthalmologists and otolaryngologists formed separate societies.

After Dr. VanDyk became chief of ophthalmology at the University of Utah, he presided over a monthly clinic. Four or five patients were interviewed by the doctors in attendance, followed by general discussion and reviews of the pertinent literature by the residents.

Monthly meetings are held from September through May, the September meeting in conjunction with the annual meeting of the Utah Medical Association, and the May meeting with the Ogden Surgical Society. For several years, a meeting has been held in Cedar City at the time of the Utah Shakespearean Festival. Similar programs have been held at Lake Powell, and recently the Society sponsored a midwinter ski meeting with invited speakers.

University of Utah

Before the conversion of Utah's two-year to a four-year medical school, the Salt Lake County Commissioners appointed attending physicians who took turns teaching and caring for patients. Dr. Vivian Parley White was doing the eye work at the time of the conversion, but Bascom Palmer was made head of the Division of Ophthalmology under Dr. Philip Price, the chief of surgery.

Drs. Palmer, Muir, and Merrill lectured. Three or four students attended the out-patient clinic for indigents one morning a week under two or three ophthalmologists who also performed needed surgery. No refractions were done, and each member of the clinical staff received one dollar per year.

Eye surgery was not considered very important, as was dramatically illustrated on one occasion when a nurse came into an operating room and took away the only operating light, requiring the completion of a cataract extraction with light from a gooseneck lamp!

The Veterans Administration Hospital was covered by the same rotating clinical staff. The VA clinic was covered by a resident in general surgery who assisted the attending ophthalmologist in surgery. The pay was $25.00 per day, regardless of the type or length of surgery.

For many years the Primary Children's Hospital, which admitted only indigent patients, had one attending ophthalmologist who served without pay. Later, paying patients were admitted and the staff was opened to other ophthalmologists.

When Bascom Palmer resigned from the University faculty, Dr. Rowland Merrill took over as chief, giving most of the student lectures. The workload in the emergency room and out-patient clinic became lighter as more ophthalmologists moved into Salt Lake City.

In 1968 Dr. Merrill resigned from the faculty and Dr. Orson White became interim chief of the division. He writes that they had 100% cooperation from the clinical staff. Dr. White and Dr. Robert Despain worked out a plan with Dr. Blodi at the University of Iowa whereby his senior ophthalmology residents rotated through a two-month stay in Salt Lake City, operating at the University and VA hospitals under the supervision of one of the clinical faculty. Many students took this tour and gained considerable experience.

When Dr. Kim Taylor came to Salt Lake City in 1967, he found that clinics were not being held regularly at the VA Hospital. He started holding a clinic once a week and operating for three hours twice a week. When the Iowa residents came, he assisted most of them. After one and a half or two years, the University residents did the surgery and Taylor assisted *them.* In 1973 the University took over the VA program entirely.

In 1967 a bequest made twenty years earlier to be used for the "care of the indigent blind" was worth $68,000, and Dean Kenneth Castleton, Keith Reemtsma (chair of the Department of Surgery), and Len Jarcho (chair of the Department of Neurology) were able to begin the search for a chair for the Division of Ophthalmology. Dr. Henry VanDyk, a neuro-ophthalmologist at the University of Oregon Medical School, was selected and assumed the position July 1, 1969.

Another bequest permitted the purchase of modern equipment for five examining rooms and $20,000 a year to recruit a junior associate. Dr. VanDyk had known Tempel Riekhof at the University of Oregon, and after taking a retinal fellowship in St. Louis, Dr. Riekhof, the first vitro-retinal surgeon, joined Dr. VanDyk in July 1970. A three-year federal grant provided funds for the new chair, a secretary, and a summer medical student.

By 1973 the rotations were pretty well established. VanDyk did neuro-ophthalmology and strabismus, and Riekhof had a good retinal service. Private practitioners helped: Joe Hatch covered corneal and external diseases; Robert Hales covered optics and the clinic; John

Nelson and Gary Stanford organized a pathology section; George Pingree and Duncan McDonald conducted the journal club. Darrell Wolfley came to Salt lake City in 1974. He developed a large oculo-plastic surgical practice and covered this field at the University. In July 1975 Dr. Michael Kottler came as a full-time faculty member specializing in glaucoma.

Each resident went to a basic science course for two or three months in the second year of the program. In January 1973 residents were doing cataract extractions using binocular loops and closing with 7-0 chromic or 6-0 silk. By 1975 they were using a microscope and 10-0 nylon sutures. The early residents did more than 100 cataract extractions in their three-year service.

For health reasons, Dr. VanDyk left Utah in 1979 for a neuro-ophthalmology position at Louisiana State University (LSU) Medical School. Dr. Randall (Randy) Olson, a young faculty member at LSU, arrived in Salt Lake City in the spring of 1979 to head the University of Utah eye program. Dr. Kottler had gone into private practice a month earlier, but Dr. Mano Swartz joined Olson shortly afterward.

The staff was rather static until the arrival in July 1981 of Drs. Alan S. Crandall, Jr., in glaucoma, Jane D. Kivlin in pediatric ophthalmology, and David J. Apple in pathology. Dr. Crandall is still a highly respected and valuable member of the University of Utah faculty. Dr. Kivlin left in May of 1990 for an appointment in ophthalmology at the Medical College of Wisconsin. Dr. Apple has been director of the Foundation for Intraocular Lens Research, analyzing specimens from all over the world, and is in great demand as a speaker at scientific meetings. In June 1988 he accepted the chair of ophthalmology at the University of South Carolina.

In 1984 Dr. Wolfley moved to an academic position at Louisiana State University and was replaced by Dr. Richard L. Anderson, who had spent nine years in oculo-plastic surgery at the University of Iowa and is now a full professor.

By 1984 the subspecialties were covered and research activities strengthened. For some time the residency program continued unchanged, accepting two residents per year for the three-year program.

An ophthalmic internship was offered which included half a year of medicine and half a year in ophthalmology. Another year added to the residency in 1987 made it a five-year commitment, including the internship.

By 1987 more than $1 million in grant support was placing more emphasis on the research side, and the lack of space had become a major problem. An effort from 1986 to 1989 to raise money for an ophthalmic building resulted in a 72,000-square-foot structure on the drawing board. The largest donation, $3.5 million, came from Mr. John A. Moran, for whom the building is named.

Some Memorable Individuals

William Bohart, and, later, Roger Harrie, have offered ultrasound determinations to practicing ophthalmologists.

Kevin Charleton, after his residency at the University of Utah, completed a one-year fellowship in corneal surgery in San Diego. He is the first in Utah to perform epikeratoprosthesis.

Mary Middleton Dahl became the first woman to practice ophthalmology in Utah since Romania Pratt. She had training in reading retinal angiograms and provided this service to the new Division of Ophthalmology after the arrival of Dr. VanDyk. She also participated in the nationwide five-year scientific Diabetic Retinopathy Study (DRS).

J. Eldon Dorman provided ophthalmic care to the people around Price, Utah, from 1941 to well into the 1980s.

After medical school, Rowland Merrill had an eye residency at Johns Hopkins, part of which he spent visiting eye centers in Vienna and Prague as well as Germany. On his return, he was the first at Hopkins to do an intracapsular cataract extraction. Later, he spent three years at Manhattan Eye and Ear before returning to Salt Lake City in 1938. He sent to Germany for glass contact lenses with which the patient could see but which were very uncomfortable.

Garth Chatterly practiced in Salt Lake City for five years, traveling to Cedar City, Utah, for one and later five days per month, finally moving there in 1961. He has helped promote the Shakespearean

Festival in Cedar City and started the annual One-Day Ophthalmological Meeting there in 1964.

Bryce Fairbanks is the physician for the Boy Scouts. He chaired the Physicians' Committee of the Utah State Medical Association (USMA) for eleven years, during which time he personally watched over physicians who had become impaired through the abuse of alcohol or drugs or through emotional illness, developing contacts that enabled physicians to receive treatment and return to practice without public embarrassment. For his service to fellow physicians and the community, he received the special USMA President's Award in 1982. The following year he received the A. H. Robins Award for Community Service Outside the Field of Medicine.

Joseph Hatch is a family man, outdoorsman, busy ophthalmologist, and active medical politician. He has always been interested in keratoplasty and has attained a high degree of competence without integrated training. On his own he discovered and developed a method of kerato-refractive surgery to aid in keratoplasty.

Tempel Riekhof, in conjunction with Drs. William Bohart and Mary Dahl, joined the DRS, the study of one of the most common causes of blindness. Beginning in 1985, with Bohart and Dr. Roy Goodart, Riekhof began participation in a second five-year study of early treatment (ETDRS). Dr. Riekhof has also served in medical society activities as speaker of the House of Delegates and as trustee of the Utah Medical Insurance Association.

Robert L. Rees trained at the University of Iowa and, following a stint in the military, joined the Salt Lake Clinic in 1953. About two years later, he left the Clinic and joined Dr. Spear for a productive, pleasant thirty-one-year partnership.

CHAPTER TWENTY-EIGHT

Urology

RICHARD G. MIDDLETON, MD

IN 1911, BEFORE ANY PHYSICIAN IN UTAH limited his practice to the field of urology, Dr. George W. Middleton, a general surgeon, performed a historically significant operation in Salt Lake City. He was responsible for the first recorded bilateral uretero-sigmoid anastomosis by a submucosal tunneling technique of Coffey. The patient was a seventeen-year-old boy born with bladder exstrophy and described as perpetually wet, smelly, and a recluse who was unable to attend school. The operation was remarkably successful.

Twenty-five years later, Dr. Middleton's son, Richard P. Middleton, a urologist in Salt Lake City, reported the event in *The Journal of Urology* in an article entitled, "Human cloaca for over twenty-five years without impairment of health." The patient led an essentially normal life, became a successful businessman, and fathered two children. After nearly fifty years of good health, he ultimately developed an adenocarcinoma of the sigmoid colon at the site of the previous ureteral reimplantation. This tumor metastasized and led to his death. Time has demonstrated that primary colon neoplasm is not uncommon many years after ureteral transplantation into the sigmoid or rectum. Prior to this time there was no reliable method for urinary diversion; the plight of the infant born with bladder exstrophy was particularly grim.

The year 1912 saw the first two self-designated urologists in Salt Lake City. Francis Goeltz from Erie, Pennsylvania, with medical training at Bellevue Hospital in New York City, joined Walter Schulte, a native of California who had previously been on the medical faculty at the University of Colorado in Denver. Goeltz and Schulte entered the newly completed Boston Building on Main Street between Third and Fourth South Streets. In that era the Boston Building and other downtown office buildings housed the majority of physicians' offices — a central location among the active hospitals: the LDS Hospital on the Avenues, Holy Cross on First South between Tenth and Eleventh East, St. Mark's in the northwest corner of the city near the railroad and across the street from Beck's Hot Springs, and the Salt Lake General (County) Hospital on Twenty-first South and State Streets.

The urologic practice of Drs. Goeltz and Schulte was dominated by venereology, while at this time most of the surgery on the genitourinary system — i.e., nephrectomy, pyelolithotomy, ureterolithotomy, suprapubic prostatic enucleation, and genital surgery — was performed by general surgeons. Gonorrhea was rampant, and there was no effective treatment for it. Patients were seen frequently, often daily, for urethral irrigation with potassium permanganate or silver proteinate. Ultimately, over a period of months, the discharge would disappear — either because of the treatment or as a result of the patient's own defense mechanisms. A urethral stricture was commonly the patient's fate following treatment. Whether the stricture was caused by the bacterial urethritis or the irritation of the chemical irrigants was never clear. Also, once cured, the patient was very likely to contract gonorrhea again and start the chain of events anew.

Richard P. Middleton began urologic practice in Salt Lake City in 1931, after surgical and urologic residency training in Worcester, Massachusetts, and the Peter Bent Brigham Hospital in Boston. At the Brigham Hospital he had been the urologic resident when Harvey Cushing was chief of the Department of Surgery. R. P. Middleton's interest was in urologic surgery, and he pioneered the transurethral resection for prostate obstruction in Utah. To quote from Dr. Middleton's reminiscences, "Our specialty was then badly stigmatized by its association with venereology. I interviewed several doctors to seek advice about whether I should stick with urology or combine it with

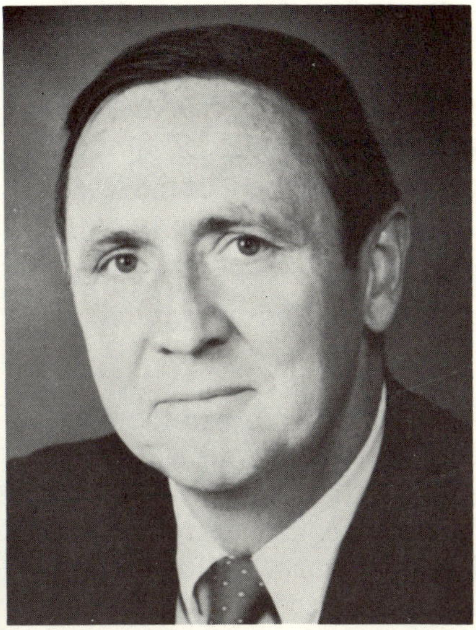

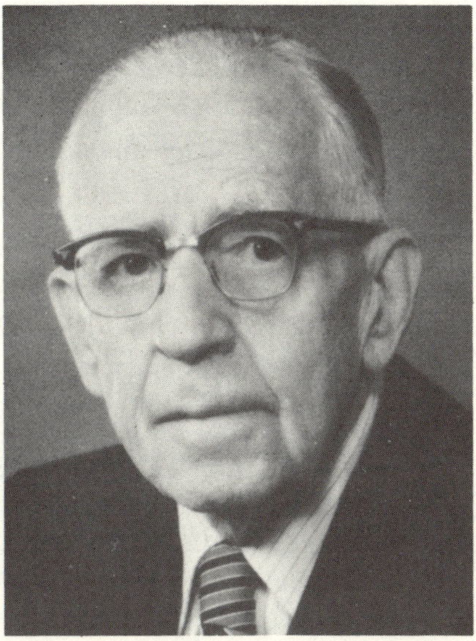

Richard G. Middleton, left. Richard P. Middleton, MD, right, the senior member of a family of six urologists, was the first well-trained urologist in Salt Lake City. He began his practice in 1931, pioneered TUR (transurethral resection of the prostate), and was appointed clinical head of the urology division in the new four-year Medical School in 1943.

general surgery, in which I had also been trained. Some older clinicians solemnly advised me to leave urology alone if I proposed to be a surgeon, since otherwise many patients would fear to be seen coming into my office lest their friends suspect they had a venereal disease."

Dr. Middleton decided to limit his practice to urology, but he also took a part-time position teaching anatomy in the Medical School to help support his family. There was no shortage of urologic patients in the early 1930s, the time of the Great Depression, but few had money to pay for medical services. The era of medical insurance had not yet arrived. In 1937 Dr. Middleton reported the largest benign prostate ever to be successfully enucleated up to that time. The prostate weighed 557 grams, and according to his report in the *Journal of the American Medical Association*, "The mammoth gland seemed to fill the true pelvis like the head of a fetus at term."

Momentous changes led to a transformation of the field of urology. The sulfa drugs (about 1936) and penicillin (about 1943) for the first time provided efficient and effective treatment for venereal and other infections. The advent of intravenous urography led to more precise diagnosis of urinary diseases. The development of the resectoscope and the necessary training and experience required to use this device effectively helped to strengthen urology as a surgical subspecialty. Dr. Middleton has described the early days of transurethral surgery in his reminiscences:

> In concept, TUR seemed tantalizingly simple and the comparison with D&C of the uterus was inevitable. In the early 30's, Salt Lake City had perhaps a dozen general surgeons with enough urologic training to do their own suprapubic prostatectomies and renal operations. Most of them bought equipment and took a crack at transurethral prostatic resection. They all soon gave it up as it became apparent that the procedure is one of the most technical and difficult in the whole domain of surgery. . . . I made frequent trips to the centers where large experience was accumulating and fought my way to competence in the new field.

The first modern urologist in Ogden was George Fister, who began urologic practice in 1929 after urologic residency training with Herman Kretchmer, a celebrated Chicago urologist and a pioneer in transurethral surgery. Fister practiced urology in Ogden for nearly forty years. He was an affable man with a huge practice, popular with fellow physicians and with his patients. Among other positions, he served as president of the Utah State Medical Association, president of the American Medical Association, and president of the Western section of the American Urologic Association. In his memory, the family of George Fister have established a fund to support an annual Visiting Professor of Urology at the University of Utah Medical Center and a Fister Memorial Lectureship at the Utah Urologic Society. This visiting professorship and lectureship have been an important event in Utah urology for fifteen years.

Anthony W. Middleton joined his brother Richard in urologic practice in Salt Lake City in 1939, after completing urologic residency training at the Mayo Clinic. Anthony concentrated his efforts at Holy Cross Hospital, while his brother carried out most of his urologic practice at LDS Hospital. Robert G. Weaver began his urologic practice in 1946, after training with Frank Hinman at the University of California at San Francisco. James Palmer, another Mayo-trained urologist, arrived in Salt Lake City in 1949, Neel Huckleberry in 1950, and Neal Natoli in 1956. Harry Fisher joined the Holy Cross Hospital staff after urologic training with Justin Cordonnier, an eminent urologist at Washington University in St. Louis. Jay Henderson, after residency at the University of Colorado, entered practice in 1950, working mainly at the LDS Hospital.

In the mid-1940s the University of Utah School of Medicine was expanded from a two-year to a four-year school able to grant an MD degree. Philip B. Price was the first full-time chair of surgery. Urology was established as a division within surgery, and Richard P. Middleton, the senior urologist in Salt Lake City, was named division chair. In the early years of the four-year Medical School, the division faculty also included Anthony W. Middleton, Robert G. Weaver, and James Palmer. Each gave medical student lectures, and each took a turn supervising the urology service at the Salt Lake General Hospital as well as the old Salt Lake Veterans Administration Hospital on the North Bench. As new urologists appeared on the scene, they were added to the faculty.

Growth at the University of Utah Medical School led to construction of a new University Hospital on the East Bench campus, which opened in 1965 and replaced the old Salt Lake General Hospital as the University's primary teaching facility. Robert Weaver became the first full-time chair of the urology division in 1963 and left his downtown private practice. He recruited James J. Yelderman to join him. Dr. Yelderman had trained in urology at the University of Iowa under the legendary Rubin Flocks.

Robert Weaver did investigative work on the regeneration of the ureter in dogs. He was also interested in renovascular hypertension; he worked on a renin assay and spent a year on a Fulbright Fellowship in Norway learning the technique of femoral artery catheterization and angiography. Dr. Weaver also gained approval for a provisional urology residency training program involving the new University Hospital and the new Salt Lake VA Hospital, adjacent to the University campus.

The 1960s and 1970s saw an influx of well-trained urologists into the state. In Salt Lake City, joining the LDS Hospital staff were Drs. Hal Bourne, Richard Lee, Ned Mangelson, Paul Clark, Douglas Dahl, A. W. Middleton, Jr., and Odell Rigby. New urologists at Holy Cross were Drs. Dahl and A. W. Middleton, Jr., and his brother, George Middleton. The city expanded greatly to the south, necessitating the construction of a new St. Mark's Hospital, Cottonwood Hospital, and Pioneer Valley Hospital. New urologists in these institutions were Drs. Richard Eliason, David Kimball, Bart Christensen, Bard Merritt, Vanez Wilson, Stephen Richardson, and James Morrell. Doctors Steven C. Hatch, Duane E. Davis, Herbert B. Spencer, Ronald I. Oldroyd, and Joseph R. Armstrong entered urology practice in Provo. New urologists practicing in Ogden were Drs. Anthony J. Lund, Dean W. Packard, and Harvey Ruskin.

Dr. Richard G. Middleton returned to Salt Lake City in 1967 after training in urology at Cornell University–New York Hospital in New York City. He joined his father, Richard P., who was nearing the end of his active practice. R. G. Middleton also joined the Medical School faculty half time, but in short order his commitment and involvement in academic urology increased. In 1968 he replaced Dr. Weaver as chair of the Division of Urology, a position he has held for twenty-three years. The urologic training program has expanded to include the Primary Children's Medical Center and the LDS Hospital as well as the University and VA hospitals.

Additional full-time urologic faculty have strengthened the training program and the stature of urology in the University. Dr. Joseph A. Smith, Jr., a former University of Utah resident, was on the faculty as a urologic oncologist for eleven years. He was recently named chair of the Department of Urology at Vanderbilt University School of Medicine in Nashville, Tennessee. Dr. Ronald L. Urry, a PhD in reproductive physiology, has directed the fertility program for the past decade; he is in charge of the University's *in vitro* fertilization program as well. Dr. Brent W. Snow, a pediatric urologist, directs the section of pediatric urology at the new Primary Children's Medical Center on the Medical School campus. Newer faculty members of the Division of Urology are Richard F. Labasky, in urodynamics and urinary tract reconstruction, and Patrick Cartwright, in pediatric urology. Doctors Labasky and Cartwright are former University of Utah urologic residents who returned following their fellowship training to begin careers in academic urology.

A total of forty-three residents have completed their training at the University of Utah and its affiliated hospitals. Of those forty-three, thirteen have entered urologic practice in the state of Utah. Doctors LaGrande C. and his sons, John C., and Ryan H. Larsen practice in Logan. Curtis Campbell is in active practice in Ogden, and Drs. Henderson and Walters are located in Davis County. Drs. Rigby, Morrell, Sorenson, and David Larsen practice in Salt Lake City, and former residents Joseph Smith, Richard Labasky, and Patrick Cartwright are on the full-time urology faculty at the University of Utah School of Medicine.

More than forty urologists currently practice in Utah. Urology is thriving with rapidly expanding technology; it is stronger both locally and nationally than the pioneer urologic forbears ever imagined.

CHAPTER TWENTY-NINE

Laser Surgery

JOHN A. DIXON, MD

LASERS ARE NOW USED AT MOST of the major hospitals in Utah. Many surgeons employ these devices routinely in their practices at laser units providing instrumentation consisting of one to as many as six lasers of different wavelengths. While the focus of this essay is surgical applications, from the point of view of the Laser Institute of the University of Utah, a low bow in the direction of ophthalmology is merited, since ophthalmic applications preceded by several years the events in this account.

Surgical laser development in Utah began in 1976 at the Department of Surgery at the University of Utah. At that time I served as vice president for health sciences and was doing endoscopy in the Division of Gastroenterology to remain active in medicine. I became interested in the possibility of laser application through endoscopes for control of gastrointestinal bleeding. Discovering that Dr. Peter Kiefhaber of Munich and Dr. Richard Dwyer of Los Angeles had treated several patients successfully by this technique, I visited both of them and returned to begin investigations in the field.

An immediate problem was the lack of equipment or funds. The crude laser devices of this time were nearly all custom-made prototypes costing from one to two hundred thousand dollars. If progress was to be made, it had to be in conjunction with a company willing to assist by providing devices in exchange for developmental information that might ultimately lead to marketable instruments.

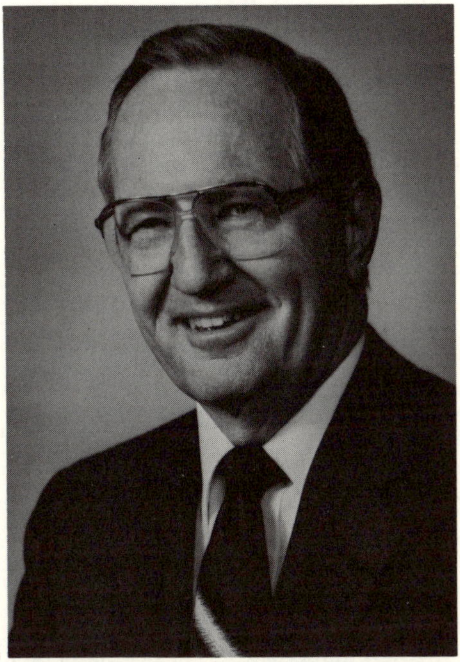

John A. Dixon.

I looked in the Yellow Pages of the Salt Lake City telephone book under "Laser" and found American Laser Company listed without any indication of what types of laser products they produced. I drove out one afternoon and had difficulty finding the address, which turned out to be an old roadhouse across from the entrance to the old Salt Lake airport. I found the president of the company, Dr. William McMahan, his secretary, and one engineer to be the whole staff. Dr. McMahan, an electrical/optical engineer, was taken aback by my animated description of gastroduodenal arteries, spurting vessels, and endoscopic photocoagulation, but he rallied somewhat during the actual discussion of technical details required for a medical instrument. It developed that American Laser manufactured small argon laser tubes that were being adapted for photocopying devices, and Dr. McMahan was interested in the possibility of applying this technology to medicine. Our first collaboration resulted in a prototype argon/neodymium:YAG laser device with an attached closed-circuit TV system for recording clinical applications.

A major problem became evident at this time which would surface on many other occasions: the difficulty in communication between a clinician and an engineer or physicist. It wasn't until each acquired enough knowledge of the others' fields that meaningful exchange could take place and instrument development begin.

Approval of the Institutional Review Board (IRB) was obtained for clinical application of the argon/neodymium:YAG. The cooperation of this body was essential in the early phases of human studies. Most of the specialty areas were almost entirely unexplored, and the IRB frequently had to act on faith and with considerable courage.

The combined argon/neodymium:YAG laser was a "breadboard" affair consisting of tubes and components scattered over various tables and benches. The numerous open-beam paths with light scattering into the room from this device would be totally unacceptable to the Food and Drug Administration today.

Other than a few cutaneous burns, no major accidents occurred during this very early period of laser instrument development. The closest call occurred one evening when a medical student who was assisting in the lab bent over an open laser beam. It very quietly and cleanly cut across the front of his polyester pants, leaving him somewhat exposed, yet unaware of his misadventure. He left to pick up his date at a sorority house down the street from the lab, where rumor has it that he was ejected by the housemother, who made some rather critical comments about his dress.

Research and clinical investigations with this primitive device began with Drs. Malcolm Berenson, John Bowers, Randy Burt, and Dale Richey from the Division of Gastroenterology playing a prominent role.

The first patient treated following IRB approval was a seventy-nine-year-old man from Ogden, Utah, who had had an esophago-gastrectomy for cancer five months earlier. Twelve hours prior to admission he began vomiting up bright red blood and was thought to have an inoperable recurrence of his tumor. His two sons (both physicians) had heard of the developmental work at the University and called me, asking only that the profuse bleeding be stopped. The first clinical laser procedure was performed in the small closet-like research laboratory where the immovable component-type laser was housed. Dr. Berenson performed the endoscopic procedure and I assisted. The patient's sons helped with intravenous lines and gastric lavage while anxiously peering over Dr. Berenson's shoulder. It was quite a way to begin human procedures. The bleeding was stopped through the endoscope with the neodymium:YAG laser; then multiple biopsies of the gastric and esophageal ulcerations were taken, which proved to be benign, and the patient was sent home the next day.

Drs. John Bowers and Ken Buchi undertook a series of very innovative investigations applying lasers in the gastrointestinal tract. They carried out some of the first experiments with coagulation of vascular malformations of the gastrointestinal tract, quantitating argon and neodymium:YAG laser applications. It was necessary to "qualify" lasers in the colon, as it had been generally assumed that the thin colon wall would perforate following laser application. After extensive research on dogs and the determination of safety parameters, many hundreds of patients were treated.

Sue Huether, RN, PhD, of the College of Nursing, played an integral role in investigation of the physiological effects of lasers on cutaneous structures, including laser Doppler-flow measurements. She later developed a laser training program for nurses that has attracted trainees from throughout the country.

The engineers at American Laser (now HGM) expressed a desire to develop an argon laser especially for medical use. Three different prototypes were designed, applied by University physicians, criticized, and returned for revision. Trial of the first such unit resulted in 108 recommendations for mechanical changes. The eventual result, however, was the HGM endocoagulator line, now the world's most successful argon laser of this type.

During this period, Dr. Gerald Krueger of the Department of Dermatology encouraged me to join him in investigating laser applications for cutaneous vascular anomalies. Since the medical argon

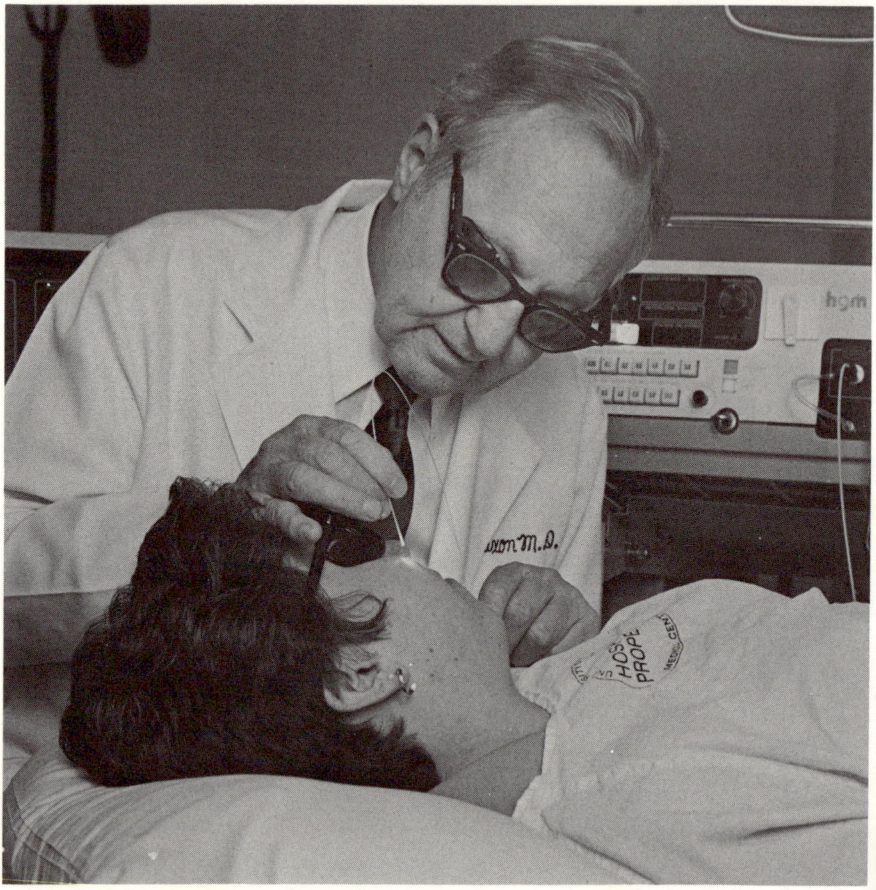

Dr. John A. Dixon treating a patient with a laser.

laser had been developed, the University group was nicely positioned for this undertaking. Treatment techniques for reducing port wine stains, telangiectasia, and other cutaneous lesions were developed. Thousands of patients were treated using these techniques, which ushered in a period of truly pioneering clinical procedures.

Dr. Mano Swartz was looking for a method for doing laser surgery close to the optic nerve and fovea centralis. The technique would be particularly important for patients who hemorrhaged following posterior vitrectomy, as their vision loss was then almost 100%. We discussed the problem and decided that a solution might be a specially clad fiber which could be inserted through a small incision in the globe into the posterior chamber to the point where it was almost in contact with the bleeding or vessel. This would allow for a very small spot size, protecting adjacent vital areas.

We made a prototype fiber and tried it on two human cadaver eyes with good mechanical results. Then we performed the procedure with apparent success on a dog under anesthesia.

The next week I was out of town at a meeting when the phone awakened me at 2:00 A.M. On the line was a very excited Dr. Swartz, who said that a patient had been referred who had had a posterior vitrectomy followed by uncontrollable bleeding, and who was almost certain to lose vision in the eye. Dr. Swartz had called all the members of the IRB and secured emergency permission to carry out the procedure. The hemorrhage was readily controlled by intravascular microsurgery. The patient recovered and retained 20/40 vision in the eye. This was the first procedure of this type published, and it initiated a whole new area of laser applications called "endophthalmic surgery." Dr. Swartz later refined the probe and patented it, and it is in general use throughout the world today.

Dr. James L. Parkin and I had been working on a technique using argon laser to control bleeding in patients with hereditary hemorrhagic telangiectasia. The technique had been successful in the first three patients with minor bleeding episodes. The fourth patient was a man with a strong familial history of telangiectasia with bleeding, and two of his siblings had died from its complications. He had had several hundred transfusions over several previous occasions, but at this time, bleeding was truly massive. Arterial ligations, including the external carotid artery, had been performed without success. Under local anesthesia Dr. Parkin identified a large arterial bleeder near the nasal septum and applied the argon laser up to its maximum power. Each time the spurting bleeding decreased somewhat, then resumed immediately. Finally, Dr. Parkin said, "The argon laser won't stop it. If we don't do something, he will bleed to death." I said, "The only thing we have left is the neodymium:YAG laser." Dr. Parkin asked what it would do to the septum and nasal bones, and I replied, "I haven't the slightest idea. It has never been applied in this region before."

We decided to go ahead with the application because of the dire circumstances. A 0.5-second application with the YAG laser at 55 W produced a loud cracking sound and almost palpable motion of the patient's head. We were encouraged to see the spurting stop and the bleeding decline to a slow ooze, and several more impacts stopped the bleeding altogether. A mucosal ulceration occurred, but no damage to the septum, and the patient recovered. We were later to quantitate experimentally the effects of argon and neodymium:YAG laser on the nasal septum and nasal bones and make its use in these regions safer, less stressful, and almost commonplace.

Dr. Jay Smith had been using the neodymium:YAG laser through a cystoscope for mucosal ablation in animals preparatory to its possible use to treat superficial bladder cancer in humans. We finally received IRB approval for this procedure. Unfortunately, Dr. Smith's patients were ambulatory patients under Veterans Administration care, and the VA would not pay for hospitalization at the University Hospital. But Dr. Smith felt that the procedure could be performed on an ambulatory basis, without general anesthesia.

Five patients with superficial bladder cancer walked into the laser lab at the University one afternoon. After obtaining fully informed patient consent, Dr. Smith put a small amount of local anesthesia in the patient's urethra and inserted the cystoscope and the laser fiber. I stood by the patient's head while Dr. Smith applied laser energy to the bladder cancer. On each application I asked the patient if any pain was present. Each responded in the negative. One had a mild sensation of warmth which was not uncomfortable. The patients then got up off the table and went home without hospital admission and without catheters. They all did well. Dr. Smith has since treated more than 500 patients using this technique, which has become a standard procedure throughout the world. Ambulatory care has reduced dramatically patients' hospital costs, loss of productive time, and suffering.

This investigative period was not without complications, however. A new, incorrectly wired laser caused an electrical shock that knocked down Sue Smith, the first head nurse in the laser unit. Fortunately, she recovered fully.

Several intratracheal fires and explosions had occurred elsewhere with bronchoscopists using the CO_2 laser on tracheal tumors. It was thought that the CO_2 laser beam had impacted on endotracheal tubes, setting them afire. Dr. Ken Casey was doing a tracheal stricture on a patient using the neodymium:YAG laser with a fiber which had been introduced several centimeters beyond the tip of the endotracheal tube. A flash explosion occurred. Dr. Casey immediately removed the bronchoscope, laser fiber, and endotracheal tube. Fortunately, the patient was not harmed. Investigation revealed that a technician had inadvertently introduced a high level of oxygen into the endotracheal tube. Dr. Casey's subsequent investigations demonstrated that the explosions were due to the characteristics of the gaseous mixture — not impact on the endotracheal tube or endoscope — and that any spark could set off the entire area. Numerous studies were conducted and published, resulting in much better safety for applications in this region.

It is remarkable that patients, physicians, and nurses suffered no ophthalmic injuries during the entire developmental period. This is probably a result of precautions suggested by the ophthalmology group as well as education and careful screening of laser physicians and nurses.

It became evident that some type of organizational structure would have to be initiated to handle the now-heavy clinical load and provide multidisciplinary University faculty input in research development. In 1985 the University of Utah Laser Institute was formed by action of the University Senate and the State Board of Regents, with myself as director, Dr. Richard Straight as associate director, and Dr. Craig Taylor (professor of physics), Dr. Robert Benner (professor of electrical engineering), and Dr. Charles Wight (assistant professor of chemistry) as associate directors.

The Institute Clinical Division was formed to supervise safety, use privileges, and clinical procedures in the hospital, and its first administrator was Dan Lundergan. The earlier clinical work had been carried out in a small laboratory on the fourth floor in the Division of Gastroenterology. Instruments had been crude prototypes built by Dr. McMahan to my specifications. Interested investigators had worked out individual relationships and schedules for using the rudimentary equipment to investigate their particular problems. The first specially designed hospital unit was on the fourth floor of the new University Hospital, next to the intensive care area, and was specially wired for the new instruments. Sue Smith was the nurse in charge, and she participated significantly in the development of techniques and instrumentation. Ultimately, three specialty operating rooms adjacent to the ambulatory surgery recovery unit were developed for ambulatory laser work, and all ten major operating rooms in the central operating suite were wired for laser applications. Privilege lists for use of each laser by individual surgeons and methods of certification for users of the unit were developed. This was one of the first such units organized in the United States.

The clinical laser facilities are used by physicians from fifteen specialties, including surgery, medicine, obstetrics and gynecology, ophthalmology, dermatology, and plastic surgery, with competence rather than specialty origin the criterion for their use. More than 15,000 patients have been treated in the clinical areas of the Institute, resulting in many seminal publications.

Because of a lack of space in the Medical Center, the research arm of the Institute under the direction of Dr. Richard Straight is housed in a building at the University Research Park. The facility includes four large multipurpose optical laboratories with laser research equipment valued at over $3 million in operation. These instruments are used extensively by almost every department and division in the University employing lasers in their investigative work. It is common to have surgeons, physicists, electrical engineers, and chemists working side by side on a project.

Grants, bequests, and other sources of revenue of approximately $1.5 million per year finance research at the Laser Institute. Initially, all support came from private foundations and commercial laser companies. More recently, a major portion of this support was from a grant by the Strategic Defense Initiative to investigate free electron laser medical applications.

Many of the organizational, safety, and technical policy procedures developed by Laser Institute members have been published and incorporated in hospital and laboratory operations manuals throughout the world.

A major function of the Laser Institute has been the education of physicians. In 1982 the first small classes were held for training four or five physicians in "hands-on" laboratory work to equip them for laser use. This endeavor was later expanded under Dan Lundergan to include almost continuous courses in laser applications for gastroenterology, surgery, obstetrics and gynecology, and vascular medicine. More than 1,500 physicians from all over the country have participated in training courses.

Utilizing Institute facilities, Dr. W. R. Keye became involved in investigating the possibility of endoscopic application of argon laser energy for the treatment of minimal to moderate endometriosis. He developed instrumentation that allowed application of the argon laser through a laparoscope and began pioneer work in photocoagulation of endometrial lesions. This work received international recognition and has resulted in a reduction in symptoms and increased conception rate in many hundreds of patients similar to or better than results noted with laparotomy and electrocoagulation methods.

As early as 1979, Drs. Peter Lawrence and Michael Vincent began investigations on cardiovascular application of lasers. Dr. Vincent felt that coronary plaque could be vaporized with lasers but that the possibility of arterial perforation was great. Subsequent premature trials at other institutions demonstrated that his concern was well founded. Dr. Lawrence proceeded, however, to develop techniques for laser removal of plaques in femoral arteries with encouraging but as yet incomplete results.

Dr. Vincent had developed innovative techniques for catheter application of mapping devices to the endocardium of the ventricle. It was hoped that this application could be utilized in humans with severe uncontrollable arrhythmias. His investigation of the histologic and hematologic effects of such applications finally led to IRB approval in 1986 of human applications during open-heart surgery. The endocardium was mapped, following which lasers were used with good results to obliterate the area of abnormal conduction. Several clinical trials are now under way.

In association with colleagues in England and Australia, Richard C. Straight, PhD, and his associates initiated a program in the study of photosensitizing agents. The group developed much new information regarding light–photosensitizer–tissue interaction and a number of new photoactive compounds.

Among the Laser Institute's many innovations was the initiation of specialized research training for residents. The first, Dr. Robert Rotering, worked primarily in the development of gastric applications. Dr. John Hunter became interested in the possibility of lasers for nonincisional interruption of vagal nerves either by laparotomy or using endoscopic techniques. Dr. J. J. Gilbertson investigated photodynamic therapy by sensitizing cells using a photosensitizer, such as Photofrin II, followed by laser light application. He carried out numerous investigations into cancer cell destruction. Dr. Scott Leckman, who reviewed the potential of dissemination of cancer cells by laser application, found that cancer cells distributed into the air and lymphatics following laser application were not viable.

Early clinical application of lasers in other Utah hospitals brought the entire state into the forefront of laser use. Residents trained at the Laser Institute, notably Drs. Dale Richey, John H. Bowers, and Gary Hunter, moved into private practice with the development of laser units at the LDS, St. Mark's, Holy Cross, McKay-Dee, and Utah Valley hospitals. Applications of the carbon dioxide, argon, and neodymium:YAG lasers are now commonplace, with strong, active programs at each of these institutions.

As a result of very early interest, research innovations, application of surgical techniques, and training of laser surgeons and nurses, Utah has occupied a unique place in the development of surgical applications of lasers. Utahns are represented by standard texts, key research papers, and important clinical studies which are milestones in the field. Many directors of laser units throughout the United States can trace their early training to participation either in Utah educational programs or with Utah-trained physicians. The program has also spun off several laser manufacturing companies in Salt Lake City that are recognized throughout the world for the quality and versatility of their products.

PART FOUR

•

OBSTETRICS AND GYNECOLOGY

CHAPTER THIRTY

Obstetrics and Gynecology in Practice and at the University of Utah

RICHARD M. HEBERTSON, MD

MANY SIGNIFICANT CHANGES HAVE OCCURRED in the practice of obstetrics and gynecology during the past four decades. A brief overview of some of them should be useful.

Richard Hebertson's first direct experience with obstetrics as a premedical student was in 1953, when his first daughter was born. His wife "fell" into labor on a Sunday morning, labored the entire day, and delivered sometime in the late afternoon. During those hours of labor he had no contact with his wife. Not until much later did he learn that during the second stage of labor she had pushed for nearly four hours before forceps were used to accomplish delivery. Isolation of the father from the laboring mother was the nature of obstetrics at that time. Within four years, however, fathers were given the opportunity to be involved in a supportive way if they desired, but that participation was still remarkably limited. Many years passed before the open involvement so common today became the rule.

Impressive changes in obstetrical anesthesia paralleled the evolution of the father's role. Trilene gas inhalers brought relief of contraction pain. "Twilight sleep" was popular in Europe before becoming the established approach for obstetric analgesia in the United States. This technique consisted of giving a mixture of demerol and scopolamine intravenously. Intravenous Nembutal was also used. These two techniques gave reasonable relief of discomfort but rendered the women essentially senseless. General anesthesia with cyclopropane was commonly used for delivery during the 1950s and 1960s. The father was not involved until well after the delivery, when the mother had regained her conscious self.

In the late 1950s local blocks were used for labor pain relief. Pudendal block became quite popular, working well for the second stage of labor and for the repair of vaginal laceration and the episiotomy. Hebertson began his obstetric experience using pudendal blocks. In the early 1960s paracervical block was used frequently for the relief of uterine pain, and when combined with a pudendal block, good vaginal and perineal pain relief occurred as well. It was not uncommon to administer two or three blocks during the harder part of the labor. More complete pain relief was available with spinal anesthesia or the saddle block. Spinal anesthesia was superb for the second stage of labor and delivery. Saddle block was used primarily for vaginal and perineal pain at the time of delivery.

In the late 1960s and early 1970s, epidural anesthesia clearly became the obstetric anesthesia of choice. The laboring mother was completely alert and pain free and could participate in social interchange with her spouse and other family members. Initially, epidural anesthesia was usually administered by the obstetrician. By the mid-1970s, it was administered almost exclusively by an anesthesiologist. Currently, in those facilities where anesthesiologists are present around the clock, epidural anesthesia is used by the majority of laboring patients. In major centers, paracervical and pudendal block and spinal anesthesia have all but disappeared, although spinal anesthetic is still used occasionally for Cesarean section.

Local perineal anesthesia is still given to women who have used natural childbirth techniques and who may need an anesthetic for the repair of a laceration or an episiotomy.

During the early 1960s, obstetric forceps use declined significantly. The decline has been associated with the more active involvement of the mother in the labor and delivery process and an attitudinal change toward abdominal delivery and Cesarean section. The decreased use of forceps has been steady for the most part, although epidural anesthesia initially produced a transient increase. However,

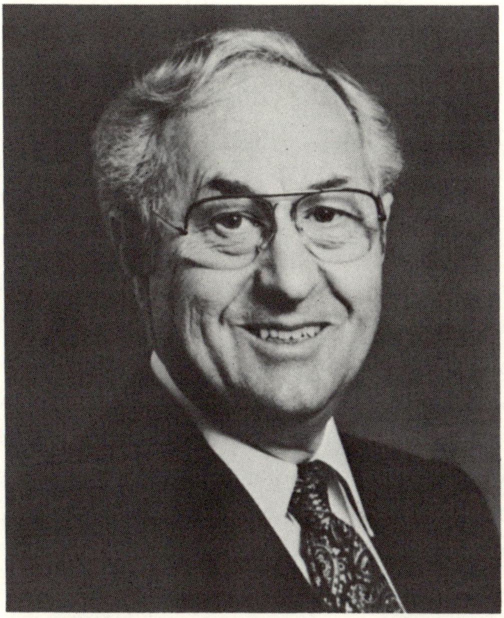

Richard M. Hebertson.

as anesthetic techniques have been refined, epidural has been used in a steadily increasing number of spontaneous deliveries.

In 1985 Dr. M. S. Sanders, an obstetrician at LDS Hospital, introduced an obstetric forceps pad for application to the forceps blade which materially reduced trauma to the newborn's head and represented the most significant change in forceps in several decades.

Oxytocin has become a tremendous asset for the laboring woman. Carefully controlled, it can enhance the quality and frequency of uterine contractions. Frequently used to induce labor, oxytocin has also played a remarkable role in diminishing postpartum blood loss.

Over the past twenty-five years, the evaluation of the fetus during labor has changed a great deal. In the late 1960s and early 1970s, the introduction of electronic fetal heart monitoring permitted a continuous evaluation of the quality of labor and the response of the fetus. Although some question its routine use, continuous electronic fetal monitoring will be used for years to come.

Another technique employed to evaluate the fetus is the fetal scalp pH, which has not been popular because of the difficulty of obtaining accurate and reproducible data. Ultrasound has contributed greatly to the management of the fetus. While its true value in the assessment of real-time physiologic changes is not yet known, the determination of anatomy and physiologic function through ultrasound is very exciting.

Cesarean section was relatively infrequent in the 1950s and 1960s, but its use began to increase during the 1970s with the introduction of continuous electronic fetal monitoring, the wider application of ultrasound, and the diminished use of forceps.

Unfortunately, fear of legal action has increased the Cesarean section rate. In the past, abdominal delivery was expected at a rate of 4 or 5%. Currently, the rate of Cesarean section varies from a low of 12 to 14% to highs of 33 to 35% nationally.

Humanization of the entire labor and delivery event has been remarkable. Extensive prenatal education of both mother and father allows significant involvement for the father as well as other relatives and friends in the labor and birthing experience. Before the early 1980s, only physicians and nursing personnel were permitted in the Cesarean section room, but changed attitudes now permit a number of nonmedical observers during an abdominal delivery.

Just a few years ago, a five- or six-day postpartum hospital stay was common. The length of the stay has been influenced by patient desire, by changes in the attitudes of physicians, by a less demanding labor and delivery process, and, significantly, by costs and changes in insurance coverage. Currently, three hospital days is the rule for an abdominal delivery and twelve hours is a common hospital stay for a vaginal delivery.

The establishment of criteria for estimating the risk of pregnancy has altered approaches in prenatal care. Attempts to reduce the risk of premature labor and premature rupture of the membranes have had a variable impact. This area remains nebulous but promising. Maternal and perinatal morbidity and mortality have been reduced appreciably, however, and further progress is expected.

Use of the computer has had an enormous impact on improving prenatal care, better documenting labor, and prompting management approaches; wider application is just a matter of time.

The Department of Obstetrics and Gynecology

The University of Utah's Department of Obstetrics and Gynecology was established in 1943 when Dr. A. Louis Dippel became its first professor. He "brought with him" a young assistant professor, Emil Holmstrom, who eventually became department chair.

Born in Texas in 1901, Dr. Dippel was a graduate of the University of Texas, where he earned his BA, MA, and MD degrees. From 1931 to 1935 he was first an intern, then a resident in obstetrics and gynecology at Johns Hopkins. He joined the faculty there in 1934 and later became an associate in obstetrics. Between 1940 and 1943 he was an associate professor at the University of Minnesota.

Dr. Dippel spent only one year as professor and chair at Utah before moving on to Baylor University in Texas. He was noted for his contribution to x-ray pelvimetry and the localization of the placenta by soft-tissue roentgenography. The technique of x-ray stereographic pelvimetry was used at Utah well into the 1960s.

Following Dippel's departure, the search committee reached again into the ranks of faculty at the University of Minnesota to select Charles Edward McLennan. Dr. McLennan was born in Duluth, Minnesota, in 1909. He obtained his BA and MA in 1934 and a PhD in 1942. At the University of Minnesota he rose to the rank of associate professor and came to Utah in 1944 as professor and chair of the department.

Dr. McLennan gained approval for a residency in obstetrics and gynecology. In those early years residents at the University came from LDS and Holy Cross hospitals in Salt Lake City and Dee Hospital in Ogden. Dr. McLennan is remembered as "a very reserved individual but an effective, methodical teacher, particularly in the clinical setting. Always a gentleman, his comments were characteristically brief, incisive."

When McLennan left the University in 1947, Dr. Holmstrom became professor and chair of the department. Also a Duluth native,

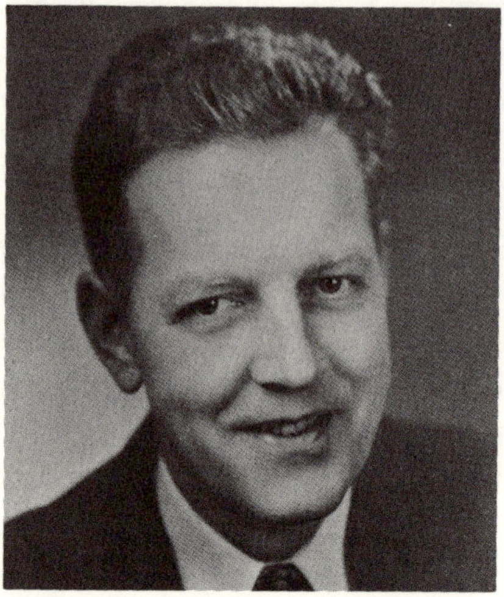

Emil G. Holmstrom, MD, one of several recruits from Minnesota, arrived in Utah in 1943. Greatly appreciated as a gentle surgeon and superb teacher, he was professor and head of the department from 1947 to 1958.

Holmstrom had received training in the universities in that state, graduating from the University of Minnesota Medical School in 1938. He began his academic career as an instructor there in 1942. He came to the University of Utah in 1943 and was promoted to associate professor in 1944.

The Department of Obstetrics and Gynecology at the old Salt Lake General Hospital occupied a one-story bungalow-type building separate from the main hospital and originally used as an isolation unit for tuberculosis patients. It accommodated all obstetric patients, an occasional gynecologic patient who desired a private room, a teaching area, and the departmental offices.

If an obstetric patient required x-ray studies or surgery, she had to be transported to the main hospital building. This was no easy task, as she had to be moved down a ramp, across a driveway, along an alley between the infirmary and the heating plant, down another ramp into the hospital emergency room area, and from there into the main hospital structure. In those days — rain, shine, or snow — the maternity patient in distress was rushed along that precarious hundred-yard route.

Dr. Holmstrom was a meticulous and very involved teacher. He had unusual skills as a gynecologic pathologist and used this knowledge extensively in teaching obstetric and gynecologic disease in the classroom as well as in the operating and delivery rooms. He guided students and residents a step at a time through the techniques required for the management of obstetric and gynecologic disease. His interaction with residents and students also brought them into his home, where he and his wife were gracious hosts.

Sometime during his student obstetric rotation, young Hebertson sprained his left ankle severely. Both ankle and foot were badly swollen, but of course this was no excuse not to be actively involved on the service. As luck would have it, he was "invited" to participate in a delivery. He changed clothes in the common changing area and then began to search through the rubber surgical shoes for one that would fit his swollen foot. The medium, which he usually wore, did not fit, nor did the large. He continued to search and found a nice large pair of white leather shoes. He slipped them on and limped down the hall to take his place at the side of the resident who was preparing the patient for delivery.

Dr. Holmstrom was the patient's attending physician. The house staff waited for him as patiently as possible while the woman bore down. The baby arrived without respect for the absence of its mother's distinguished obstetrician. Just as the baby was being delivered, Dr. Holmstrom entered the room properly attired in his scrub suit, cap, and mask but in his stocking feet. It became apparent to whom the very clean white leather shoes belonged. In his very gentle and patient way he asked, "Has anyone seen my operating room shoes?" Fortunately for young Hebertson, Dr. Holmstrom was also a very understanding man.

Dr. Holmstrom left Salt Lake City rather suddenly in 1958. He moved to Los Angeles, California, as head of Ob-Gyn at Kaiser Permanente. Many years later he died tragically and unexpectedly. The University community was stunned.

Once again the Medical School began a search for a replacement for this distinguished teacher. In 1959 Dr. Irwin Kaiser came to Utah as professor in the Department of Obstetrics and Gynecology, the fourth chair recruited from the University of Minnesota. Born in New York City, he received his BA from Columbia University and in 1942 his MD from Johns Hopkins. He served an internship in obstetrics and gynecology, followed by another internship in internal medicine at Sinai Hospital in Baltimore, Maryland, where he completed his residency in obstetrics and gynecology. In 1950 Dr. Kaiser joined the University of Minnesota obstetrics and gynecology faculty as an instructor. Over the years he rose to the rank of associate professor, and in 1953 he also earned a PhD. In 1957-58 he studied at the Karolinska Institute in Stockholm, Sweden. The thrust of that year was broadening his understanding of radiation techniques for the management of gynecologic malignancies.

Dr. Kaiser, like his immediate predecessors, was a distinguished teacher. Didactic sessions, walking rounds, personal instruction in the pathology laboratory, and weekly chart rounds were high points in the education of his residents. Careful and specific questioning were techniques which sharpened the residents' understanding of obstetric and gynecologic disease. Each and every chart was reviewed meticulously, from the patient's admission through her management while in the hospital to discharge and follow-up care. The resident who managed the patient and completed the chart had to defend its contents. The resident's signature meant the chart was ready for Dr. Kaiser's scrutiny, criticism, and signature — the gaining of which was no easy task.

Under Dr. Kaiser's leadership the first resident was recruited directly to the University's own Obstetrics and Gynecology training program. Kaiser brought significant improvements to the management of gynecologic malignancy in the entire Intermountain West. He had energetic therapeutic approaches especially for the therapy of cervical malignancies. He reached for the highest level of cure, and his expertise brought patients with tumors of all types to the University. He also established the first Ob-Gyn postgraduate education course in the Intermountain community. From very humble beginnings, that postgraduate course has become one of the oldest and most successful continuous education programs in the United States.

During Kaiser's tenure the department sent its first resident to Philadelphia to study reproductive endocrinology. That resident, Dr. Marsh Poulson, returned about a year later to become the first reproductive endocrinologist in the Intermountain area, and he is still a member of the department.

Kaiser's scholarship and interest extended beyond departmental demands. He was a moving force in many social issues related to the specialty. He was instrumental in introducing "humanizing" concepts to obstetric care, including patients walking about during labor, fathers being actively supportive during labor and being allowed in the delivery room, and the use of local anesthetics as opposed to "twilight sleep" and general anesthetics. Spontaneous delivery with a diminished use of forceps characterized his approach. He also had great concern for the proper application of contraception and the right of women to make independent decisions concerning abortion. Many of his views were advanced for his time.

Kaiser had as his first associate Dr. Thomas Kirshbaum, a very promising young academician, well informed and astute. He was completely confident and not infrequently would challenge the professor. Dr. Kaiser readily responded to that challenge, and their discussions were very informative and stimulating for all.

Dr. Kaiser brought visiting professors to Utah. Dr. George Enhorning came from Sweden on a sabbatical. He had been deeply involved in the early studies dealing with stress urinary incontinence, the evaluation of intravesical and intraurethral pressures, and the changes which are characteristic of stress urinary incontinence. Dr. Enhorning also had considerable skill in the surgical management of gynecologic malignancy, and he and Dr. Kaiser instructed the residents in radical gynecologic pelvic surgery. It was not until several years after Kaiser left Utah that subspecialists and gynecologic oncologists came on the staff.

During Kaiser's tenure, plans were made for, and construction completed on, the new University Medical School and University Hospital. This project was time-consuming, but it marked a critical step in the development of the department.

During his administration the School of Nurse Midwifery was established, and Dr. Kaiser was very supportive of this concept of obstetric care.

In a very sophisticated circadian laboratory at the new Medical Center, Dr. Kaiser began experiments on rodents. He introduced solid clinical and bench research into the department, expanded the faculty, and attracted interested researchers from other departments and disciplines. He was involved with Dr. Leo Samuels, a pioneer in biochemistry research at the University who made significant contributions to the expanding literature. Eventually two biochemists, Drs. Max Sweat and Melvin Bryson, were given appointments in the department, and laboratory research became a departmental activity. In particular their studies dealt with metabolically active gynecologic tumors.

Dr. Kaiser began efforts toward affiliating other hospitals with the University training program, a goal which was not achieved until after his departure. He established a foundation which allowed continued, solid expansion.

When Kaiser moved from the University in 1968, he left many good friends and a faculty that bridged the gap between his departure and the recruiting of Dr. Morton Stenchever.

Dr. Richard Hebertson, a 1958 graduate of the University of Utah Medical School and instructor in the department from 1964 to 1968, was promoted to assistant professor and acting chair from 1968 to 1970. He became associate professor in 1971, when he assumed the position as full-time chief of a very active service at LDS Hospital, with 4,863 deliveries and 2,062 gynecologic procedures that year.

In 1970 Dr. Morton A. Stenchever came to the University of Utah from Case Western Reserve Medical School. From the outset he established himself as a community leader strongly committed to an extended base for the residency program, and soon after his arrival LDS Hospital became an affiliate. The added staff and clinical material contributed significantly to the recruitment of residents to the combined program.

Dr. Stenchever stimulated expanded departmental research activities. He established the Cytogenetics Laboratory, which was the first of its type in the Intermountain region. A clinical prenatal testing laboratory introduced precision into the evaluation of fetal lung maturity, and techniques for evaluating placental function began.

Cytogenetics and prenatal testing established the department as a major referral center for high-risk obstetrics. As a result, perinatology and maternal transport became departmental activities. Neonatologists became part of the improved care for the newborn. Electronic fetal monitoring was also begun during this period, and he added additional staff to the Division of Reproductive Endocrinology.

Expanding on Kaiser's work in gynecologic oncology, Stenchever soon recruited the region's first gynecologic oncologist — Dr. Gary Johnson from UCLA — in 1972. Johnson was joined later by Dr. Gary Smith from M. D. Anderson Hospital in Houston, and both moved from the University to LDS Hospital in 1981. They have developed a busy practice there, with referrals from the entire Intermountain area, and they have participated actively in the national gynecologic oncology group. Dr. Chris Jolles was appointed at the University in their place.

Stenchever's personal interest in the education of students and residents established him as a national leader in the methodology of medical education. He was also involved in organizations responsible for developing educational goals for the discipline of obstetrics and gynecology and established educational outreach for the region. The surge in research, application of innovative clinical management techniques, and innovative education programs greatly enhanced the recruitment of residents and, for the first time, the University residency gained a national reputation.

Dr. Stenchever was recognized as a cordial and gentlemanly ambassador within the Salt Lake and Intermountain community. In 1977 he accepted the chair at the University of Washington in Seattle.

The next department chair, Dr. James R. Scott, came to Utah in 1977 from the faculty of the University of Iowa, where he also had attended medical school. After several years of family practice, he took a residency in obstetrics and gynecology there as well. He completed a fellowship in immunology at the University of Texas

Southwestern Medical School and served on the faculty of that school before returning to Iowa.

During Dr. Scott's tenure, the department faculty has more than doubled in size, with commensurate expansion of clinical, laboratory, and administrative facilities. Soon after his arrival, the detailed planning phase for the new University Hospital was begun, and this permitted major departmental input into the final form of the innovative perinatal facility, which has been occupied since 1981. Total remodeling of the Ob-Gyn outpatient area was completed in 1984. This has furthered a primary commitment to high-quality patient care. Remarkable growth in basic and clinical research productivity within the department has taken place. The immunology laboratory enjoys an international reputation as a leading unit in reproductive and tumor immunology research, and each division has added programs to provide breadth and depth to the total research endeavor.

Commitment to teaching remains a top priority at student, resident, and postgraduate levels. The Utah residency is now among the most sought-after in the country, fostering selection of an outstanding group of trainees.

PART FIVE

•

PEDIATRICS

CHAPTER THIRTY-ONE

Department of Pediatrics at the University of Utah

L. GEORGE VEASY, MD

THE DEPARTMENT OF PEDIATRICS BEGAN WITH a full-time faculty of two individuals in the fall of 1943. The first chair of the department was John A. Anderson, MD, PhD, who came from the University of Minnesota Department of Pediatrics, where he was an assistant professor. At age thirty-five he assumed the dual role of professor and chair of the Department of Pediatrics and head of the Department of Pediatrics at the Salt Lake General Hospital. Dr. Anderson brought Dr. Robert H. Alway as the only other full-time member. Dr. Alway was just completing his tour as head resident in the Department of Pediatrics at the University of Minnesota Hospitals, and he was appointed instructor. For a brief period in 1945 and 1946 a third full-time member, Dr. C. Harrison Snyder, was in the department. Dr. Sophie Alway, Robert Alway's wife, was also a pediatrician and, while not a full-time faculty member, she carried the bulk of the load for the well-baby clinic.

"Downtown" pediatricians gave considerable support in medical student teaching and in covering a large part of the clinical service. Most prominent in this group was Dr. L. Paul Rasmussen, but Drs. Spencer Snow, John Mason, and William Young were also heavily involved in the activities of the embryonic department.

Dr. Anderson was an unusually charismatic and persuasive individual who successfully won the support of the entire pediatric community. He became well known for his investigative efforts in

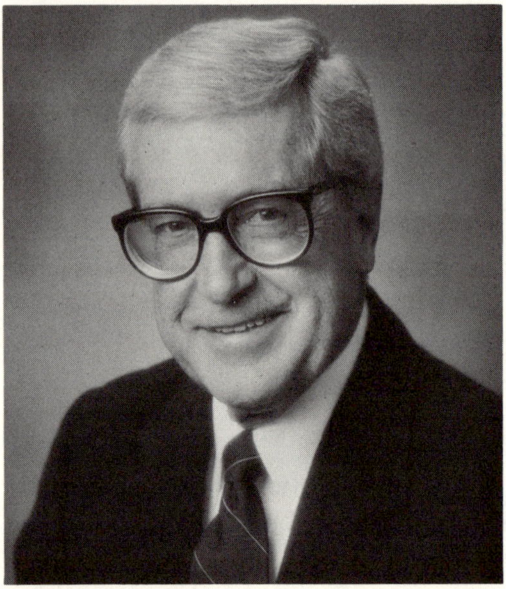

L. George Veasy.

management of poliomyelitis victims. Perhaps his most significant contribution was pointing out the increased risk of bulbar poliomyelitis following a tonsillectomy.

As a teacher he had a strong conviction that disease and its manifestations should be explained in terms of basic science. Pure empiricism was his pet peeve, which resulted in a firm scientific basis for all his teaching. He was well known for citing metabolic pathways during his rounds and would, at the drop of a hat, run through a metabolic cycle — much to the dismay of house staff and medical students, as well as attending physicians.

His impact on the community was profound. He created an impressive board of community leaders and also obtained legislative support to establish a children's hospital in Salt Lake City, which was funded and built in 1949 at a cost of $623,000. One-third of the cost was covered by the Federal Hospital Survey and Construction Act. The remainder was raised successfully through the hospital corporation, which he had founded, and by contributions from the National Foun-

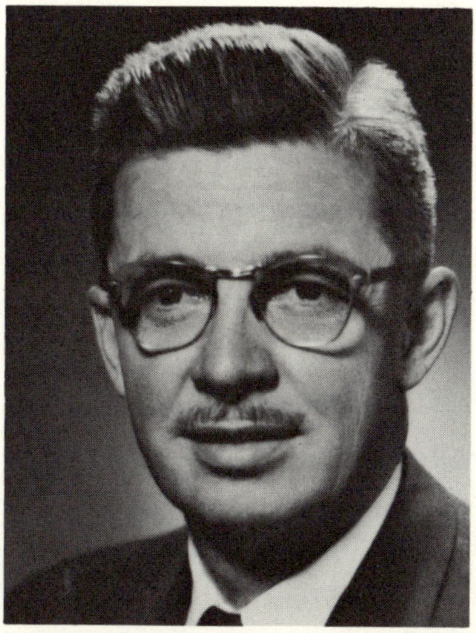

John A. Anderson, MD, PhD, arrived at the Medical School in 1943 as the first chair of the Department of Pediatrics. Known for the scientific basis of his teaching and for his investigations into poliomyelitis, Anderson was also very active and effective in the community.

dation for Infantile Paralysis (now birth defects), the Lions' Club, and several affluent donors in the community. The hospital was to have opened in 1950, but Governor J. Bracken Lee vetoed the maintenance appropriation, saying that Primary Children's Hospital and Shriners' Hospital were functioning in the community and that a fifty-bed hospital primarily for poliomyelitis patients did not seem justified.

The structure that was to have been the children's hospital became instead the headquarters for the Crippled Children's Services of the State of Utah (now Handicapped Children's Services) and served as the state bacteriology and virology laboratory for nearly two decades. Few people realize that the yellow-brown brick building just below the University of Utah Medical Center was indeed designed to be a children's hospital. It is quite remarkable that the structure housing the University of Utah School of Medicine and University Medical Center was erected adjacent to this building some twenty years later. It is more remarkable that four decades later a new Primary Children's Medical Center (PCMC) was occupied in early 1990, less than a block away.

Dr. Anderson left Utah in September of 1949 to chair the Department of Pediatrics at Stanford University School of Medicine, then located in San Francisco. Five years later he left Stanford to head the Department of Pediatrics at the University of Minnesota, his old alma mater, a post he held until his retirement in 1967.

When Dr. Anderson left for Stanford, he took Dr. Alway with him. Alway eventually became dean of Stanford's Medical School from 1958 to 1964, guiding the School through a very stormy period in its move from San Francisco to its present location in Palo Alto. The administrative building at Stanford University Medical School was renamed the Robert H. Alway Building in 1988.

Dr. Alway was particularly proud of the fact that he had been a two-pound premature who had miraculously survived without the benefit of modern-day support, being placed in a shoe box and surrounded by cotton batting and an attentive, anxious family.

From September 1949 to January of 1950, the Department of Pediatrics had no head. Dr. John Waldo of the Department of Medicine, who headed the infectious disease section, served as acting chair during this shaky interlude. Dr. Eugene Lahey, who later became department chair, was serving the last year of his fellowship in hematology under Dr. Maxwell Wintrobe, and he and Dr. Waldo were essentially the only full-time faculty members. Once again, the community pediatricians rallied to support the teaching and clinical programs of the School.

The second department chair was Dr. James F. Bosma, who was also a graduate of the University of Minnesota program. He brought his Minnesota colleague Dr. Vincent C. Kelley with him. Like his predecessor Dr. Anderson, Dr. Bosma was particularly interested in poliomyelitis and was intrigued by the ravaging effects of bulbar involvement. He became increasingly interested in the complex neuromuscular interaction involved with swallowing and devoted his life to the study of the swallowing mechanism.

Dr. Kelley established an energetic young group of investigators, including Drs. Robert Ely and Thomas Good. Their particular interest was the pituitary adrenal axis, and they became leaders in investigat-

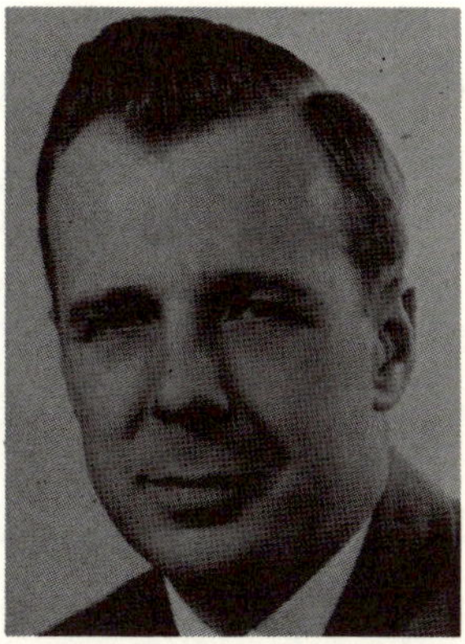

James F. Bosma, MD, recruited from the University of Minnesota as professor and chair of the Department of Pediatrics in 1949, served in that capacity until 1958. He devoted his life to research into poliomyelitis and problems in swallowing and phonation.

ing the alterations seen in children with auto-immune disorders, particularly acute rheumatic fever.

During the first years of Dr. Bosma's term as chair, the department grew rather impressively and rapidly with the addition of pediatric neurologists Drs. Neils Lowe and Patrick Bray and pediatric cardiologists Drs. Harry Stoeckle and Lorin Ainger.

As a result of funding problems and some personal dissension in the department, several members left for positions elsewhere — Dr. Lowe to Columbia, Dr. Kelley to the University of Washington, Dr. Ely to the University of Arkansas, Dr. Good to the University of Maryland, Dr. Stoeckle to the University of Missouri, and Dr. Ainger to Le Bonheur Children's Hospital in Memphis, Tennessee. Dr. Bosma, discouraged by the lack of support from his faculty members, elected to step down as department chair in 1958. In a most fervent and productive manner, he continued to study the complex mechanisms of deglutition at the University of Utah for an additional eighteen months and then took a sabbatical leave to continue his studies on a fellowship in Sweden. In 1961 he returned to the U.S. to become chief of the Oral and Pharyngeal Development Section of the Dental Research Institute, a division of the National Institutes of Health. He continued his studies on swallowing and phonation until his retirement in 1980. Although Dr. Bosma had asked to step down as department chair, he continued to direct departmental affairs until Dr. M. Eugene Lahey assumed the chair in the summer of 1958.

Dr. Lahey was an exceptionally popular choice, since he was well known to both the Medical School faculty and the community pediatricians. He had completed a National Research Council fellowship in hematology under Dr. Max Wintrobe in 1951. He had also been an assistant professor in the department from 1951 to 1952. He was well respected for his fundamental work in copper metabolism and became known as an exceptionally astute clinician. In 1952 he left for the University of Cincinnati, where he became highly visible on the national scene as an authority on copper metabolism and hematopoiesis.

He returned to Utah as chair in 1958 to a hero's welcome. There probably has never been a department head selected who was more popular with the full-time faculty and downtown pediatricians. A small nucleus of dedicated academicians remained at the time of his return, including Drs. Bosma, Alan K. Done, who was interested in pharmacology and toxicology, and Pat Bray.

Dr. Done served as a research associate under Dr. Kelley in 1955 and was appointed an instructor in the department in 1956. In December 1971 he left to assume a position with the Federal Drug Administration, where he remained until 1975, when he moved to Wayne University and Children's Hospital of Michigan to head the Division of Toxicology.

Dr. Bray worked during the first half of 1958 with Dr. Lahey and then spent a year at Stanford University and a year in neurology at Babies Hospital associated with Columbia University in New York. He returned in 1960 as associate professor and became chair of the Division of Neurology.

Needless to say, with the department in limbo for such a long time, morale was low despite the remaining stalwarts. Dr. Lahey began turning this around by his very arrival, and he embarked on an orderly program to recruit bright young faculty members to meet the teaching, research, and patient-care needs of the department.

As had been the case with his predecessors, Dr. Lahey brought with him the brightest young man with whom he had been associated. This was Dr. Jack Wilson, who was just finishing his term as chief resident at Cincinnati Children's Hospital. Dr. Lahey had served as his mentor during the time that Dr. Wilson developed an intense interest in pediatric hematology. Working together, these two made significant clinical observations and confirmed the presence of protein-losing enteropathy in iron deficiency anemia. Dr. Wilson's interest in hematology ultimately stimulated him to take a pathology residency, primarily to increase his skills in laboratory research. However, he decided to finish the entire pathology residency to become a board-certified pathologist. In 1969 he became head of pathology at PCMC, where he remained for the next twenty years.

Dr. Douglas Heiner, a pediatric cardiologist from Boston Children's Hospital, also joined the faculty in 1960. This superbly trained and skilled cardiologist became involved with Drs. Lahey and Wilson in the investigation of protein-losing enteropathy associated with exclusive oral intake of milk. He also became fascinated with a gel diffusion technique which demonstrated the presence of serum antibodies to gluten in celiac disease. Dr. Heiner became so involved with the immunology entailed with this disorder that he left the field of cardiology and Salt Lake City to obtain additional training in protein metabolism at the University of Quebec. He then took a position at UCLA, where he remains at the present time.

Dr. Marvin Rallison joined the department in 1963 and remains as professor and head of the Division of Endocrinology. He wrote a textbook on pediatric endocrinology and has become recognized as a leading authority on thyroid disease in children.

In 1964 Dr. Lahey resigned his University appointment and went to Children's Hospital of East Bay in Oakland, California, where he served as director of research. Dr. Bray, chair of the Division of Neurology, was acting chair for the year of Dr. Lahey's absence (August 1964 to August 1965), and the department continued to thrive under his leadership. During this twelve-month period some problems between Dr. Lahey and the Department of Surgery and PCMC were resolved. Much credit is due Dr. Bray for guiding the department smoothly through what could easily have been a very stormy period.

Dr. Lahey was reappointed professor and department chair and resumed his duties in August 1965. During the course of the next two years, an agreement was made with PCMC for the Medical School to have increased house staff and medical student rotation there. The stipulation was that a full-time faculty member would have to be based at the hospital to supervise educational activities.

Dr. L. George Veasy was approved by the University to hold the rank of associate professor and begin his duties at PCMC as the director of pediatrics, education, and research in January of 1968. Dr. Veasy was a University of Utah graduate who obtained his training in pediatrics and pediatric cardiology at the University of Minnesota. He had been a member of the faculty as instructor in the department in 1952 and 1953 before entering private practice in Salt Lake City.

The Division of Neurology added Drs. Jack Madsen and Fred Ziter in 1965. Dr. Madsen became interested in seizure disorders and established the Epilepsy Center, based initially at the American Fork Training Center and now at PCMC. Dr. Ziter developed a particular interest in neuromuscular disease and now serves as director of the Electromyography Laboratory at the University Medical Center.

In 1967 Dr. August L. (Larry) Jung, also a University of Utah Medical School graduate and former pediatric resident, joined the department as an instructor. After taking a neonatology fellowship at the University of Colorado, he returned in 1968 to head the Division of Neonatology and established the first neonatal intensive care unit in the Intermountain area. The unit began with just five beds, but the demand was so heavy that it was rapidly expanded to twelve beds and to thirty beds within a five-year span. The unit became the showpiece of the University Hospital. Even with expansion, the demand for neonatology intensive care services could not be met, and many babies had to be sent to out-of-state facilities. Planning for a sister unit at PCMC was begun in 1975, and it was completed in 1978 with twenty-two beds. This unit continues to be directed by the Division of Neonatology.

Dr. James Overall joined the department as chair of infectious disease in 1968. He remains as professor and chair of the Division of Infectious Disease and enjoys a well-established national reputation. He currently serves as vice-chair of the department under Dr. Michael Simmons.

The year 1969 saw three appointments. Dr. Herbert Ruttenberg came from UCLA to head the Division of Cardiology. (The clinical services for the cardiology division moved to PCMC in 1975 with the research labs continuing at the University.) Dr. Joel Thompson joined the Division of Neurology and has been based at PCMC. He was appointed chair of the Division of Neurology in 1988 and continues to serve in that capacity. And, finally, Dr. John Herbst joined the faculty that year as a subspecialist in gastroenterology. He established a cystic fibrosis clinic and remained active on the staff as professor until 1987, when he left to chair the Department of Pediatrics at the University of Louisiana in Shreveport.

Dr. Richard Siegler joined the department in 1972, after completing his pediatric residency at the University of Utah and an additional year of fellowship in nephrology. He has been chair of the Division of Nephrology since 1974, and he served as acting head of the department from 1982 to 1983.

Dr. Harry Hill joined the staff in 1974 from the University of Minnesota, where he had completed an infectious disease fellowship and was serving as instructor. He currently holds a professorship in pediatrics and pathology and is head of the Division of Immunology and Allergy.

Dr. Lowell Glasgow, a graduate of the University of Rochester School of Medicine, was appointed chair of the Department of Microbiology at the University of Utah in 1973 and was given a joint appointment in pediatrics at that time. He had served his residency in pediatrics at Rochester and later had been appointed a research associate at the National Institute of Allergy and Infectious Diseases. Dr. Glasgow was remarkably successful as an investigator, teacher, and administrator and was able to procure a planning grant for cancer research for the University of Utah School of Medicine which did not come to fruition until he was being diligently pursued by several institutions to head their departments of pediatrics as well as microbiology. Dr. Lahey feared that should Lowell Glasgow leave, Dr. Overall, an irreplaceable faculty member, would likely move with him, since the two had become very good friends while collaborating in several projects. Therefore, in 1972 Dr. Lahey proposed to Dr. Frank Tyler, then dean of the School of Medicine, that he should step down as chair of the department and that Dr. Glasgow should be appointed in his stead.

Dr. Tyler appointed Dr. Glasgow chair in 1973. While this was an ideal solution for all concerned, the action initially stirred up considerable controversy, with feelings that Dr. Lahey had been pressured inappropriately and that proper University protocol had not been followed in Glasgow's appointment. All furor died down, however, when the facts were known, and Dr. Glasgow was then able to assume his chairmanship with strong faculty support.

Dr. Lahey continued on as professor, remaining active in teaching and investigating his number-one interest, the poorly understood storage disease histiocytosis. He became professor emeritus in 1983 but continues to be active in departmental affairs.

Dr. Glasgow expanded the full-time faculty rapidly and effectively. During the nine years that he was department chair, the full-time faculty membership grew from fourteen to more than fifty, with nearly all subspecialties represented. Dr. Glasgow continued to contribute to his chosen field of infectious diseases and served on many national scientific advisory bodies, including the virology subsection of the National Institute of Allergy and Infectious Disease, and chaired the committee on toxic shock syndrome of the National Academy of Sciences. He won the Squibb Award of the Infectious Disease Society of America in 1977. Dr. Glasgow worked arduously with an ad hoc committee from the University and PCMC to obtain a more comprehensive agreement between the two institutions. Through this agreement he became medical director in PCMC, and Dr. Veasy's title was changed to physician-in-chief at PCMC in 1975.

The Medical School and the entire pediatric community were shocked by Dr. Glasgow's sudden and totally unexpected death on

February 4, 1982. At forty-nine, while sitting at his desk at home reviewing grants in the early morning hours, he succumbed to a massive myocardial infarction.

Dr. Richard Siegler was appointed interim chair of the department, which was able through his hard work and special interpersonal skills to weather a rather stormy period. Dr. Glasgow had handled virtually all of the administrative duties of the department, and many management details died with him. Departmental affairs were briefly in disarray until Dr. Siegler could stabilize the many pressures upon him from the faculty, other University departments, and PCMC. He managed to keep the situation under control, despite the fact that he was in the uncomfortable position of being responsible for decisions without having full authority to make them.

The search committee for a new chair selected Dr. Michael A. Simmons early in 1983. Dr. Simmons was clearly the obvious choice, and all concerned were extremely relieved when he accepted the appointment. A 1967 graduate of Harvard Medical School, Simmons completed his pediatric internship and residency at Johns Hopkins in 1969. He then moved to Colorado for a fellowship in neonatology and was appointed instructor in the Department of Pediatrics in 1972 and co-director of newborn services in 1974. He had moved to Johns Hopkins in 1977 as an associate professor of pediatrics and obstetrics and co-director of newborn services, and in 1981 he was made deputy director of the Department of Pediatrics.

Dr. Simmons's reputation as an energetic, charismatic, and effective leader proved to be well founded, and the department has experienced truly phenomenal growth since he assumed the chair. Sagging morale and lack of cohesiveness turned around dramatically and emphatically with his arrival. He instilled a new sense of commitment and confidence. He achieved this primarily as an exemplary role model, assuming more than his share of mundane tasks and clearly working harder and more effectively than anyone else in the department. He also delegated division chairs to assume complete management of their own divisions and to share more responsibility for the department as a whole.

Dr. Simmons engineered an even stronger affiliation agreement between the University and PCMC, which committed the parties to mutually supporting the development of a unique program to provide optimal pediatric medical care. This agreement made it possible for the new PCMC to be built on the University campus.

The move in April of 1990 into the beautiful, up-to-date Primary Children's Medical Center next to the University of Utah School of Medicine helped in the recruitment of many promising young faculty members who are able to embark upon a wide range of basic science as well as clinical research projects. Their presence will provide the opportunity to develop an unmatched center for the care of children.

The full-time faculty currently comprises eighty-one staff positions and three PhDs. A clinical faculty of ninety-nine participates as attending physicians at the University of Utah and at PCMC.

The founders of the University of Utah Medical School in their most ambitious moments would not have dreamed that the School would attain such size and prestige. This certainly holds true for the Department of Pediatrics, which had such a shaky and inconspicuous beginning. While the faculty can take pride in what has been achieved, they look forward with excited anticipation to a promising future for the specialty and the care it will provide for the next generation of children.

CHAPTER THIRTY-TWO

Primary Children's Medical Center

L. GEORGE VEASY, MD

WITH CHILDREN'S HOSPITAL OF PHILADELPHIA established in 1855, Children's Hospital in Boston opening in 1869, and virtually all long-standing children's hospitals in North America operating by 1900, Primary Children's was a late arrival on the scene. The hospital's origin is attributable to the efforts of Mrs. Louie B. Felt and Miss May Anderson, who were serving as President and First Counselor of the Church of Jesus Christ of Latter-day Saints' Primary Association (the children's division) in 1911, when an encounter with a crippled boy prompted them to go to the church's general authorities to seek support to provide care for such children under Primary sponsorship. They were successful, and for more than a decade funds were provided for care for a limited number of children in the orthopedic ward at the LDS Hospital. The prolonged period necessary for full convalescent recovery proved to be an enormous load for the few available beds.

The Hyde Home, a large house on North Temple Street, was purchased and remodeled and opened its doors in 1922, marking the beginning of the Primary Children's Hospital. During that first year, 212 children were cared for.

The hospital continued to function at the North Temple site for the next three decades, while its reputation as an institution that provided compassionate and concerned care in an exemplary manner grew steadily. Nurse Anna Rosenkilde headed the administrative staff.

She was "Mama Rose" to her charges, and her kind demeanor was legendary.

Dr. Samuel Baldwin, a skilled and gentle orthopedic surgeon, headed the medical staff until 1937. By 1950 the staff had expanded to include seven orthopedic surgeons, eight pediatricians, three general surgeons, three otolaryngologists, five dentists, two urologists, a neurosurgeon, a thoracic surgeon, and a plastic surgeon, but all major surgery continued to be performed at the LDS Hospital. During the three decades of the "Convalescent Home," as it was first known, 5,907 children were treated, and the average length of stay was 158 days.

As the demand for facilities increased, LDS Church President Heber J. Grant authorized the purchase of land at 12th Avenue and D Street. Construction of a new hospital building started in 1949, and it was completed and occupied in February 1952. The Primary Association raised half of the $2 million cost, and half was donated by the LDS Church. The names of all the children and Primary workers who contributed a dime for a brick in the "brick fund" were placed in the cornerstone of the new building. The cornerstone was opened on "Legacy Day," just before the patients were moved to the present facility on the University of Utah campus on April 23, 1990.

The original capacity of the 12th Avenue facility was seventy-two beds, double the number in the Hyde Home. The census increased each year, and in 1961 the fifth floor was completed. The bed capacity was now eighty-four, and inpatient days increased to 18,873. A new "West Wing" was completed in 1966, doubling the bed capacity once again to 170 and providing badly needed space to update the radiology department and the clinical laboratory. The pediatric ward at LDS Hospital was then closed, making Primary Children's the largest pediatric care facility in the Intermountain area.

From the outside the building looks much the same today as it did in 1966, but the inside has continued to undergo constant revision, with child psychiatry occupying the entire third floor ward area and the southwest corner. In 1974 the schoolrooms on the third floor gave way to the Special Procedures Laboratory, and in 1978 the Four South ward was remodeled to accommodate the newborn intensive care area. In 1980 the emergency room was expanded and a CT scan unit added. That same year, additional remodeling on the fifth floor permitted outpatient surgery for the first time. The curved areas on the east and west ends of the original building were covered to provide waiting areas on the west for families with patients in ICU and on the east to expand outpatient surgery. Virtually every area of the building has undergone remodeling, and expansion of services was possible only by moving personnel to the "Annex" in the Old Veterans Administration facility to the north or into not-so-temporary trailers to the south.

In 1971 the LDS Church authorities decided to centralize the management of the fourteen Church-owned hospitals in the Intermountain area. The agency was called Health Services Corporation (HSC), and Dr. James Mason was appointed director. Ownership of the children's hospital was transferred to HSC from the Primary Association, and the Primary Association Board no longer served as the hospital's governing board. All hospital boards in the new HSC organization were chaired by presidents of the LDS stakes located near the individual hospitals.

The year 1973 inaugurated an extremely troublesome and turbulent period for Primary Children's. To further consolidate hospital management, HSC chose to eliminate the board altogether and have the LDS Hospital Board, with Primary representation, serve for both institutions. In addition, the administrator of LDS Hospital became the administrator of Primary Children's, whose former head was made assistant administrator.

In 1975 the LDS Church transferred the ownership of its hospitals yet again to a newly formed and independent organization, Intermountain Health Care (IHC), headed by Scott S. Parker. One of the new organization's first administrative actions was to restore the independent board and administration of the children's hospital, now Primary Children's Medical Center (PCMC). Richard Van Winkle accepted the board chairmanship, and Donald Poulter was appointed administrator.

In less than five years, PCMC had been owned by three different organizations and had had four distinctly different boards and four administrators. After 1975 the stability of the hospital and the support it received resulted in phenomenal growth. The association with the University's Department of Pediatrics has been openly encouraged and allowed to flourish, resulting in the move to a new $70 million facility on the University of Utah campus.

The Medical Staff

Through the years, the medical staff of Primary Children's has experienced remarkable growth, paralleling the hospital's increase in size and capability. In 1936 there were 27 medical doctors on the staff. By 1950 the total was 34, 8 of whom were pediatricians, including Drs. Merritt Egan, W. L. Felt, Esther Gross, William McMain, Robert Rothwell, Paul Rasmussen, Spencer Snow, and William Young. A decade later in 1960, the staff had grown to 126 members. In 1970 there were 244 members, increasing to 341 by 1980. Currently in 1990 there are 438, including board-certified members in every specialty and virtually every subspecialty related to pediatrics.

In 1960 the Primary Hospital Board decided to change the hospital's mission from providing convalescent and custodial care to more acute care, with the goal of becoming a complete total-care hospital. In keeping with this decision, Dr. John Caffey, the "father" of pediatric radiology, was recruited as the first radiologist in 1961, sharing his time with St. Mark's Hospital and the University of Utah. Caffey, a native Utahn who had recently retired from Babies Hospital in New York City, was persuaded by Dr. Henry Plenk and the radiology community to accept this position. His appointment must surely have raised many an academic eyebrow in the East, but it brought broad smiles to the pediatric community in Utah.

In that same year, Dr. Richard Elwyn became the first pediatric anesthesiologist to be based at Primary and to limit his practice to children. Now there are nine. Dr. Garth Myers started the Birth Defects Center, a multi-specialty clinic primarily to manage patients with myelomeningocele defects.

In 1962 Dr. Virgil Condon replaced Dr. Caffey as the first full-time chief radiologist when Dr. Caffey opted to return to the East for personal reasons. Dr. Condon proved to be a remarkably gifted and knowledgeable radiologist. His presence was pivotal to the subsequent growth of the hospital, which now includes five full-time pediatric radiologists. The department of medical imaging now includes magnetic resonance imaging (MRI), computerized tomography, special procedures room, and full ultrasound capability. In 1960, 2,132 x-ray examinations were done compared with 28,080 in 1989.

Pediatric resident rotations also were begun in 1962 and then extended through an agreement with Dr. Eugene Lahey, chair of the University of Utah Department of Pediatrics. As part of that agreement, in 1967 Dr. L. George Veasy, a pediatric cardiologist on Primary Children's staff, was selected to fill the position of full-time director of Pediatric Education and Research.

In 1968 Dr. Paul L. Whitehead was appointed full-time chair of child psychiatry. The program grew rapidly and currently requires five full-time psychiatrists headed by Dr. Richard Ferre, who supervises the care of 40 inpatients at PCMC, 16 at Cottonwood Hospital, 14 at the residential treatment center in University Park, and 14 in the old VA hospital.

Open-heart surgery was initiated in 1968 by Dr. J D Mortensen. In 1970 Dr. Conrad B. Jenson assumed the directorship of the thoracic and cardiovascular division, and since 1984 the program has been directed by Dr. Ed McGough. In 1989, 132 patients underwent open-heart surgery and 131 had closed-heart surgery.

In 1968 Dr. Jack Wilson joined the hospital-based staff as chair of pathology. Dr. Wilson was uniquely qualified for this position, since he was board-certified in both pediatrics and pathology and had previously been a faculty member in the Department of Pediatrics at the University of Utah. He chaired the Department of Pathology at PCMC for twenty years until his retirement in 1988. During his tenure, he was successful in recruiting Drs. Manford Gooch and Ted Pysher to join him in establishing an outstanding laboratory service. Gooch and Pysher were also doubly Boarded in pediatrics and pathology.

The number of laboratory examinations increased dramatically from 21,211 determinations in 1960 to 398,639 in 1980.

In 1969 Dr. Joel Thompson joined the full-time staff in neurology, expanding the hospital's clinical services. He holds joint appointments in pediatrics and neurology and has been chair of the Division of Pediatric Neurology since 1988.

Dr. Dale Johnson became chair of the Department of Surgery at PCMC in 1972. He was concurrently named chair of the Division of Pediatric Surgery at the University of Utah. Dr. Keith Reemtsma, then chair of the Department of Surgery at the University, was extremely helpful in recruiting Dr. Johnson, who enjoyed an excellent national reputation for his work at Children's Hospital of Philadelphia. Dr. Johnson's expertise resulted in a large referral practice for PCMC, and he has been joined by surgeons Drs. Michael Matlak and Richard Black.

Dr. Herbert Ruttenberg, chair of the Division of Pediatric Cardiology, moved his clinical practice from the University Medical Center to PCMC in 1975. The Special Procedures Laboratory had been completed the year before and provided PCMC with a state-of-the-art facility for studying infants and children with heart disease. During that same year, Dr. Martin Palmer joined the staff to direct outpatient programs. He continues in this position and also serves as chair of the Division of General Pediatrics at the University.

In 1976 Dr. Garth Orsmond joined the staff as a pediatric cardiologist. He directed the development of the echocardiology service at PCMC. Since 1984 he has served as chair of the Division of Pediatric Cardiology at PCMC and at the University.

In 1977 an even stronger and closer affiliation between PCMC and the University's Department of Pediatrics was achieved under the direction of Dr. Lowell Glasgow, Dr. Lahey's successor as department chair. Under the terms of this agreement, Dr. Glasgow became the medical director and Dr. Veasy was made physician-in-chief. The president of the staff, secretary-treasurer, chair of medicine (pediatrics), the medical staff, and the executive committee remained unchanged.

Dr. Richard O'Brien, coming from Yale, where he had held a similar position, assumed the direction of the hematology-oncology program at PCMC in 1981. He currently is head of the Division of Pediatric Hematology–Oncology, which includes a total of six specialists: Drs. Blair Bybee, Richard Lemons, Greg Thomas, Roberta Adams, and Eugene Lahey, Emeritus.

In cooperation with Dr. August L. (Larry) Jung, chair of the University's Division of Neonatology, a six-bed newborn intensive care unit was opened at PCMC in 1978. Because of the demand, it was expanded to twenty-two beds within a year. This unit remains part of the Intermountain Newborn Intensive Care Program and functions as a sister unit to the intensive care unit at the University Medical Center. Patients with congenital birth defects and those requiring neonatal surgery are selectively referred to the PCMC unit. University neonatologists continue to provide twenty-four-hour medical staffing.

Under the direction of Drs. Jack Walker and Richard Black, a transport team of MDs and RNs was trained and activated in 1979 specifically to handle the air transport of critically ill pediatric patients. During its first year of operation, the team transported 232 patients and logged more than 20,000 miles.

The Newest Hospital

In 1981 discussions were undertaken by the staff and administration concerning the need to expand the hospital on 12th Avenue to accommodate the ever-increasing patient load and expanding programs. It was readily apparent that the hospital had literally run out of space. The remodeling and expansion of the emergency room and outpatient surgery, expansion of intensive-care facilities, and the addition of psychiatry beds in the Veterans Hospital Annex clearly were not keeping pace with the demands, and a major building program was inevitable. Consideration was given to building a new hospital on the University campus, a concept strongly supported by Drs. Johnson and Glasgow. An independent study by a consulting group sponsored by Intermountain Health Care recommended expan-

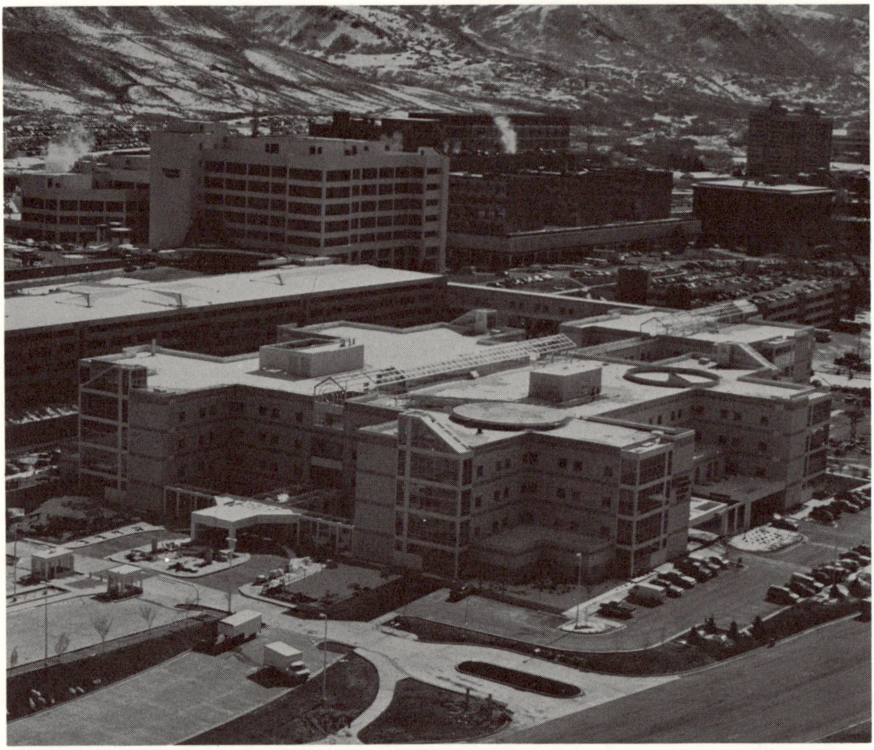

Aerial photograph of the new Primary Children's Medical Center by Colleen Clark, March 16, 1990.

sion on the 12th Avenue site, since the expense of a move to a University site was, in their opinion, prohibitive.

The untimely and totally unexpected death of Dr. Glasgow on February 4, 1982, was a severe loss sorely felt by the medical staff. In addition, the door was closed to further consideration of a new hospital at the University, since the chief advocate for the move had been lost.

While serving as a member of the IHC board of trustees in 1983, Dr. Chase Peterson, the University of Utah's vice president for health sciences, challenged the consulting group's figures and proposed to the medical and administrative staffs of PCMC that the advantages of moving to the University campus would far outweigh the trivial differences in estimated cost — and, indeed, that the move would actually prove less expensive over a twenty-year period.

While reassessment was being conducted by the IHC and PCMC administrative staffs, Dr. Michael Simmons accepted the University's invitation to become chair of the Department of Pediatrics. He assumed this duty and that of medical director of PCMC in October of 1983.

Under Dr. Simmons's guidance, a new and more complete affiliation than that represented by the 1977 agreement between PCMC and the University of Utah School of Medicine was initiated. A major component of this historic affiliation contract was that the chair of the Department of Pediatrics at the University would automatically become the medical director of PCMC. The department chair, however, could be appointed only with the approval of the PCMC board of trustees. This most remarkable concession by both parties ultimately resulted in the decision to build a new Primary Children's Medical Center on the University campus. The agreement was signed in December 1985, after the board of trustees of Intermountain Health Care, as well as the Institutional Council and the Board of Regents of the University, voted affirmatively.

New programs and staff were being added even while the new hospital was under construction. In 1986 Dr. Ed McGough started a program for extracorporeal membrane oxygenation (ECMO), and that same year Dr. Jack Walker introduced the surgical procedure of dorsal rhizotomy, which effects a dramatic functional improvement in selected patients with cerebral palsy.

In 1987 three pediatric intensivists — Drs. Michael Dean, William Banner, and Donald Vernon — joined the staff to direct patient management in the pediatric intensive care unit. Dr. Richard Molteni joined the neonatology staff and started the six-bed bronchopulmonary dysplasia unit (BPD).

On April 23, 1990, patients were transferred in a remarkably short time (eight carefully organized hours) from the "old" hospital on 12th Avenue to the beautiful new hospital on the University campus. This facility of 525,000 square feet more than doubles the size of the

PCMC. All beds except those in intensive care areas are housed in private rooms. The surgical suite has been expanded to eight rooms, with an additional room for endoscopy. Pediatric intensive care has been expanded to twenty-six beds with 155 square feet per bed (nearly double the space in the previous unit). The newborn intensive care unit contains a total of fifty-two beds, including a special room for three patients on ECMO, and offers adjacent family sleeping space (nearly 500 newborns are transferred to PCMC each year). Child psychiatry has a total of forty beds and a large gymnasium for play therapy.

At this writing, this facility is the newest children's hospital in the world and provides the children of the Intermountain community with unrivaled state-of-the-art technology and medical expertise.

CHAPTER THIRTY-THREE

Pediatric Neurology

JACK A. MADSEN, MD

PEDIATRIC NEUROLOGY IS A YOUNGSTER among the giants of medical specialties. The parent fields were neurology and pediatrics. Bernard Sachs (1858–1944), Bronson Crothers (1884–1959), and Frank R. Ford (1892–1970) are honored as the field's "establishment." They were the first to define the bases of pediatric neurology comprehensively through their interest, study, and publication of the first texts of nervous system diseases in children and adolescents. Training in the field largely was a matter of special interest and individual fellowship contact until the late 1950s. Conference among pediatric and neurology leaders of the day, pushed by Pearce Bailey, Jr. (1902–76), who was then head of the National Institute of Neurological Diseases and Blindness (NINDB) resulted in the present concepts of training. The NINDB began funding fellowships in pediatric neurology in 1957. From that point, multiple site-reviewed programs for training pediatric neurologists developed. The American Board of Psychiatry and Neurology began offering "Special Competence in Child Neurology" certifications in 1969, establishing pediatric neurology with the qualifying standard of knowledge and ability recognized for all of the certified specialties.

At Utah, neurological interests were a major focus from the beginning of its four-year College of Medicine, fondly called "the Johns Hopkins of the West." Louis Goodman's interest in antiepileptic drugs and other neurologically active agents is well recognized. Two of Dr. Goodman's students, Ewart Swinyard and Dixon Woodbury, are still very active in the field. Woodbury has labored long in the pharmacology, biochemistry, and physiology of epilepsy and has been a major figure in national epilepsy research policy and direction. Swinyard directs a major drug screening program for the National Institute for Neurology, Communicative Disorders and Stroke (NINCDS) — formerly NINDB — and to date has screened more than 12,000 such agents, approximately twenty of which have undergone human testing, with several approaching FDA approval for marketing.

Gordon Millichap arrived in Utah in 1954 to work with Goodman. He did specific work with acetazolamide, later pronouncing that drug the choice agent for petit mal (it was upstaged the same year when ethosuximide proved even better). Utah's pharmacological impact on epilepsy is well appreciated internationally. The pharmacology department supported the evolving pediatric neurology program strongly, and its support through research in epilepsy continues.

Frank Tyler, the metabolism guru of internal medicine, and Marvin Armstrong of the Department of Biochemistry were pioneers in the identification and treatment of phenylketonuria through studies first done at the Medical School in 1954 and 1955. These and other projects provided background development in pediatric neurology research and set the stage for research and formal training in pediatric neurology in Utah.

Utah's pediatric neurology program was influenced directly by the division of pediatric neurology at Columbia Presbyterian Medical Center. Sidney Carter was the third chairman of this division, first established by Bernard Sachs in 1934. Patrick Bray and Neils Lowe were fellows of Carter in 1954 and 1955. They returned to Columbia to complete "ped-neuro" training under new guidelines in 1957 and 1958. Both played important teaching and research roles in the Department of Pediatrics at Utah in the mid-fifties when they were "between" fellowships. Dr. Lowe remained at Columbia after completing his fellowship, and Dr. Bray returned to Utah in 1960 to establish its first Division of Pediatric Neurology, under Drs. Leonard

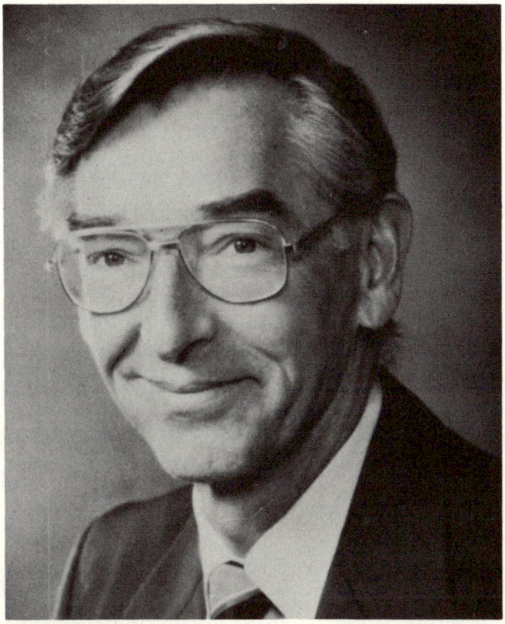

Jack A. Madsen.

Jarcho and Eugene Lahey, chairs of the University's departments of neurology and pediatrics, respectively.

Dr. Garth Myers was pediatrician with the Utah State Health Department's Crippled Children's Service in 1954. Later, with the encouragement of Dr. Madison Thomas (a pioneer neurologist in Utah), Myers' interest in neurologically handicapping conditions solidified, and he trained in pediatric neurology at Bowman Gray School of Medicine in Winston-Salem, North Carolina. In 1961 he returned to develop and head the neurology program at Primary Children's Hospital and to continue his association with the State Health Department's handicapped children's programs.

Dr. James F. Bosma, chair of Pediatrics at Utah from 1951 to 1958, deserves special mention. He was very interested in neurological problems of children, especially epilepsy and poliomyelitis. While he never took formal neurological training, Bosma was an important figure in Utah pediatric neurology of the fifties. His love for children and compassionate understanding for the trials of their parents was appreciated by hundreds of families in the area. His departure, with the entire pediatric department (except for Paul Rasmussen, who patiently held together some tendrils of care and training as acting chair), was abrupt. The administrative catastrophe which led to the departmental rupture serves only to highlight a major point of redirection. Dr. Bosma took sabbatical in Sweden and subsequently joined the National Institutes of Health.

Dr. Eugene Lahey was recruited from Cleveland to head the new department, and it was his vibrant collection of new faculty which Pat Bray joined in 1960. In 1959 Dr. Leonard Jarcho returned from neurology training at Harvard's Massachusetts General Hospital under Raymond D. Adams and a fellowship at Queen's Square, London, to head the Division of Neurology under the Department of Medicine.

Thus, four new programs, the Department of Pediatrics Division of Neurology, the interdepartmental Division of Pediatric Neurology at the University of Utah College of Medicine, the Neurology Division at Primary Children's Hospital, and their related program with the State Division of Health, began in the two-year period from 1959 to 1961. The programs embarked on their struggle to establish themselves, to become the entities their directors' visions foresaw, and each has had its problems and successes.

Pat Bray and his long-standing secretary, Dorothy Holmgren, began the Division of Pediatric Neurology based on hard-core teaching and credible clinical research. An observation Bray had first made in the mid-fifties was the phenomenon of focal seizures and certain characteristic focal EEG discharges in children whose families had epilepsy. He spent the next four to five years studying this phenomenon with Nick Wiser, biochemist and geneticist; Walt Needham, psychologist; and Shirley Pusey, social worker. Theirs was the first genetic cohort of "Benign Rolandic Epilepsy," defined in 1967 by Lombroso and in 1975 by Lerman and Kivity. Unfortunately, an approved but non-refunded NINDS grant shifted Bray's attention from epilepsy and broke up the study team he had developed.

Bray had an intense and, in the end, somewhat disappointing year in 1965, when he was chosen acting chair of pediatrics. Dr. Lahey had resigned his position and then chose to return. Bray, to everybody's benefit, concentrated on his ped-neuro training program and wrote a textbook, *Neurology in Pediatrics*, published in 1969. He supervised a funded NINCDS training program in pediatric neurology during the entire twelve years of its existence (1965-77). He trained twenty-three pediatric neurologists during his chairmanship of the division, fourteen of whom are in academic positions. Collectively they have had major impact on the nation's ped-neurology programs. Five are in hospital-based positions and four are in private practice. This highly commendable record of training reflects Pat Bray's dedication of purpose. Utah's influence is felt nationally and internationally because of him. Bray's further work on the American Board of Psychiatry and Neurology, his ongoing research in demyelinating processes and virology, and his new effort to develop a stand-alone computer database for neurology are all of importance.

Other significant elements in the development of pediatric neurology include the evolution of Primary Children's Medical Center, now in its new location next to the University Medical Center. Joel Thompson is head of the program at PCMC and has recently been made chief of the Division of Pediatric Neurology. Most of the future clinical work and training in ped-neuro will emanate from PCMC.

Fred Ziter has made a career commitment to the neuromuscular diseases of childhood, and his Thursday neuromuscular clinic is prized by pediatric and neurology trainees as one of the finest teaching experiences in the program. Chris Jones has developed a sleep disorders program at the University Medical Center, both adult and pediatric in its orientation. Vera Frances Tait is the prime mover in pediatric neurology rehabilitation. Located at the new PCMC, this program promises to be the major ped-rehab unit in the Intermountain West. Phil Chance, a pediatric neurologist in the genetics unit of the pediatric department, is making some major inroads in research of neuromuscular disease genetics. New additions to the pediatric neurology faculty are Fran Fillioux and Marsha Litzinger. The potential of their research in neurotransmitters and calcium channel function in the developing nervous system is significant.

In 1970 Jack Madsen and Nick Wiser began a service and teaching program at the Utah State Training School (USTS) which evolved into a significant training experience in mental retardation and epilepsy for both pediatric and neurology trainees. It is currently under the medical direction of David Green and John Esbenshade in the pediatric department; Jack Madsen directs the neurologic program. The past ten years have seen a major movement of persons formerly at USTS into community group home programs. Medical assessments and follow-up of patients is now more difficult, but Drs. Marsha Litzinger and Patricia Gay are developing innovative programs in long-term medical care for persons with intractable epilepsy and other handicaps.

Epilepsy evaluation, medical treatment, surgery, and research are in stages of rapid development. The advent of long-term video-EEG monitoring, intracranial EEG monitoring, new drug-testing programs, and dedicated interest in advancing neurosurgery facilities for intractable seizure disorders are examples of these advances. New antiepileptic drug testing is in concert with the National Drug Testing Program through NINCDS and is carried out with adult and pediatric populations through Drs. Fred Matsuo, John Foley, Patricia Gay, and Jack Madsen. The new PCMC facility will have four monitoring beds for detailed investigation and treatment of difficult epilepsy in children.

Pediatric neurologists in private practice provide extremely important components in the overall pediatric-neuro programs for Utah. Drs. Gerald Moress, Michael Goldstein, Craig Banta, Julie Meyers, and, most recently, Phil Savia round out the Utah group of pediatric neurologists who bring to this area some of the highest quality care in the nation.

The general direction for future pediatric neurology is established, largely by Dr. Bray. The challenge is to sustain his principles of dedicated work in research and teaching, while bringing the most effective patient care possible to the population of the Intermountain West.

CHAPTER THIRTY-FOUR

Neonatology

AUGUST L. JUNG, MD

NEONATAL MORTALITY, defined as death in the first 28 days of life, was extraordinarily high through all of the first half of this century. For example, in Utah in 1927, the rate was 38 deaths per 1,000 live births. Immunizations, sterilization of formulas, and antibiotics accounted for a major change, and by 1955 the percentage had decreased to 15 deaths per 1,000 live births. At mid-century, most deaths in newborns were caused by prematurity, respiratory distress, birth asphyxia or injury, congenital anomalies, infection, or metabolic disorders.

The accepted standard of care for sick newborns emphasized isolation, delayed feeding, and minimal handling. As an intern in 1961, Dr. Jung remembers being asked to see a premature infant weighing about three pounds in the Obstetrics Pavilion, an old barracks building at the Salt Lake County General Hospital (SLGH) at 21st South and State Streets. The baby was placed in an isolette and wheeled across the campus to the building where the pediatric ward was housed. One room was available for newborns, and this isolette contained the sole occupant of the room. The baby labored with hyaline membrane disease, his chest sinking to the spine. As cyanosis appeared, oxygen was turned into the isolette and restricted to no more than 40% to prevent blindness. However, as cyanosis deepened and respiratory distress increased, up went the red flag on the isolette, signifying that greater than 40% oxygen was being given with disregard for retrolental fibroplasia, as a life was at stake. As this baby labored on, fluid was withheld as long as possible. By the third day, fluids were offered by clysis. However, all the staff's efforts were to no avail.

While Jung was serving on rotation at the LDS Hospital newborn nursery, Dr. Ray Rumel, an imaginative thoracic surgeon quite renowned in Salt Lake City for his bold and innovative style, devised a steel cage that could surround a premature infant in an isolette. The chest was suspended in this cage by placing sutures under the sternum to prevent the deep sternal retractions so characteristic of preemies laboring with hyaline membrane disease. Futile as the effort was, Rumel's dedication to preserving these lives left a lasting impression on many.

Three things changed care for newborns in the second half of the century. First, scientists took an interest in the physiology and pathophysiology of newborns, and second, from this science came technological innovations and equipment scaled to newborn needs. Last, the emergence of specialists in newborn medicine and their concentration, with the science and technology, at regional centers — often university or children's hospitals across the U.S. — had an impact on newborn care. Management of respiratory distress of the premature is a perfect example.

Early recognition that temperature regulation, a neutral thermal environment, was critical to sick prematures led to better isolettes. Respiratory Distress Syndrome (RDS) was long known as hyaline membrane disease. In the late fifties it became apparent that the hyaline membranes seen at necropsy had little to do with RDS. Rather, a deficiency of surfactant secondary to unfinished lungs precipitated RDS, and this discovery led ultimately to the introduction of replacement therapy. The first surfactant drug was approved by the FDA in 1990. In the interim, however, adult respirators were scaled down to newborn size and the designs better adapted to RDS management.

The gathering of the sickest RDS babies in regional centers allowed the concentration of all resources to bear on their illness. In 1949 one of the first units in the country was established at the University of Colorado by Dr. Lula O. Lubchenco. By 1968 Maternal and Child Health Services of the Department of Health, Education

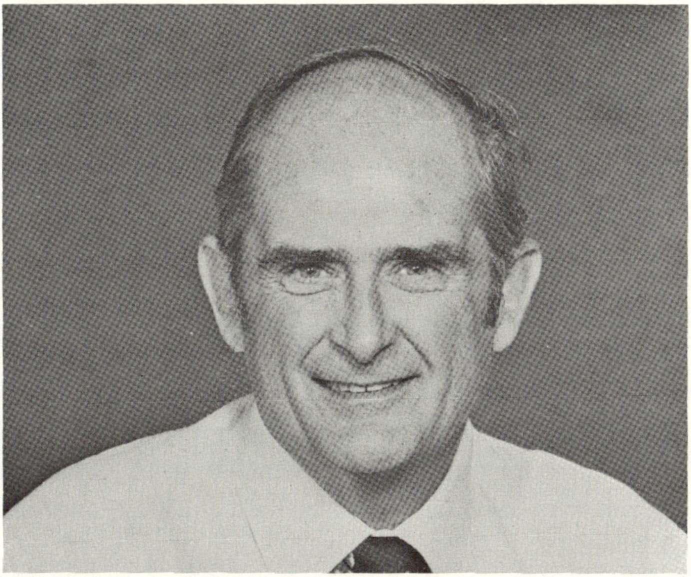

August L. (Larry) Jung.

and Welfare was funding nine newborn intensive care centers nationwide. However, no center existed between Denver and the West Coast or from Phoenix to the Canadian border — a vast area with approximately 60,000 births annually.

One example of how far science, technology, and the regionalization of newborn care have brought the field is isoimmunization with Rh antigen-antibody, now virtually nonexistent. Hydrops fetalis from Rh incompatibility is rarely seen, owing to recognition of blood types and identification of the disease, Coombs testing, exchange transfusion, amniocentesis for optical density measurements of pigment to determine severity, intrauterine transfusion, RhoGam, and phototherapy. Management of diabetes in pregnancy and care of the newborn have improved. Aggressive preventive measures also minimize meconium aspiration syndrome.

Regionalization of newborn care began in Utah and the Intermountain West in 1968, and Dr. Jung was pivotal in the development. He was born in Chicago in 1935, the son of a pumpernickel baker, and came to Utah in 1953 as a forestry major at Utah State Agricultural College (now Utah State University). He switched to medicine, graduated in 1961, and finished a pediatric residency at the University of Utah. After completing a year-long developmental pharmacology fellowship in 1967, he became the ninth full-time member of the Department of Pediatrics.

The opportunity to develop the center at the University of Utah came quite fortuitously. In 1967 Dr. M. Eugene Lahey, then chair of the Department of Pediatrics, received a call from Dr. Lubchenco at the University of Colorado inquiring whether any of the faculty would like to use a six-month neonatology fellowship. Jung's interest in neonatology had been influenced by his many experiences with neonates in the Army and by his mentor, Dr. Alan K. Done. From January to July of 1968 he completed the clinical fellowship under Dr. Lubchenco.

On July 1, 1968, a small area of the University Hospital's pediatric ward, 2 East, was set aside for the first newborn intensive care unit in Utah. The total capacity was five babies, primarily inborn distressed infants. Financial support came from University, hospital, state, and private funds. The nursing staff consisted of one registered nurse, Patricia C. Isaacs (the first head nurse of the unit), two licensed practical nurses, and several part-time nurses from the pediatric floor. In addition to the director, the medical staff consisted of rotating pediatric residents, with other pediatric faculty available for special problems. Modest amounts of equipment were purchased, other items borrowed from units in the hospital and medical equipment companies. For the first heart-rate monitor, the Newborn ICU nurses and doctors sold doughnuts, raising enough money to buy this vital piece of equipment. The service grew rapidly, with more and more inborn infants admitted, as well as a gratifying number of referrals from area physicians.

Infant ventilators were virtually nonexistent in Utah in 1968-69. When an infant was born with respiratory distress, an adult-size respirator was borrowed with the promise that if an adult in need came along, the baby would be taken off. Fortunately, that never happened in spite of many close calls. It was quite a sight to see a huge Bennett MA1 ventilator next to an isolette, its enormous bellows barely lifting to give the tiniest tidal volume the staff could squeak out of this goliath. The full-sized Bird respirator also was used at times. What a triumph it was when the Newborn ICU had its first survivor on the ventilator! A determined Dr. Robert Kechley, the first pediatric resident to work in the Newborn ICU, sat hour after hour with this baby until she finally improved enough to come off the ventilator. He is currently practicing pediatrics in Helena, Montana, and that first survivor, Janie Ballard, returned twenty years later to work as a clerk in the Newborn ICU.

Shortly after the unit opened, the Bourns volume ventilator, designed specifically for newborns, became available. A manufacturer's demonstrator was kept in use despite requests for its return. Eventually, the Salt Lake Chapter of the March of Dimes came to the rescue and bought it — the first of many of their valuable and timely equipment purchases. In the first six months, fifty patients were treated in the new unit.

Late in 1968, Dr. William Jordan, pediatric anesthesiologist and member of the anesthesiology faculty at the Medical School, shared medical responsibility for the unit. His knowledge of ventilation, monitoring equipment, and respiratory physiology proved essential to the emerging Newborn ICU. In 1972 he was made acting chair of anesthesiology. His help during those formative years assured the success of the unit.

Referral of sick babies from community or regional hospitals was pivotal to a regionalized newborn intensive care program. That first referral came in late 1968 from Dr. Neil Spring at Holy Cross. A transport team of a nurse and Dr. Jung used a standard isolette and a Gold Cross ambulance. Thereafter, a great effort was put into formalizing transport.

On a mid-winter day in 1969, the unit received a call to pick up quadruplets in Jerome, Idaho. A couple of isolettes were mustered, one a transport and the other a regular model, and an airplane. Pat Isaacs, RN, Carol Kirgis, RN, and Dr. Jung flew to Twin Falls, where they were met by an ambulance and driven on a wild ride in a blinding

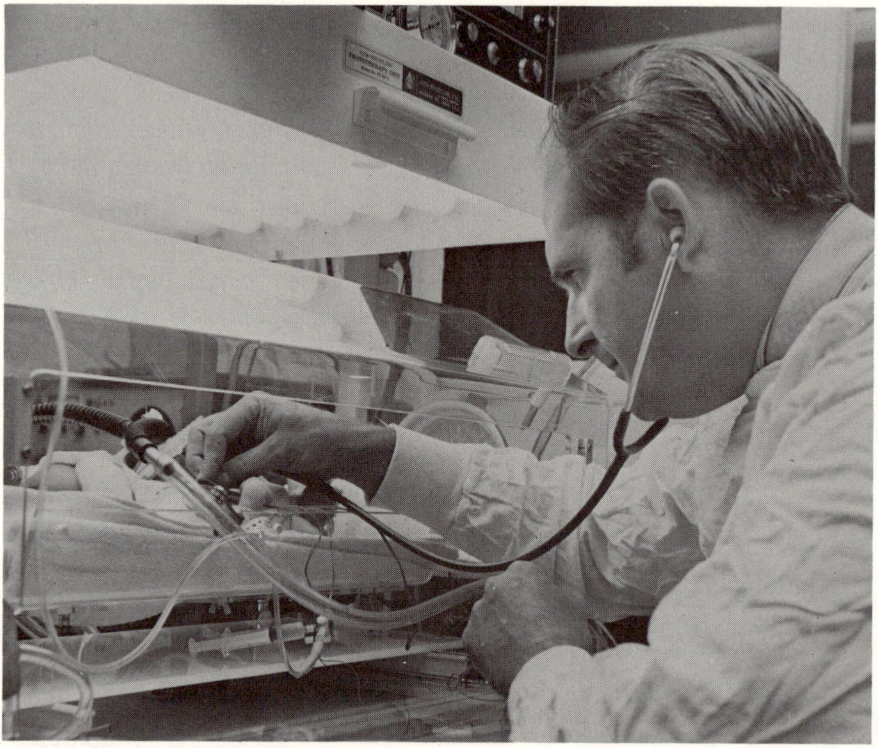

August L. Jung, MD, medical director and founder of Utah's first newborn intensive care unit, at the University of Utah in 1968. Photo courtesy March of Dimes.

storm to Jerome by a young driver with instructions to rush, as the babies were not doing well. On arrival, three had already died, and the fourth infant was moribund. The team worked feverishly to resuscitate the baby and transport him back to the Newborn ICU. The staff there worked for three days and nights, but to no avail; on the third day this baby died. However, the transport represented one of the first by fixed-wing aircraft. In 1969 ninety-two infants were brought to the Newborn ICU by ground ambulance, fixed-wing, or helicopter. The first transport isolette was an Air Shields model with a monitoring console fabricated from sheet metal by Dr. Jung's father to fit a Holter infusion pump, an oxygen analyzer, a Yellow Springs temperature monitor, and a Parks heart-rate monitor.

The first helicopter transport of a newborn was from Brigham City in 1969. Often a case of oil cans would be placed in front of the three-man seat of the helicopter to support the isolette while a transport physician or nurse occupied the middle seat between isolette and pilot.

A grant from the Maternal and Child Health Services of Health, Education and Welfare, Region VIII, for support for the development of the concept of regionalization of care for newborns came to the University of Utah Department of Pediatrics in May 1970 and continued for five years. Nearly $100,000 annually enabled the University of Utah Intensive Care Unit to assume Intermountain significance. Dr. Carlyle Thompson, director of the State Department of Health, was very supportive of the program and provided significant state support.

More was expected of nurses in this unit than was traditional. Approval of nurses for bag and mask ventilation and postural drainage, let alone intubation, aspiration of pneumothoraces, and placement of umbilical arterial catheters, caused a major confrontation with the Medical Board. A clinical specialist, Carolyn Hargrove, RN, MS, joined the staff to help with the many necessary in-service and educational programs.

By 1972 the new center had grown precipitously. Referrals came from throughout the Intermountain West, including all of Utah, much of Wyoming, Idaho, Montana, the western slope of Colorado, and the eastern slope of Nevada, and admissions totaled 400 annually. The space had been remodeled once, and the unit was still bulging at the seams, continually encroaching upon pediatric ward bed space.

Dr. Stephen Atherton, a new graduate of the neonatology program at the University of California at Irvine, became co-director of the unit in 1972. He was a long, lanky, fun-loving young man with a keen intellect and a burning desire to study the psychosocial aspects of neonatology. He would weep openly when a baby died. During the ensuing years, significant focus was placed on the psychosocial aspects of newborn medicine. Dr. Atherton and the social work staff, Katie Paulsen, Pam Grant, and Tom Coleman, put together a number of family support programs, including a parent support group, Parent to Parent, which was the forerunner of the national support group Parent Care. One of the first parents, Becky Hatfield, serves today as the Parent to Parent program coordinator.

Head nurse Pat Isaacs originated a foster grandparent program in 1969. Mildred Miles was the first official "grandparent" to give additional personalized tender care. More grandparents were assigned to the unit to hold and feed the babies, which relieved the nurses to care for other seriously ill infants. They became an essential part of the Newborn ICU service.

Nurse Isaacs also developed a home health care service for oxygen-dependent babies. A parents' orientation booklet to the Newborn ICU was published that became a model for similar publications at other centers and is now in its fourth revision. The initial custom of excluding parents from nurseries had given way to an emphasis on bonding.

Expansion of the Transport Program

A formal newborn transport team of registered nurses was developed in 1975. This highly skilled team, using sophisticated transport equipment, including ventilator and vital signs monitoring equipment, has grown to twelve specially trained registered nurses who currently transport 1,000 neonates per year throughout the Intermountain West.

The transport team served as the model for the present critical care air evacuation services provided by Air Med and Life Flight to Utah patients of all ages.

Outreach Education

Nan Sherman Streeter, RN, was the first nursing coordinator of the neonatal outreach education program, later expanded with the addition of Diana Doerr, RN, as assistant outreach coordinator.

Outreach education has continued to grow into an integrated neonatal/obstetric and pediatric curriculum which spans the Univer-

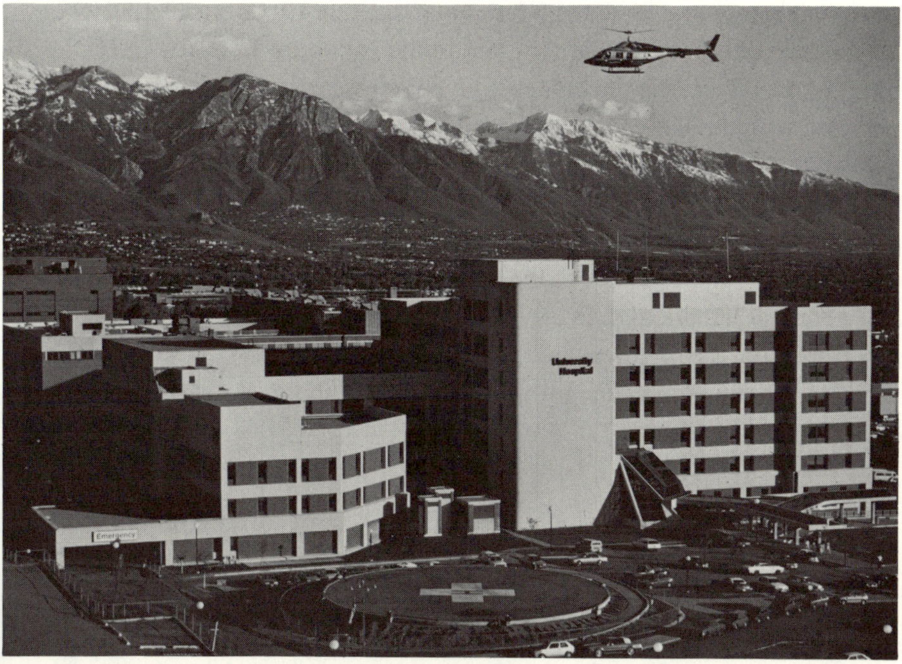

New University Hospital with the helipad that became an important part of hospital operations, photographed in 1981.

sity of Utah, Primary Children's Medical Center (PCMC), LDS Hospital, Intermountain Health Care, and the Bureau of Maternal and Infant Health of the state health department. Regional conferences, grand rounds on videotape, teleconferences, and nationally developed educational packages have been added to the diverse educational offerings.

Neonatal Nurse Practitioner Program

In 1974, under the auspices of Drs. Jung and Atherton, a University of Utah College of Nursing master's student, Pat Johnson, completed her training as a neonatal nurse practitioner (NNP) with a clinical internship in the Newborn ICU. The quality of primary care delivered during her internship provided much support and validation for the NNP role.

There was a hiatus of NNP care in the late 1970s until 1979, when Nancy Shaw joined the program in the Newborn ICU at PCMC. Dr. Thomas R. Harris developed an NNP master's program in collaboration with the University of Utah College of Nursing. Four of the first seven graduates began their practice at PCMC in the summer of 1981, and the program continues.

Recognition of the need for and difficulty in providing nutrition to high-risk infants led to the employment of Laurie Moyer-Mileur, a neonatal nutritionist, in 1979. The incorporation of a neonatal nutritionist in the medical team has resulted in improved growth and overall nutrition status for infants admitted to the Newborn ICU.

House Staff

House staff have always been a vital part of care for infants at the University's Newborn ICU. In return they have had an opportunity to learn newborn medicine. The majority of pediatricians in the Intermountain West today were trained in this unit. In the past twenty-three years, about 150 pediatric residents have rotated through the unit. While long hours and hard work have characterized their time there, many considered it a most valuable experience. During the past fifteen years obstetrics, family practice, and anesthesia house staff have rotated through the unit as well. The unit's teaching mission includes medical and nursing students, respiratory therapists, and medical social workers, to name a few.

Neonatologists

Many early neonatologists stayed on staff for several years and then moved on to important positions in practice or academia. The following are current staff members: Drs. Dave Coulter (1982), medical director, NBICU, LDS Hospital; Robert Kimura (1983), research scientist in gastrointestinal metabolism; Michael Simmons (1983), chair, Department of Pediatrics; Jerald King (1984), medical director, NBICU, University of Utah; Robert M. Ward (1985), medical director, NBICU, PCMC; Richard Molteni (1986), director of medical services, Division of Neonatology, and vice chair for clinical affairs, Department of Pediatrics; J. Ross Milley, MD, PhD (1988), research scientist investigating protein metabolism in the fetus and newborn; Michael Trautman (1988), research scientist studying cell development; Richard Bland (1989), Field's Professor of Pediatrics, research scientist studying the movement of fluids and protein in the fetal and newborn lung; David Carlton (1989), research scientist studying pulmonary physiology at the cellular level; and John Britton (1990), medical director, NBICU, Holy Cross Hospital. Four more research scientists were appointed in 1990: Drs. Candice Fike, studying pulmonary vasculature micropuncture for fluid movement; Susan Wiedmeier, studying white cell immunology; Diane Lorant, studying neutrophil endothelial cell adhesion; and Carolyn Rich-Denson, researching the effects of oxygen delivery on GI metabolism.

The Division of Neonatology currently has eighteen members and manages care for approximately 1,200 sick infants annually at the University of Utah, PCMC, and LDS Hospital Newborn ICU's, and at Holy Cross Hospital Nursery. The division maintains a research scientist fellowship in neonatology and has trained twenty-seven fellows between 1973 and 1991.

Perinatology

In 1985 a new University Hospital was built. The second floor was dedicated to perinatal care. The obstetrical high-risk unit with antepartum and delivery suites was integrated with a newly designed Newborn ICU with three ten-bed rooms. One of these rooms is immediately adjacent to the delivery rooms. Sick or extremely premature infants can be passed directly from the perineum to a Newborn ICU bed, and management begins immediately. Because the inborn high-risk population is so large, the thirty beds are generally filled with inborn babies.

In the past year, the unit has taken on an identity as the regional center for "Very Very Low Birth Weight Babies" or micropreemies. Medical and nursing staff have dedicated themselves to the special needs of this population with gratifying results.

NEWBORN CARE AT THE PRIVATE HOSPITALS

Primary Children's Medical Center (PCMC). In 1977 Donald R. Poulter, hospital administrator, and Richard Van Winkle, chairman of the Board of Governors, approved Dr. Jung's request to develop a Newborn ICU at PCMC. It was their foresight which would see PCMC's unit become a premier facility for neonates in the Intermountain West. The new twenty-six-bed Newborn ICU was opened in February of 1978 to provide additional beds for the ever-growing numbers of infants being referred to Salt Lake City. The unit's affiliation with the University of Utah School of Medicine and the Division of Neonatology has continued. Dr. Margaret Watkins was appointed medical director, and Afton Bowman, RN, was the first head nurse.

On April 23, 1990, PCMC moved to its new facility on the University of Utah campus. This ultramodern children's hospital now has fifty-one neonatal beds, eight of which comprise a bronchopulmonary dysplasia (BPD) unit. The BPD unit is a concept pioneered at PCMC which addresses the special needs of neonates with chronic lung problems. It was developed through the efforts of Drs. Richard Molteni and Felipe Gonzales of the Division of Neonatology, and Dennis Nielsen, chief of the Division of Pulmonary Medicine. Extracorporeal membrane oxygenation (ECMO) technology was introduced into the newborn unit at PCMC by Drs. Ed McGough and Richard Molteni in 1986. To date, about 5,000 newborns have been cared for in the PCMC Newborn ICU.

LDS Hospital. After developing the fledgling Newborn ICU at the University Hospital in 1968, Dr. Jung was often called to LDS Hospital to consult on infants. At the request of the medical staff there, a small area for four Newborn ICU beds was remodeled in 1969. Marjorie Saylor, RN, was the head nurse of this unit. A Plexiglas shield on an outside wall was devised so that x-rays could be taken overhead through the shield and isolette, since the room was too small for the machine. Sick infants born at LDS were transferred to the

University as a practical matter of resource utilization, and the unit closed in about 1971.

In 1980, with the development of an expanded LDS Hospital and more than 5,000 deliveries per year, a new fifteen-bed nursery ICU was constructed in close proximity to the delivery rooms. Dr. Rick Bucciarelli, who played a significant part in planning this nursery, became the unit's first medical director through an affiliation agreement worked out with the Division of Neonatology and the University of Utah. Later, Drs. Larry Eggert, Joan Hulme, and Jerry King became medical directors of the unit.

In 1986 a firm affiliation of the Division of Neonatology and LDS was negotiated. In mid-1987, Dr. David Coulter assumed responsibility as medical director of the NICU at LDS and remains in that position.

The Division of Neonatology staffs the unit with a neonatologist on a rotational basis. Sally Dosier, RN, was the first head nurse in the NICU at LDS, and the current head nurse is Rob Nichols, RN. Pediatricians provide a significant portion of the care for sick newborns.

McKAY-DEE HOSPITAL. Following completion of his neonatal fellowship at the University of Utah in 1978, Dr. Rick Weeks joined the staff of the McKay-Dee Hospital in Ogden, Utah. In 1979 a formal agreement was reached for the hospital to employ Weeks and Dr. Michael Clark (also a graduate of the University's neonatal/perinatal fellowship program) to develop a Newborn ICU. Started as a twelve-bed unit in 1984, the NICU has since been remodeled as a twenty-three-bed unit averaging about 350 admissions annually. Referrals come from surrounding hospitals, including Logan and Brigham City, Utah, and Evanston, Wyoming. In 1981 Dr. Benjamin Hart joined the staff, followed in 1982 by Drs. Mac Wright and Larry Eggert.

ST. BENEDICT'S HOSPITAL. In October 1987, a commitment was made to develop a Newborn ICU at St. Benedict's Hospital in Ogden, Utah. Drs. Rick Weeks and Ben Hart left McKay-Dee to become the first neonatologists at St. Benedict's. In April 1990, Dr. Nick Harper joined them as chief of the neonatology service. Their first head nurse was Bart Chournos, RN, who was recruited from the University's Newborn ICU.

The six-bed unit started in 1988 has been enlarged to twelve beds, and admissions per year average 120 to 150 patients.

UTAH VALLEY REGIONAL MEDICAL CENTER. In 1979, UVRMC recruited its first neonatologist, Dr. Stephen Minton, and escalated its nursery from a Level II to a Level III center. The unit's first head nurse was Darlene Pickup, RN. Earlier, UVRMC's pediatricians had established a relatively sophisticated nursery for the care of sick babies. The Newborn ICU has been remodeled and expanded three times to its present twenty-nine beds. In 1986 Dr. Ronald Stoddard joined the staff. A transport team was established in 1979 to carry high-risk mothers and babies from area hospitals; they presently transport 190 patients per year. The UVRMC Newborn ICU averages 325 babies annually.

Pediatricians have remained involved in the care of the patients at UVRMC's Newborn ICU. The nursery has also made a dedicated effort at outreach education.

Utah Perinatal Association

The Utah Perinatal Association (UPA) was incorporated in April 1978 to promote optimal perinatal health care in Utah. The organization joined the National Perinatal Association (NPA) later that same year. The first annual conference was held in the summer of 1978 at Snowbird and officers were elected. Dr. Margaret Watkins was elected the first president. Conferences have been held annually since then, with increasing attendance and an excellent reputation.

The UPA's first lobbying effort was for legislation regarding car seat safety for children. The group also participated in legislative lobbying for a prenatal care initiative passed by the state legislature in 1987.

In the same year an annual UPA award was established to recognize the contributions of individuals or programs working to better the status of childbearing-aged women in Utah and/or their infants. The first Annual Award was presented to Dr. Neil Kochenour, division chief of perinatal medicine at the University of Utah, in gratitude for his influence on perinatal practice in Utah.

In 1988 the second Annual Award was presented to Dr. August L. Jung, director of neonatology at the University, for his twenty-one years of effort in building the foundation for Utah's perinatal care by opening the Intermountain NBICU.

Summary

The impact of neonatology as we know it today — incorporating science, technology, neonatologists, and the regionalization of perinatal care offered by highly skilled personnel — can, in part, be portrayed in neonatal mortality. Utah's neonatal mortality in 1955 was 15 deaths per 1,000 liveborn babies. This rate had not changed by 1968, the year the first newborn intensive care center in the Intermountain West opened at the University of Utah. Thereafter, however, it declined steadily to a 1988 rate of 3.7 deaths per 1,000 live births.

PART SIX

•

INDEPENDENT DEPARTMENTS

CHAPTER THIRTY-FIVE

Anesthesiology

HARRY C. WONG, MD

PRIOR TO WORLD WAR II, FEW PHYSICIANS considered anesthesiology as a medical specialty. Although physicians interested in anesthesia had been organized as early as 1905 in New York, the American Society of Anesthesiologists was not founded until 1936, with 487 charter members. In 1940 anesthesiology became a recognized specialty when the American Medical Association House of Delegates unanimously approved a section on anesthesiology. In 1941 the American Board of Anesthesiology was established as an independent specialty board. In the same year Dr. Noel Gillespie published his book *Endotracheal Anesthesia*, and Dr. Harold Griffith discovered the properties of curare as a muscle relaxant to be used as an adjunct for anesthesiology.

During World War II, multiple deaths directly attributable to anesthetic complications occurred with war casualties. Vomiting, aspiration, and postoperative pneumonias were all commonplace complications that frequently produced fatal results. Pentathol used for anesthesia also produced many fatalities most likely due to hypotension and hypovolemic shock. As a result of these unfortunate events, the Surgeon General of the United States encouraged the passage of the Bolton Act in 1945 to encourage and subsidize training in anesthesia.

Concurrently with World War II, the history of anesthesiology for Utah began in 1940 when a young surgical resident named Scott

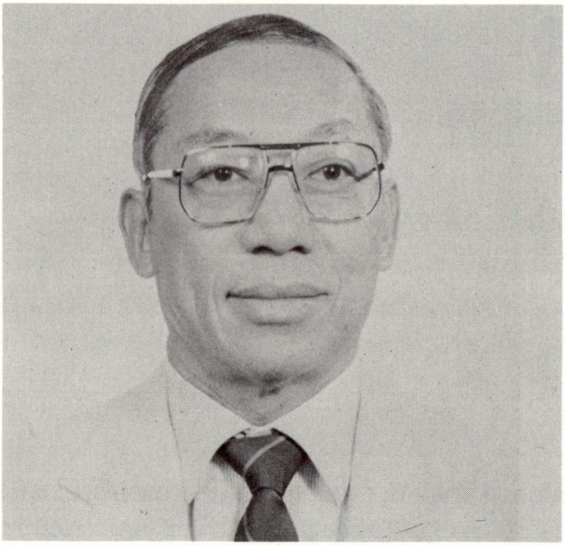

Harry C. Wong.

Meadows Smith spent three months on an orthopedic rotation at City Hospital in St. Louis, Missouri. During this rotation, Dr. Smith reduced multiple fractures under fluoroscopy and in a few weeks began to notice pain, tenderness, and edema of his left hand. Eventually the skin on his fingers broke down and open sores developed. The fluoroscope was found to be defective and was emitting excessive amounts of radiation. The severe radiation burns required multiple surgical procedures and skin grafts which terminated Dr. Smith's surgical residency but meant the birth of anesthesiology for Utah. In an effort to stay close to the practice of surgery, Dr. Smith searched for and found a position in anesthesiology at the University of Minnesota under the direction of Dr. Ralph Knight. Upon completion of his anesthesia training in 1943, and on his way to California to seek a position, Dr. Smith had a train stop in Salt Lake City. He spoke with a few surgeons about opportunities for an anesthesiologist.

Dr. William Ray Rumel, who was practicing in Salt Lake City and Ogden as the state's first thoracic surgeon, was anxious to have an anesthesiologist who could provide endotracheal anesthesia for his

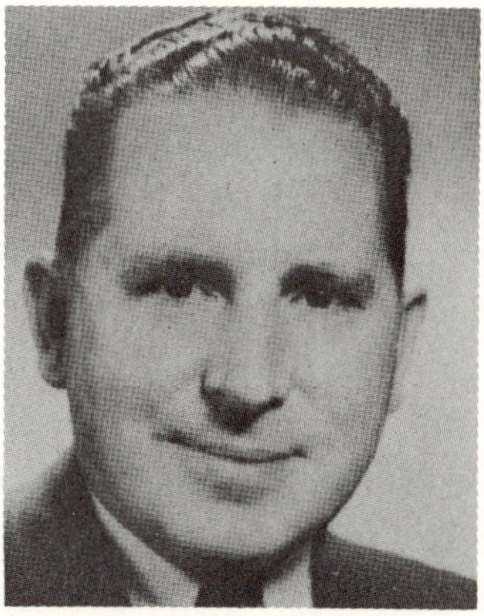

Scott M. Smith, MD, came to the Medical School from the University of Minnesota in 1943, becoming Utah's pioneer anesthesiologist.

surgical patients. In addition, the University of Utah had just become a four-year medical school and was seeking a faculty member in anesthesiology. Dr. Smith, unsure how his hand would hold up in actual practice, accepted the faculty position at the University with a feeling that he could be a teacher of anesthesia if his hand proved inadequate for its practice.

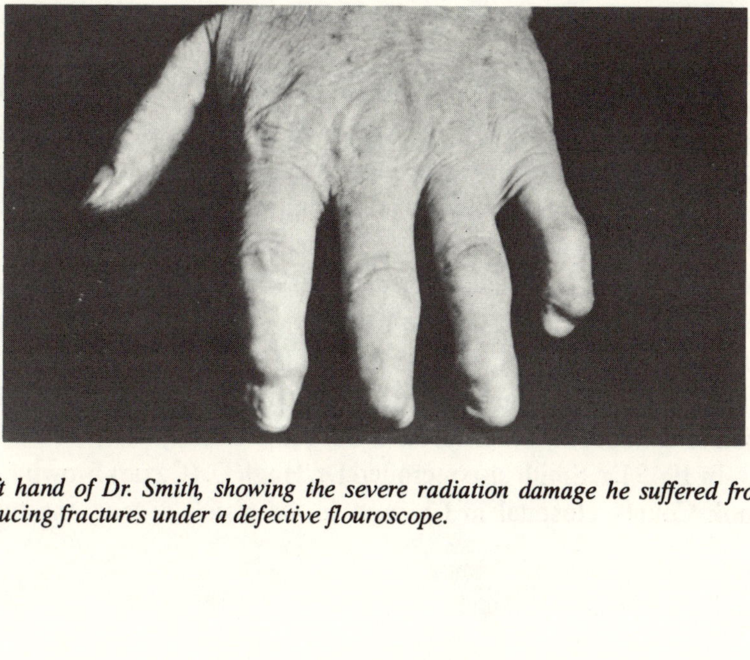

Left hand of Dr. Smith, showing the severe radiation damage he suffered from reducing fractures under a defective flouroscope.

When Dr. Smith began practicing in Utah he was not readily accepted, and only a few surgeons gave him any support at all to achieve a livelihood for his wife and family. The fees he received for his anesthesiology services at that time were $10 for a major anesthesia such as thoracic or intra-abdominal surgery and $5 for minor anesthesias, which included tonsillectomies and adenoidectomies and extremity surgery. No consideration was given to the duration, complexity, or extent of the anesthesia service provided. At that time anesthesia was usually administered by the referring physician, family practitioner, pediatrician, or nurse anesthetist and was mostly open-drop ether.

Dr. Smith represented a potential economic threat to the physicians who used anesthesia services to supplement their office practice income. As a result, he practiced anesthesia with the few surgeons who recognized the significant additional skills a trained anesthesiologist could provide their patients. These surgeons were Dr. William Ray Rumel and Dr. Preston Cutler in thoracic surgery and Dr. N. Frederick Hicken, the first board-certified general surgeon in Utah. They were able to keep Dr. Smith solvent, but he had to travel with them a great deal throughout the state with his anesthesia machine, endotracheal equipment, and laryngoscopes in tow. He accompanied these surgeons to such places as Panguitch, Heber, Provo, Ogden, Logan, and Tremonton to provide anesthesia care.

By 1945, Dr. Smith had managed to raise the level of consciousness in the community enough to convince the Utah State Industrial Commission to allow time considerations for anesthesiology service. This was ultimately accepted by other health insurance companies, and an additional $5 was awarded for the second hour of anesthesia. By the late 1940s the schedule for anesthesia reimbursement had been changed from one-hour to one-half-hour increments. Anesthesiologists were paid $15 for the first half hour and $5 for each half hour thereafter. (By 1964 the current time increment of twelve minutes had been established by the Utah Relative Value Guide.)

In 1945 Dr. Smith also recruited Dr. Hugh O. (Ozzie) Brown from Cook County Hospital in Chicago as the state's second anesthesiologist. Dr. Brown was Mayo-trained under Dr. John Lundy and had been Director of Anesthesia at Cook County Hospital since 1941. Dr. Smith provided anesthesia services at LDS Hospital and at Salt Lake General Hospital for the University of Utah, and Dr. Brown covered St. Mark's and the Veterans Administration hospitals.

As early as 1943 Dr. Smith had developed a great interest in the use of curare and the great debate in the anesthesia literature on its various actions. Many claimed curare, in addition to providing muscle paralysis, had analgesic and central nervous system depressant effects and could, therefore, be used for general anesthesia without supplement of inhalation anesthetic agents. To resolve this controversy, Dr. Smith undertook one of the most classic bits of human pharmacologic research, assisted by Dr. Brown and by Drs. Louis Goodman and James Tolman of the University of Utah Department of Pharmacology and Physiology, respectively.

They performed their experiment on January 10, 1946, and the results were published in *Anesthesiology* in January of 1947 under the title, "The lack of cerebral effects of d-tubocurare." Dr. Smith had himself totally paralyzed with d-tubocurare to prove its lack of analgesic or central nervous system depressant effects. I remember very vividly the first time I asked him about that experience, soon after I joined him in Salt Lake City. His comments on the experience were not as benign as those related in the publication. Dr. Smith vividly described his anxiety and panic when unable to breathe, to swallow, to cough, or to talk. Loss of any one of these four functions in a conscious person would be sufficient to produce a psychotic break in many people. The fear and anxiety of being paralyzed and conscious in our present-day environment has produced significant financial awards in the malpractice courts. It is hard to believe that anyone had the intestinal fortitude to subject himself to such an ordeal.

In 1946, while still on the part-time clinical faculty, Dr. Smith was able to achieve departmental status for anesthesiology at the University of Utah, and he began a residency training program. Dr. Leland O. Learned was the first resident and Dr. Edward J. Hruska the second. Others who followed the first year were Drs. C. J. Christensen, Tunnie

Lee, and Erwin Dritz. In addition, under the Bolton Act, Dr. Smith was training nurse anesthetists for the military services and continued to do so from 1946 until 1951. The faculty for these early residents consisted of Dr. Smith at LDS and Salt Lake General hospitals, Dr. Brown at St. Mark's Hospital, and Dr. Bryce Ozanne, who covered the VA and Holy Cross hospitals.

Dr. Ozanne was the third anesthesiologist in Utah but practiced only about eighteen months before returning to the Midwest in 1947. In that same year, Dr. Paul A. Clayton came to Salt Lake City and became the first full-time anesthesiologist at Holy Cross Hospital. Dr. Clayton was also Mayo-trained. He served on the first Board of Directors of the American Society of Anesthesiologists in 1948 and later became president of the Utah State Medical Association. Dr. Clayton also contributed significantly in the early years to the development of Blue Cross and Blue Shield and to the first Utah State Medical Association Relative Value Guide in the 1950s.

The number of anesthesiologists increased in the late 1940s, as most of the early residents remained in Utah to practice after they had completed their residencies. Dr. Learned became chief of anesthesia at the VA, Dr. Hruska joined Dr. Smith at LDS, Dr. Tunnie Lee joined Dr. Clayton at Holy Cross, and Dr. C. J. Christensen joined Dr. Brown at St. Mark's. Other well-known early residents who stayed include Drs. Esther M. Buchanan, Reynolds Cahoon, Dee Dickson, Joe Allen, and Clel Jensen.

During the 1940s, anesthesiologists relied on nitrous oxide, ether, and cyclopropane as their inhalation agents. Curare was the only muscle relaxant available, and because of the flammable properties of ether and cyclopropane, electronic monitoring was neither available nor possible. Anesthesiologists kept constant contact with their patients for two reasons: to palpate pulses and to avoid the potential of developing a differential static electric charge from the patient that could produce a spark and a fatal anesthetic explosion. Monitoring anesthetized patients was purely noninvasive — using information from pulse, blood pressure, color, respiration, temperature, and muscle tone — and was limited to the anesthesiologist's clinical judgment.

During the 1950s, many changes occurred in anesthesiology in Utah. In 1953 the University of Utah moved to an all full-time faculty. When Dr. Smith chose to remain in private practice, he was relieved as department chair. Dr. Paul Clayton became acting chair while the University search committee sought a full-time faculty member. In 1954 Dr. Carter Ballinger accepted the full-time position at the University of Utah in anesthesiology, but as a division of surgery. This was a reduction in status for anesthesiology that Dr. Smith was never able to accept. He continued to be politically active and became president of the American Society of Anesthesiologists in 1956, the only Utah anesthesiologist ever to achieve that prestigious distinction.

Dr. Ballinger continued the residency program and began the first postgraduate anesthesiology meeting in conjunction with the Utah State Society of Anesthesiologists in 1955. He remained the sole faculty member until Dr. Robert Loehning joined him in 1956. Dr. Norman Bergman came in 1957 to become chief of anesthesiology at the VA Hospital. Dr. Ballinger remained chair of the Division of Anesthesia at the University of Utah until 1973. Throughout his tenure at the University, Dr. Ballinger relied heavily upon the community anesthesiologists, and the residents received much of their clinical training at Primary Children's Hospital, LDS, Holy Cross, and St. Mark's in addition to the University and the VA.

Some of the darkest hours for Utah anesthesiology occurred in the mid-1950s, when the anesthesiologists at LDS Hospital were told by the LDS Church's Presiding Bishopric that they could not form an anesthesia group and that a percentage of their incomes must be paid to the hospital for the privilege of practicing there. Anesthesiologists were actually denied staff privileges during this debate, which ultimately involved input from the American Society of Anesthesiologists and their legal counsel, Mr. John Landsdale. The anesthesiologists at LDS remained firm and unified in their conviction that, as medical specialists, they had the same rights as other private-practice physicians on the LDS medical staff. The hospital's medical staff officers also supported the anesthesiologists, and the debate reached the public through the newspapers. Eventually, the Presiding

Bishopric relented, and the private practice of anesthesiology as a medical specialty was preserved.

The introduction in 1956 of halothane as the first potent nonexplosive inhalation agent was a major breakthrough in the practice of anesthesiology. With the elimination of the potential hazards of explosive agents, significant advances in the electric monitoring of electroencephalography, electrocardiography, and an invasive vascular monitoring were possible. In addition, succinylcholine, an ultrashort-acting depolarizing muscle relaxant, was discovered, which facilitated the ease and safety of endotracheal intubation. Other technical advances in the 1950s that improved the practice of anesthesiology greatly were mechanical ventilators and the precursor of the angiocath, the Rochester blunt intravenous needle. These advances made other developments possible in major surgical specialties such as thoracic, cardiovascular, and neurosurgery.

Ironically, in December of 1959 one of the pioneers of Utah anesthesiology, Dr. Hugh O. Brown, suffered a complication of aspiration while undergoing emergency surgery for postoperative bleeding following a cholecystectomy and met an untimely demise. Dr. Brown was a very colorful character who had contributed greatly to the field in Utah. Dr. Hruska loved to relate a story about him. As a frugal man, Dr. Brown raised pigs to help feed his large family. To feed the pigs, he arranged to have the slop and garbage from the St. Mark's Hospital kitchen saved for him in a container that he collected daily. Unfortunately, many times he had to return to the hospital for an emergency after he had fed the pigs. Dr. Hruska used to relate how, as a resident, he often had to explain to patients or their families that Dr. Brown really was a very skilled physician and not a pig farmer passing himself off as a doctor. Dr. Brown assisted Dr. Smith in his classic curare research. Brown injected the drugs and recorded the findings, providing Dr. Smith's endotracheal intubation, artificial ventilation, and reversal of the curare at the end of the experiment. He also published on continuous caudal anesthesia for obstetrics in the 1940s, decades before the now-current popularity of epidural obstetrical anesthesia. After his death, the Utah State Society of Anesthesiologists dedicated the Anesthesia Library at the University of Utah in his name.

In the 1960s technical advances in anesthesiology increased the safety for high-risk patients to tolerate surgical procedures of increasing complexity. Extracorporeal heart-lung bypass replaced the total body immersion in ice water for hypothermia and the atrial well technique for heart surgery at the LDS Hospital. Invasive direct arterial and venous monitoring became reliable and routine with the development of indwelling plastic catheters and needles, many of which were designed and developed in Utah. Improvements in blood gas analysis proved to be of vital importance in the management of anesthetized and critically ill patients. In addition, a continuous low-flow flush device was developed through research performed at the LDS Hospital to replace the pressurized glass flush bottles. Flush volumes administered by stopcocks from flush bottles had produced fluid overloads to pediatric cardiac surgery patients, which stimulated the research.

During this time, intensive care units were developed, and computer applications for hemodynamic cardiovascular monitoring were undertaken at LDS Hospital under the direction of Dr. Homer Warner. Using computerized monitoring and direct arterial pressures on patients undergoing cardiac surgery, computer anesthesia records were developed from the mid-1960s. Early reports of these computer applications in anesthesiology were made by Dr. Harry Wong at the New York Post-Graduate Assembly of Anesthesiology in 1969 and the World Congress of Anesthesiology in Kyoto, Japan, in 1972.

Dr. Richard Elwyn became the first specially trained pediatric anesthesiologist at the Primary Children's Hospital in 1963 and was soon joined by Drs. Wallace Ring and John Adair. Dr. Ring invented a special mouth gag after seeing tonsillectomy and adenoidectomy surgery being performed dangerously without an endotracheal tube in place. Surgeons complained that the tube obstructed their surgical field. The mouth gag held the endotracheal tube out of the surgeon's way for all oral surgery. In addition, Dr. Ring holds several other patents on medical devices, including the preformed RAE (Ring Adair

Elwyn) endotracheal tube, which is still commonly used throughout the world.

Additional nonflammable inhalation anesthesia agents were added to the armamentarium during the 1960s, including fluoxene and penthrane, but neither of these agents survived the test of time. Newer muscle relaxants with fewer side effects were also introduced, including pancuronium, which nearly replaced curare as the standard nondepolarizing muscle relaxant used by anesthesiologists. The use of controlled hypotensive anesthesia reduced blood loss during surgery, and hypothermic anesthesia techniques were extended from cardiovascular surgery to neurosurgery to reduce oxygen requirements to vital organs.

In the 1970s, increasingly sophisticated monitoring techniques were developed. Pulmonary artery catheters allowed an indirect evaluation of left ventricular heart function and became a valuable adjunct in critically ill patients subjected to surgery and anesthesia. The introduction of reliable oxygen monitors, along with oxygen fail-safe interlocks in the new anesthesia machines, nearly eliminated the possibility of hypoxic anesthesia mixtures being administered to patients. Not only would the newer machines not allow hypoxic concentrations to be delivered, if no oxygen pressure was in the system the other agents would automatically turn off. Pressure disconnect alarms were developed for ventilators, as well as more accurate measures of pulmonary function in ventilation. Positive-end expiratory pressure was found to be an extremely valuable adjunct in certain critically ill patients with pulmonary disease. Another nonflammable inhalation agent, enflurane, was introduced in 1972; it rapidly became one of the favorite nonexplosive agents because of much adverse publicity related to rare cases of hepatic failure that developed following some halothane anesthesias. (A national study revealed that halothane was actually extremely safe and that hepatic failure had been noted to occur following anesthesia from nearly all agents.)

The movement to balanced anesthesia, eliminating or reducing the halogenated inhalation agents in favor of a balance of muscle relaxants and narcotics, stimulated the development of newer and more potent synthetic narcotics. The term 'neurolept analgesia' was coined to describe this type of balanced anesthesia technique. Fentanyl, a potent synthetic narcotic, became a favorite for cardiovascular anesthesia in the late 1970s, and much of the initial research and publication of this technique was performed by Dr. Theodore Stanley, professor and acting chair of anesthesiology at the University of Utah. Dr. Stanley has become nationally and internationally known and continues to contribute significantly to research on potent synthetic narcotics for anesthesiology applications. He is also currently investigating alternative drug delivery systems.

It was in 1973 that the Division of Anesthesiology was able to achieve departmental status at the University of Utah Medical School. The search committee for the new department chair searched for two years before appointing Dr. K. C. Wong in 1975. Continuing in this position, he has improved the status of the department both locally and nationally and, through his leadership, the residency program is now one of the most prestigious and sought-after in the United States. It was also in 1973 that Dr. Robert Hall, a well-known Salt Lake City obstetrician, returned to LDS Hospital following an anesthesia residency at the University of Washington to become the first full-time obstetrical anesthesiologist in Utah. Dr. Hall made his skills available to the anesthesiology residents for a rotation dedicated to obstetrical anesthesia. Other residents at LDS Hospital had rotations in cardiovascular anesthesia under the direction of Dr. Harry Wong and an ICU rotation under the direction of Dr. Terry Clemmer. By 1975, Dr. Hall had obtained additional anesthesiologists, and they began to provide the first twenty-four-hour, seven-day-a-week coverage for obstetrics in Utah. Since that time, obstetrical anesthesiology coverage has been provided at nearly all hospitals along the Wasatch Front.

In the eventful 1970s another major contribution to Utah health care was made through the pioneering efforts of three Utah anesthesiologists, Drs. John Adair, Wallace Ring, and Harry Wong, who developed the Salt Lake Surgical Center, the first licensed free-standing ambulatory surgical facility in the state, which opened in 1976.

The facility provided the first alternative to hospitals for certain surgical procedures and was designed thoughtfully and innovatively to allay patient apprehension associated with a surgical experience. The Salt Lake Surgical Center was dedicated to the private practice of medicine and was operated under administrative and medical control of the anesthesiologists to provide efficient utilization of operating rooms by the surgical staff. Under the direction of these anesthesiologists, the Salt Lake Surgical Center staff grew to more than 200 surgeons, representing every hospital staff in the community.

The success of the Center in escalating ambulatory surgery eliminated the need to build more hospital beds, as all the hospitals improved or developed their own ambulatory surgical programs to compete. When the Center reached maximum operating capacity in 1980, a Certificate of Need was awarded to expand the facility despite opposition from nearly all the hospitals in the community. At the present time, more than 50% of all surgery performed in the Salt Lake metropolitan area is now performed on an ambulatory basis. When the SurgiCenter was sold by the three original anesthesiologist owners in 1988, Dr. Wong joined the full-time University faculty to devote more of his effort to teaching and clinical research.

In the 1980s, technical advances in anesthesia continued with the development of reliable pulse oximeters, mass gas spectrometry, and capnography, which have allowed anesthesiologists to provide more sophisticated and, it is hoped, safer anesthesia. A new nonexplosive inhalation agent, isoflurane, renewed interest in inhalational anesthesia. Anesthesiologists have also become more involved in acute and chronic pain management at the University of Utah and some community hospitals. Epidural and intrathecal narcotics provide long periods of pain control with small doses of drugs to allow more pleasant recovery from surgery and Cesarean sections. Intravenous patient-controlled analgesia (PCA) devices are also finding much greater use. In the 1980s anesthesiology also played a very important role at the University with the first patient to receive an implanted artificial heart, separation of Siamese twins joined at the head, and development of the premier cardiac transplant program in the United States.

While the use of invasive monitors, computer applications, drugs, and mechanical devices has increased the sophistication of anesthesia care, many older anesthesiologists voice their great concern that these devices rather than the patient have become the focus. While these new tools are valuable aids to provide safer anesthesia, they are only adjuncts to good clinical judgment.

The 1980s have also brought the same problems of health care delivery faced by all Utah physicians with the escalation of malpractice claims and the emphasis on cost containment in health care. Confusion reigns as multiple HMO's and PPO's and other managed systems have entered health care in Utah, all with promises yet to be fulfilled. Hospitals are exerting more pressures and controls on their medical staffs. The hospitals and HMO's and PPO's, as confused as the physicians, have tried to market health-care services, believing that health care is a free market. Unfortunately, organization and development of these managed plans and their marketing has done little but expend economic resources at a cost to providers without benefit to patients, and the cost to the health care system continues to escalate.

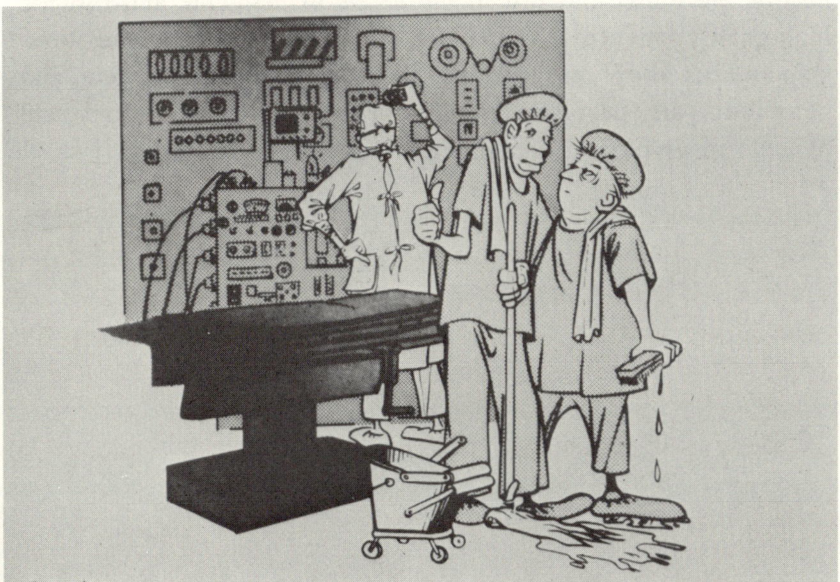

"I DON'T HAVE THE HEART TO TELL HIM THEY HAVE ALREADY TAKEN THE PATIENT AWAY".

Anesthesiologists have contributed significantly to the history of medicine in Utah. Utah has one of the highest ratios of anesthesiologists to the total physician population in the country. Thomas Carlyle wrote that "the history of the world is but the biography of great men." The 1980s have seen the retirements and the deaths of some of the great men who contributed to the history of anesthesiology in the state. In 1986 the Utah State Society of Anesthesiologists honored Dr. Scott Smith with its Distinguished Service Award for his pioneering efforts as the first anesthesiologist and the first professor of anesthesiology in Utah. The only other Distinguished Service Award the Society has made was to Dr. Carter Ballinger. In addition to Dr. Hugh Brown, pioneering anesthesiologists who are deceased are Drs. Scott Smith, Edward Hruska, Leland Learned, William Dillon, and Paul Clayton. Other early anesthesiologists who have retired but are still living are Drs. Eric Simonson, Joe Allen, Reynolds Cahoon, and Clel Jensen.

It is imperative that physicians look to leadership from their medical associations and specialty societies to meet the challenges of the future. If anesthesiology and medicine are to continue to have a history, we must hold fast to the ideals of medicine and provide high-quality patient care and a close, direct physician-patient relationship and not allow managed health-care systems, government, and other third-party payers to intervene in that relationship or to dictate patient care on purely economic grounds.

CHAPTER THIRTY-SIX

Artificial Organs Research at the University of Utah Medical Center

TRUDY McMURRIN • BASED ON DOCUMENTS PROVIDED BY WILLEM J. KOLFF, MD, PhD

WHILE RESEARCHERS OF THE UNIVERSITY OF UTAH Medical Center have won worldwide acclaim for literally hundreds of discoveries, new procedures, and new instruments, no area of inquiry has generated more excitement than the Division of Artificial Organs and its internationally acclaimed head, Willem J. Kolff.

When Dr. Kolff left Holland for the Cleveland (Ohio) Clinic in 1950, he had years of solid work behind him. He had invented the artificial kidney under very difficult circumstances — the German occupation of The Netherlands. Materials for his work in Groningen, beginning in 1939, were hard to obtain and had to be procured without the knowledge of the Germans. The first person to be saved by the artificial kidney underwent treatment in 1945. Kolff himself, who earned his MD in Leyden in 1938 and his PhD in Groningen in 1946, credits three American scientists, Abel, Rowntree, and Turner, with describing the artificial kidney at a physiological conference in Groningen in 1913, when he was two years old. Crediting others is characteristic of the charismatic pioneer, who has put his own name first on review articles but not on any of the hundreds of publications resulting from his research with younger coworkers.

Kolff left the University of Groningen when the Germans appointed a National Socialist as head of the department of medicine. He settled in the small town of Kempen, and there he "induced" an industrialist named Berk to construct the first clinically useful version of the kidney. "And so it has been during the rest of my very interesting life," says Kolff. "I have induced other people to make and invent things, and in many cases I have assisted with the invention." Now 450,000 people are dialyzed worldwide — a quarter of a million in the U.S. alone. The University of Utah has its dialysis center, with three satellites.

Based on their experience with artificial kidneys, Kolff and his associates, first in The Netherlands and then in Cleveland, pioneered in the development of the heart-lung machine, followed by the procedure of elective cardiac arrest, which allows much more effective heart surgery than was previously possible. In 1955 they made the first clinically used membrane oxygenator. Heart-lung machines are now being used in 300,000 cases per year in the United States alone, and membrane oxygenators are gradually taking over.

In 1961 Moulopoulos, Topaz, and Kolff developed the intra-aortic balloon pump. Kolff still remembers how difficult it was to have the pump accepted. Dr. Adrian Kantrowitz introduced the balloon pump clinically, and it is now the most widely used cardiac-assist device in the world.

Early Artificial Hearts

In 1937 a Russian scientist named Demichov had implanted an artificial heart in the chest of a dog, with the drive shaft protruding through the sternum. In December of 1957, Kolff and Dr. Tet Akutsu implanted their first artificial heart into a dog, the first such implantation in the Western world. Since that time, hundreds of scientists have assisted Dr. Kolff, and those who helped to develop artificial hearts have had their models named for them. "Thus, we have had Akutsu hearts, Norton hearts, Nose's giant atria, Lyman hearts, Donovan hearts, Kwan-Gett hearts, Unger hearts, and Jarvik hearts," says Dr. Kolff. "The only thing we have not had is a Kolff heart."

The 1957 model was made of a thermosetting polyvinyl chloride called Plastisol inside hollow molds so that there were no seams. This artificial heart was driven with compressed air and used a principle the researchers have honored ever since: to provide sufficient pressure

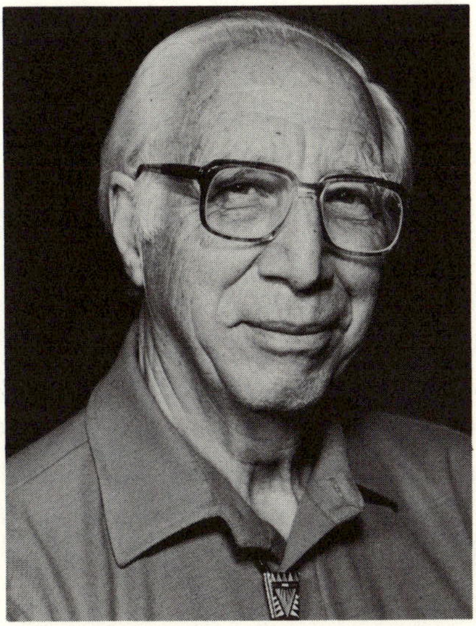

Willem J. Kolff.

to expel the blood from the ventricles and use as little suction as possible so that the venous filling determines the cardiac output (Starling's Law of the artificial heart). Shortly thereafter, they made hearts driven by electric motors and, with S. Harry Norton, an electrohydraulic model driven by solenoids.

Kolff and his associates became "restless" with what they considered slow progress, and then Dr. Kirby Hiller of NASA urged a return to the compressed air-driven devices. They built a drive system in which one could program the shape of the air pressure waves, the rate, and the duration of systole and diastole, and it could be guided by linear position transducers which would, at least in theory, prevent the crushing of blood cells. "The drive system was magnificent," says Kolff, "but one needed a pilot's license to drive it. It would fail from time to time due to such simple things as a surgical suture sticking in a programmed air valve. We began to look for simpler drive systems. From then on, simplicity has been the hallmark of our major attempts. . . . This made funding very difficult because it is relatively easy to obtain funding for complicated computerized drive systems with which one can simulate a thousand things. It is nearly impossible to obtain funding for something simple. Therefore, over the years my laboratory has teetered along, always on the rim of bankruptcy, always having too many ideas and too little money to carry them out."

Westward Ho

Happily for Utah and the region, Kolff brought his ideas and his yearning for simplicity to the University of Utah Medical Center in 1967. Dr. Clifford Kwan-Gett accompanied him from Cleveland, and Dr. Ted Stanley came from Michigan that same year. Work on the artificial heart continued at an accelerated pace, but it was for further improvements in the artificial kidney that the residents of the area first appreciated Kolff's presence.

The team kept forging ahead with improvements. "We sent patients home with a little winding machine with which they could wind their own coil artificial kidneys," says Kolff. "Four of these coils were placed in a Maytag washing machine." Despite the increased portability and lower cost of the washing machine and "wind-them-yourself" kidneys, Kolff has fought a losing battle against the increased cost of dialysis, which many physicians prefer to have administered in dialysis centers or hospitals rather than in the patients' homes.

The Wearable Artificial Kidney (WAK) was ready for use in 1979. It was designed in the University laboratory of Dr. Steve Jacobsen, whose coworkers included Todd Johnson, David Knutti, Barry Hanover, and many others. The WAK, which does not need conventional electrical and water connections, allowed hemodialysis patients the freedom to explore the Western wilderness in specially planned expeditions, so-called Dialysis in Wonderland trips. Administrator John Warner at one time organized twenty-eight of these trips per year. As Kolff says, "It was very important to prove to those patients what they could do, to restore their self-confidence and happiness."

With the advent of better immunosuppression drugs, which make kidney transplantation easier and more successful, chronic dialysis for end-stage renal disease is, according to Kolff, "on the way out."

Membrane plasmapheresis, closely related to dialysis, deserves to increase, however. Cascade membrane plasmapheresis has been developed in the Kolff laboratory by Dr. Udipi R. Shettigar. It removes toxic substances from the blood, returning everything else to the patient. Plasmapheresis offers future applications for rheumatoid arthritis, myasthenia gravis, cancer, and burns, to name a few.

Artificial Heart Beats

When Kolff and his team implanted an artificial heart in Dr. Barney Clark, a Seattle dentist, on December 2, 1982, the entire world

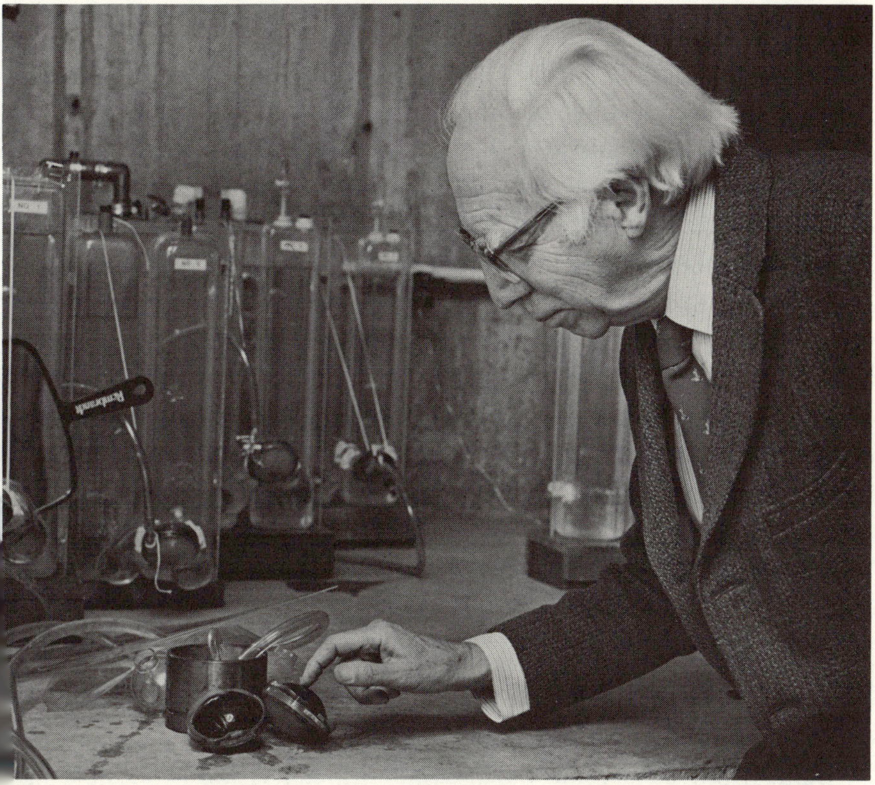

Dr. Willem J. Kolff developed the first artificial kidney and numerous models of the artificial heart.

began to watch for twice-daily updates from Salt Lake City. Dr. Clark survived, gamely and with great good humor, for 112 days, making a remarkable contribution to research and to human hopes for the future.

At the time of this writing, 160 artificial hearts of the Utah type have been implanted in humans, mainly as a bridge to transplantation, yet there is little clinical progress today. This is partly because emphasis has shifted toward heart transplantation, but there are still only 2,000 donor hearts available, while the need is for 35,000 per year in the U.S. alone. Lack of further progress is also due to lack of funding. "Our priorities are wrong," says Kolff. "We are wasting our money on 'Star Wars.'"

Institute for Biomedical Engineering of the University of Utah

When Dr. Kolff arrived in Salt Lake City in 1967, he wrote a program for an Institute of Biomedical Engineering. The plan called for collaboration among medicine, engineering, computer science, chemistry, physics, and other disciplines. A number of exciting medical advances were anticipated, including the artificial heart, and, later, the artificial eye, ear, and arm.

The Institute needed advanced electronics, and so Kolff's associate Dr. William Dobelle induced General Instruments to donate its microcircuit laboratory in Salt Lake City to the University. The laboratory became a major source of income for the Research Institute (not the Institute of Biomedical Engineering), and it lives on as the Hedco Laboratory in the University's Merrill Engineering Building.

Continuing Research

THE ARTIFICIAL EYE: With the artificial eye, developed under the direction of Dr. Dobelle, the optical cortex of the brain is stimulated, and a blind person sees silvery white points of light floating in air! The Utah artificial eye was far ahead of any other artificial eye program. It proved definitely that some artificial vision is possible in people without eyes and that the blind person can understand what he "sees."

THE ARTIFICIAL EAR: Developed by Dr. Donald Eddington and his associates, the artificial ear stimulates the acoustic nerve in the cochlea. Clinically, it is far more developed than the artificial eye. Dr. James L. Parkin has implanted more than fifty of these artificial ears in totally deaf people, one third of whom can now use the telephone.

THE ARTIFICIAL ARM: One of the Institute's most practical projects is the Utah Arm, developed under the direction of Dr. Steve Jacobsen. The arm picks up myoelectrical signals from the wearer's own stump which move the arm automatically. The hand is strong enough to crack a nut and gentle enough to slice a ripe tomato. Dr. Jacobsen's design laboratory has become a leader in the nation and is currently building all the automated puppets for Walt Disney.

Conclusion

In a special Fall 1990 issue of *Life* magazine, Dr. Willem J. Kolff was honored as one of the 100 Most Important Americans of the Century — an indication that we have seen only the beginning of the significance and contribution of artificial organs.

A dearth of funding from the National Institutes of Health, difficulties with the Food and Drug Administration, and a lack of interest on the part of American industry are retarding the development and application of artificial organ technology in the United States. Other countries are moving forward on this front and beginning to reap the benefits of Utah research.

Kolff has always had one guiding principle: "Artificial organs should restore lives to a happy existence. If that is not possible, artificial organs should not be used; certainly they should not be used to prolong misery." After Leif Stenberg — his artificial heart beating inside and his drive system on his shoulder — had served himself four times from a smorgasbord, he sent a telegram to the United States saying, "I am the happiest man in Europe."

CHAPTER THIRTY-SEVEN

Genetic Epidemiology

HENRY P. PLENK, MD, MS
MARK H. SKOLNICK, PHD

MARK H. SKOLNICK WAS BORN IN Temple, Texas, in 1946. His father is a psychoanalyst and his mother is described as a "social activist." As an undergraduate at Princeton, Skolnick majored in economics, with a focus on demography — the study of human populations, emphasizing analysis of fertility, mortality, and migration. He was particularly interested in world health and decided to combine this field with genetics. Skolnick was attracted to Stanford by Nobel Prize–winning Professor Joshua Lederberg, chair of genetics, who introduced him to population geneticist Dr. Luca Cavalli-Sforza, a professor at the University of Pavia, Italy, who was spending a sabbatical at Stanford in 1968–69 before moving there permanently. Cavalli-Sforza suggested the topic of automated reconstruction of genealogies of the Parma Valley in Northern Italy as Skolnick's thesis subject.

In order to pursue this topic, Lederberg arranged for Skolnick to join Cavalli-Sforza in Pavia in September of 1969. One of the first people he met there was Angela Gilberti, Cavalli-Sforza's librarian. They were married that June.

Skolnick's project required analysis of a collection of parish records assembled by Cavalli-Sforza and his colleague Antonio Moroni. The collection consisted of about 100,000 records of Catholic baptisms, marriages, and deaths dating back as far as 350 years for 40 parishes in the Parma Valley covering an area inhabited by fewer than 10,000 people. He linked families to each other and reconstituted

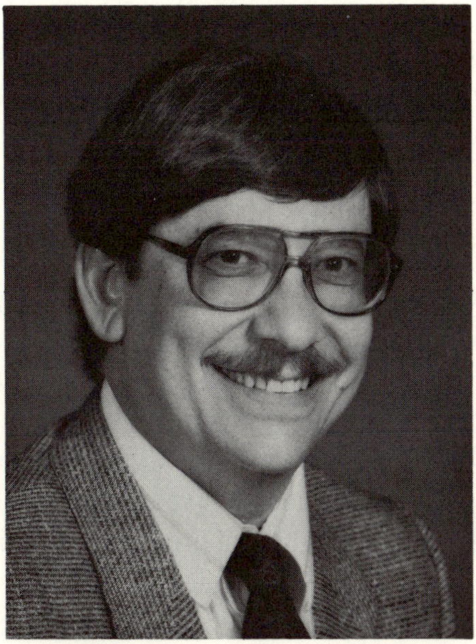

Mark H. Skolnick.

genealogies to analyze the genetic evolution of the population.

In 1973 Dr. Robert Stewart of the University obtained an NCI planning grant to prepare an application for a Regional Cancer Center. Dr. Charles Smart, the first surgical oncologist at the University, had started to organize the Intermountain Cancer Registry. As an international authority in population genetics, Dr. Cavalli-Sforza was asked to Utah to evaluate the use of the genealogical records held in the Genealogical Society of Utah to enhance the Cancer Center research base.

While Skolnick was working in Parma in 1970, the head of the Genealogical Society of Utah came to negotiate with Professor Moroni (who is also a priest) for permission to microfilm historical records from the region, and Skolnick became aware that Utah possessed the material for continuing his research interests. After Dr. Cavalli-Sforza's visit, Skolnick was also invited to Utah to discuss the use of the genealogical library for cancer research. In 1973 he met Drs. Charles Smart, Homer Warner, and Henry Plenk — who were all at

LDS Hospital at that time — as well as Dr. Frank Tyler, chief of endocrinology at the University of Utah, who was much involved in the study of genetic diseases. Skolnick accepted an offer for a newly created position with minimal temporary "creative" funding from the Cancer Society and the Cancer Center planning grant.

Skolnick's preference was to obtain a University appointment in Dr. Warner's Department of Biophysics and Bioengineering (now Medical Informatics) located at the LDS Hospital. Before he had even completed his PhD, he applied for his first National Cancer Institute (NCI) grant of about $400,000 through the LDS Hospital to computerize the entire genealogy of the state of Utah. The application was received with disbelief because of the magnitude of the task and the young applicant's lack of academic experience, as well as the size of the grant request. It was nearly dismissed by the study section. A site visit took place in August 1974. A high-priority score was the result, and funding started in February 1975. Skolnick received permission to photocopy some 200,000 family group sheets from the Genealogical Society of Utah's library and proceeded to create a computer database. The records were linked by name and birthdate to the Utah Cancer Registry, Utah death certificates, and other medical records and data. Dr. Lee Bean, then chair of the Department of Sociology at the University of Utah, is a demographer. He and Skolnick started a study group and then wrote another successful grant application for a major exploration of Utah demographic history from the same records.

Homer Warner had started to hire promising high school students for the summer to stimulate their interest in scientific investigation. One of the first was Peter Cartwright, son of the chair of the Department of Medicine. Dr. George Cartwright was interested in the study of Wilson's disease and hemochromatosis, diseases of abnormal storage of copper and iron, respectively, and both highly fatal if not diagnosed and treated early in life. In both conditions a genetic basis was known. Peter brought Drs. Cartwright and Skolnick together, and a close personal relationship developed. In regular weekly meetings, Cartwright taught Skolnick a great deal about medicine and learned a lot about genetics from Skolnick.

When Cartwright first became interested in hemochromatosis in the fifties, it was thought to occur in one in 10,000 patients. The frequency of the disease is much greater than was imagined, however, and the present incidence is suggested to be more like one in every 200 patients. More than a million Americans are now estimated to have genetic hemochromatosis, and many will eventually die if their disease is not treated.

If presently available screening methods are used to discover hemochromatosis in an early state, late consequences of the disease, such as cirrhosis of the liver, can be avoided. The treatment consists of frequent, on average quarterly, drawing of blood from the patient — which can be utilized by blood banks. Revenue from selling the blood could be used for screening the entire population.

Impressed by the power of genetic analysis, Cartwright suggested developing the study of genetic predisposition to heart disease. He, Skolnick, Homer Warner, and Dr. Hiroshi Kuida (chair of the University cardiology division) formed a committee. They recruited Dr. Roger Williams, a former student and house officer doing epidemiologic research at the National Institutes of Health. Williams accepted the call and set up a vigorous program in cardiovascular genetics.

Dr. Cartwright became a strong believer in the role of genetics in medicine. At age sixty he resigned his position as chair of the Department of Medicine with the expectation of devoting his remaining years to the application of genetics to medicine. Tragically, he died of heart disease at sixty-one, as had his father, despite his being an ardent skier, hiker, and outdoorsman without an ounce of excess fat (but certainly not without considerable stress associated with his position). His genes were his undoing.

At a meeting in 1978 in Alta, Utah, Skolnick and Drs. David Botstein of MIT and Ron Davis of Stanford came to the conclusion that genetic markers derived from cloned DNA were needed to map various diseases in which the biochemical defect was still unknown. This realization was one of the beginnings of the "genome project." The need to recruit an expert who would dedicate his career to discovering these markers led them to Dr. Ray White at the University of Massachusetts. White was recruited by Dr. Cartwright with funds from the Howard Hughes Medical Institute and eventually became the co-chair of a newly created Department of Human Genetics at the University of Utah, described further in the following chapter.

To understand the genetics of cancer, a precancerous phenotype was needed. Dr. Randall Burt of the Division of Gastroenterology introduced Skolnick to the concept of incorporating the solitary adenomatous polyp, a precursor to colon cancer, in genetic studies. Dr. Eldon Gardner and others had studied known familial polyposis associated with subcutaneous sebaceous cysts developing into colon cancer (Gardner's Syndrome). The presence of associated bony tumors (osteomas) had been discovered by Dr. Plenk (Plenk-Gardner's Syndrome). The Skolnick-Burt collaboration demonstrated that a genetic predisposition to a single microadenoma possibly in one-third of the population is apt to lead to colon cancer when combined with dietary factors.

This model attracted attention to dysplastic nevi, which may be either markers or precursors of the malignant melanoma likely to develop after early and/or excessive sun exposure.

Cancer of the breast became the third site of study. Fine-needle aspirations of asymptomatic breasts revealed evidence of proliferative breast disease in some genetically susceptible individuals.

Skolnick accepts the hypothesis that by combining the large pedigrees in Utah with the good markers created in the eighties, huge headway will be made in determining predispositions to various cancers. Selective screening of genetically susceptible individuals may detect their cancer much earlier and could be the key in both cancer prevention and cure. Predictive medicine may be the best way to utilize medical dollars to the greatest advantage.

Skolnick now presides over his own group of some twenty-five researchers in genetic epidemiology within the Department of Medical Informatics located in University Research Park. He has been able to attract ample funding for his projects and plays a prominent role in national and international organizations and meetings. Cooperation with the Department of Human Genetics has been of great advantage to both groups.

CHAPTER THIRTY-EIGHT

Human Genetics

MARK F. LEPPERT, PHD
RAYMOND F. GESTELAND, PHD

HUMAN GENETICS AS A FIELD OF STUDY at the University of Utah had its beginnings with clinicians who came to teach in the Medical School soon after its founding in 1942. George Cartwright, for example, became interested in the inheritance of hemochromatosis in a number of Utah families whose members came to him for treatment. Two other early faculty members, Frank Tyler and Eldon Gardner, also initiated studies in genetic diseases. Over a period of many years, these and other early genetic studies laid the groundwork for research on the incidence and etiology of a number of inherited human diseases. Utah provides excellent resources for genetic studies, because families tend to be large and emphasize the importance of keeping personal records. Such records have become the cornerstone for genetic linkage studies that are of crucial importance to the Department of Human Genetics as it is now constituted.

The department can trace its particular roots to a commitment engineered by Peter Gardner under President James C. Fletcher to make molecular biology a focus of special interest at the University. As a result of this decision, programs in molecular genetics were crafted in various departments of the University during the 1970s and have continued to grow under the encouragement of subsequent presidents Alfred C. Emery, David P. Gardner, and Chase Peterson.

K. Gordon Lark, who had studied genes involved in the replication of DNA in bacteria, came from the University of Kansas in 1970

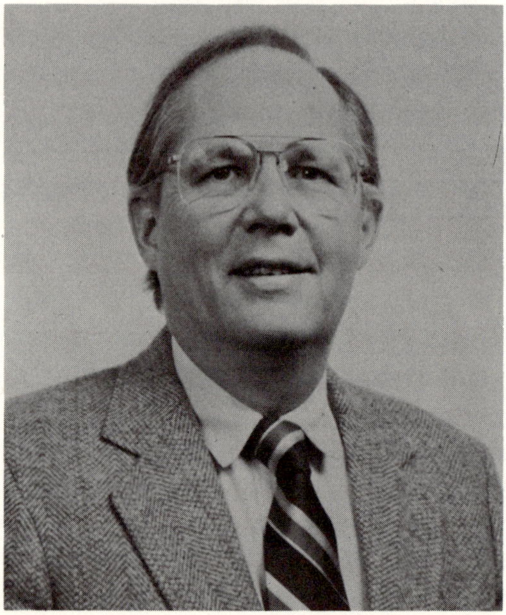

Mark F. Leppert.

to chair the Department of Biology. A major commitment was made to new positions and to new space in the "South Biology" building, which had been used by the U.S. Army for biological research. Dr. Lark recruited to his faculty a number of outstanding basic researchers in cellular and molecular biology; among them were Toto Olivera, David Wolstenholm, Mario Capecchi, now a member of the human genetics department, Martin Rechsteiner, now co-chair of biochemistry, and John Roth, who is now chair of the department and a member of the National Academy of Sciences.

In 1974 Donald F. Summers, a virologist from the Albert Einstein College of Medicine in New York City, replaced Dr. Lowell Glasgow, who switched from chair of microbiology to chair of the Department of Pediatrics. Dr. Summers restructured his department and facilities to accommodate new technology that was opening the field of molecular genetics, and to develop research in nucleic acid biochemistry in bacterial and viral systems. The Department of Microbiology, renamed

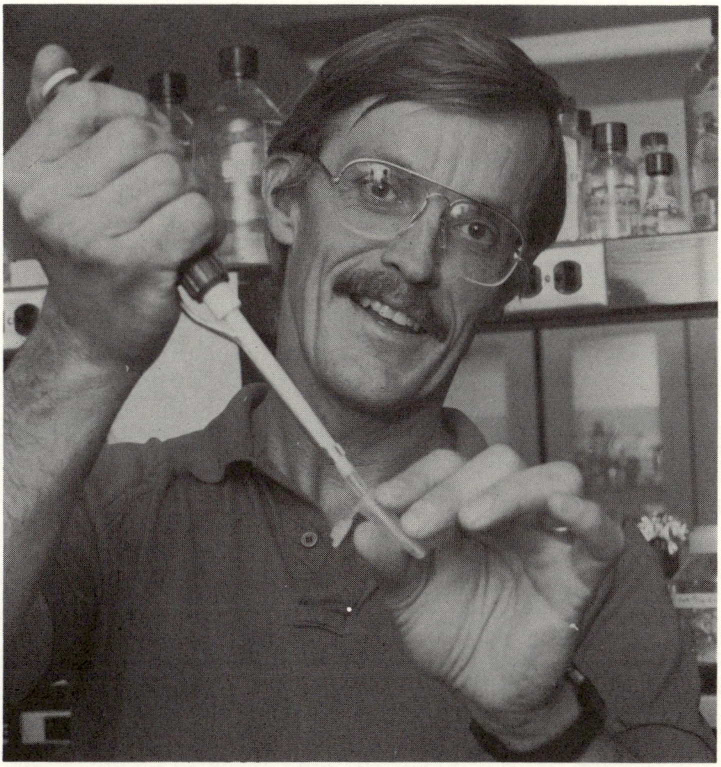

Raymond F. Gesteland.

Cellular, Viral and Molecular Biology (CVMB), attracted outstanding young virologists and biochemists like Dana Carroll (now co-chair of biochemistry), Costa Georgopoulos, Sherwood Casjens, Wai-Mun Huang, and Daniel Kolakofsky. Dr. Summers became one of the first influential voices for molecular biology in the Medical School during the era of transition when the pathogenesis of microbial diseases could begin to be studied at the molecular as well as the biochemical level.

From a key meeting during these years, Leo Samuels, Gordon Lark, Henry Eyring, and Maxwell Wintrobe emerged with the consensus that Utah's unique genealogical records might be exploited to study the genetics of cancer. Mark Skolnick, who was about to receive his PhD from Stanford University, where he had worked with Dr. Luca

Cavalli-Sforza, came to Utah in 1973 to join the biophysics department (now the Department of Medical Informatics) and began to build a database derived from genealogical records kept by the LDS Church. Dr. Skolnick serves as a resource for identifying families with genetic predispositions to various types of malignancies. His database has been valuable also for investigation of a variety of other diseases.

Another major development during that decade was the establishment of a genetics unit at the University of Utah by the Howard Hughes Medical Institute (HHMI). This privately funded institute maintains facilities and investigators in a number of medical schools around the country for research in medically related disciplines; HHMI investigators also serve on the faculties of their host institutions. HHMI chose to place a genetics laboratory here because of Utah's national reputation for molecular biology and genetics. The unique family resources already mentioned also provided an intriguing opportunity for studying molecular genetics in the human biological system.

HHMI had supported individual investigators at the University of Utah Medical School for many years, including Don Nelson, Gerry Rothstein, R. E. Lynch, Harry Hill, and Jim Overall.In the late 1970s, HHMI's directors decided to concentrate the Institute's research nationally in three fields of biology — one of which would be genetics — and to develop funding for larger laboratory groups. In response to a proposal nurtured and guided by Dr. Cedric Davern, then dean of the Medical School, HHMI agreed to make a much larger commitment to Utah. Ray Gesteland was chosen in 1978 to head the first of the new HHMI laboratories at Utah; he came from Cold Spring Harbor Laboratory in Maine, where he had worked with Nobel Prize winner Dr. James Watson. Gesteland's faculty appointment was in the biology department; laboratories were reconstructed for him in the basement of the old Life Sciences Building, which had been the home of the Medical School from 1920 to 1965.

The meeting that was to revolutionize human genetic studies took place at Alta, Utah, in April of 1978, when a group of scientists, including Mark Skolnick from Utah, Ronald Davis from Stanford University, and David Botstein from MIT, among others, developed a new concept: using small pieces of human DNA that do not necessarily have a genetic function but can vary among individuals — that is, polymorphisms in anonymous DNA segments — as genetic "markers." The inference was clear: because many human phenotypes are caused by genes whose biochemical products are unknown, one should be able to find and ultimately isolate such genes by following the inheritance of an identifiable version of a DNA marker that lies close to the unknown gene on a chromosome. Studies in lower organisms had implied that the human genome was likely to contain a great number of polymorphic sites that could be developed as genetic markers. Ray White, then on the faculty of the University of Massachusetts Medical School at Worcester, entered these discussions and made the crucial decision to commit his energies to proving experimentally that the revolutionary approach was feasible for the identification of unknown genes in humans. Four scientists — Botstein, White, Skolnick, and Davis — presented their conclusions in a landmark paper in the *American Journal of Human Genetics* (1980).

In undertaking those experiments, Ray White wanted to know in particular if anonymous DNA markers could help to locate genes in which mutations lead to disease by finding "linkage" (i.e., co-inheritance) between a marker and the disease locus (as defined by the phenotype) in an affected family. In 1980, HHMI invited Dr. White to establish a laboratory in Utah, where he would launch a massive effort to develop hundreds of DNA markers and to map them to chromosomes with sufficient density that any disease-causing version of an unknown gene could be localized and eventually isolated. A few years into the project, physician-geneticist-statistician Jean-Marc Lalouel came to Utah from France as a new HHMI investigator, to develop and conduct the statistical analyses required for assigning markers to their places in the genome and for constructing the chromosomal maps. Dr. Lalouel had already collaborated with White in mapping markers and had helped to establish an internationally accessible center in Paris, called CEPH, that maintains cell lines and DNA from a panel of normal reference families (two-thirds of them from Utah) whose structure is ideal for mapping new markers.

When Dr. White came to HHMI-Utah in 1980, he joined the faculty of CVMB. His laboratory was established in the new Wintrobe Building in the Medical Center, dedicated in 1981; soon afterward, Ray Gesteland's laboratory was moved there from its original quarters on lower campus so that the HHMI groups could be together. Mark Leppert joined White's group, and as new genetic markers were developed he supervised linkage studies in families that came to the attention of clinicians treating family members for a variety of inherited diseases.

As a growing number of DNA markers were mapped to chromosomes, the linkage studies began to pinpoint the locations of important disease genes. The accelerating pace of such localizations occurred not only in Utah but elsewhere, because the maps constructed by Dr. Lalouel's group from Dr. White's markers were made available to medical researchers around the world who were studying families that carried genes for many different diseases. The approach developed by the Utah group, in conjunction with the interest of clinicians in families carrying predisposition to genetic diseases, has resulted in remarkable progress in understanding how altered genes cause disease. The work has resulted in the localization of genes for cystic fibrosis, von Recklinghausen neurofibromatosis (NF1), familial adenomatous polyposis (FAP), familial benign neonatal seizures, Usher's type II (a deafness syndrome), and several other disorders.

Genetic mapping and inheritance studies of disease can only be done in families whose pedigree structure is clear. New techniques of molecular biology and the development of genetic markers for human chromosomes came together in the 1980s to exploit information from the family studies that had been going on in Utah for many years. Frank Tyler's group in the Division of Endocrinology had studied hundreds of patients with various inherited forms of muscle diseases. Beginning in the early 1950s, Eldon Gardner had documented large pedigrees with a high incidence of colon cancer; Roger Williams has ascertained numerous families for genetic studies of early coronary disease; James Kushner follows families with hemochromatosis and Wilson's disease. A clinical genetics division, which provides genetic counseling to families and training for postdoctoral fellows in genetics, functions primarily in the pediatrics department under the direction of John Carey.

In 1990 Ray White's group identified and cloned the NF1 gene and characterized its function as a participant in the chemical signal pathways that control growth and differentiation in cells. White's interest in cancer genes stems from the early 1980s, when he and his postdoctoral fellow Webster Cavenee showed by means of genetic markers that the loss of both copies of a gene on chromosome 13 was responsible for retinoblastoma, a cancer of the eye. Their findings represented the first demonstration of tumor suppressor genes in human cancer and led to their being awarded the General Motors Mott Prize for Cancer Research in 1990.

By the mid-1980s the increasing importance of genetic studies to the medical community had become the incentive for creation of a Department of Human Genetics within the Medical School. Drs. Gesteland and White were named co-chairs. The "Human" part of Human Genetics is interpreted very broadly in the faculty of the new department. A coterie of faculty do work primarily on the human system: Ray White; Jean Marc Lalouel; Ryk Ward, an epidemiologist from Vancouver; Lynne Jorde, a statistical geneticist from New Mexico who is studying isolated populations; and Sandra Hasstedt, a mathematical geneticist from Michigan who is modeling complicated genetics systems with computer technology. Mark Leppert, a molecular geneticist from the University of Minnesota, is mapping disease genes, and Peter O'Connell, a molecular geneticist from Brandeis University, is working to isolate some of them.

Much of the department, however, is concerned with nonhuman systems that are often experimentally and biologically better suited to answering certain basic questions in genetics. Shige Sakonju from the University of California at Berkeley and Carl Thummel from Stanford University use the fruit fly to dissect the molecular mechanisms involved in development. David Grunwald from Princeton is developing a new system in the zebra fish, an animal that is ideally suited for studying early neural development. John Atkins from Cork,

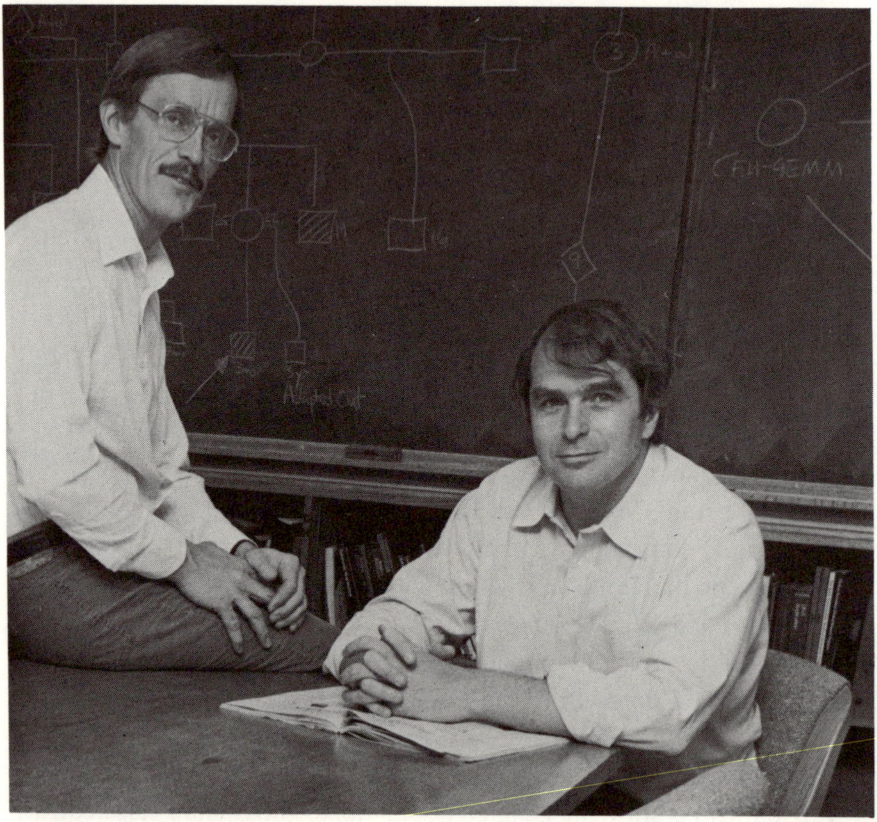

Drs. Raymond F. Gesteland (left) and Raymond L. White, co-chairs of the Department of Human Genetics.

Ireland, Robert Weiss from the University of Washington, and Ray Gesteland use bacterial, yeast, and plant systems to study the molecular mechanisms involved in deciphering the genetic code. Mario Capecchi from Harvard is developing the mouse as a model system for studying how to move altered genes in and out of chromosomes and the effect of these genetic changes on development.

The success of all these programs would not have been possible without key funding from the community or without the continuing support of the University administration, especially President Chase Peterson. A gift to the Medical School permitted establishment of the

Thomas Dee Chair of Human Genetics; generous funding also established the George and Delores Doré Eccles Institute of Human Genetics. Together with HHMI, the Eccles Foundation provided the funds for the recently completed genetics building within the Medical Center complex, which currently houses three major programs: (1) the Department of Human Genetics; (2) the Human Molecular Biology and Genetics Program (HMBG) directed by Stephen Prescott, which recruits investigators with academic appointments in various departments of the Medical School to provide a unique research environment that brings both medical and molecular expertise to bear on problems of human disease; and (3) the Utah Center for Human Genome Research, one of six centers for the Human Genome Project of the National Institutes of Health, which will develop technology and tools for the complete sequencing of the human genome.

The University of Utah is now an internationally recognized center for genetics research, where a creative and powerful blend of clinical and basic science forms a cohesive program that is perhaps unique in the world.

CHAPTER THIRTY-NINE

Medical Informatics: Application of Computers to Medical Science

HOMER R. WARNER, MD, PHD

THE DEPARTMENT OF MEDICAL INFORMATICS at the University of Utah originated from the interests and activities of Homer R. Warner. Warner was born in Salt Lake City in 1922. Playing football at the University of Utah was more interesting than his pre-med studies, so he was turned down when he applied for admission to the Medical School. He joined the Navy and was trained as a carrier-based fighter pilot, but the war ended before he saw combat. After the war he completed his bachelor's degree in zoology, applied to medical school again, and this time was accepted.

Warner's class of old veterans, whose average age as medical school freshmen was twenty-seven, graduated on the accelerated war-time program in 1949. Being the only student in his freshman class to answer a difficult midterm question in physiology correctly had given Warner self-confidence and represented an important turning point in his life.

After Warner's graduation, Dr. Max Wintrobe arranged for him to intern at the University of Texas in Dallas with Tinsley Harrison, a very dynamic teacher and role-model, who could make a routine stroke case sound like the most challenging diagnostic problem in the world. Warner's belief that a teacher's principal role is to arouse interest and intellectual curiosity stems from his time with Harrison.

Harrison sent Warner to the University of Minnesota, where he spent the next year as a resident in medicine with Cecil Watson. After

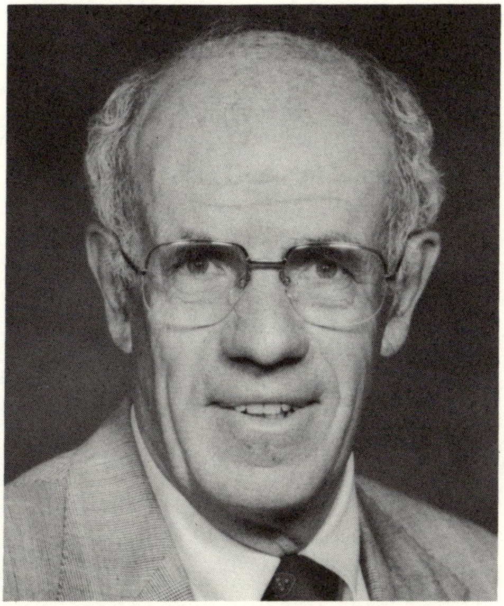

Homer R. Warner.

a year, he continued his residency at the Mayo Clinic in Rochester, where he was stimulated by physiologist Earl Wood to develop a real interest in research.

During these very early days of heart catheterization and diagnostic physiological testing, Mayo Clinic researchers were injecting a blue dye into people, mostly children, with different kinds of right-to-left and left-to-right shunts, trying to detect and quantitate the degree of shunt from the shape of the indicator dilution curve recorded downstream. Warner got so interested in these exciting new developments that he applied for a year in physiology to work with Dr. Wood. Credit for this year was to be applied toward his Board requirements in internal medicine, but he never got back to completing the residency.

Wood got Warner interested in writing and also in developing a method for estimating stroke volume from the shape of aortic pressure waves. He worked out an equation which could be calibrated against the dye dilution or the Fick method and tested it on a series of normal subjects. The stroke volume estimation method performed so well that

Wood suggested the work could become a doctoral dissertation. As a result, Warner returned to the University of Minnesota and spent one more year with Maurice Vissher completing work in mathematics and engineering to fulfill the requirements for a PhD in physiology.

In 1953 Warner returned to the University of Utah to work with Dr. Hans Hecht in the Department of Cardiology at the old Salt Lake General Hospital. He didn't really have a job, but he had applied for a one-year American Heart fellowship, and Hecht was willing to take him since he brought his own support. He helped Hecht set up the catheterization lab using many of the techniques that Mayo had developed. About half way through the year, Dr. Ray Rumel, the only heart surgeon in Salt Lake, and Clarence Wonnacott, the administrator of the LDS Hospital, asked Warner to set up a heart catheterization lab at LDS. In July of 1954 Warner went to the LDS Hospital, where he was to work for the next thirty-two years.

That first laboratory was in a little room on Six West, just outside the doors to surgery. On a budget of $10,000, Warner bought a used fluoroscope and table and the necessary equipment. One end of the room was sealed off and painted black to house the homemade recording equipment. On a table made from a slab door, he mounted a recording camera and a light source on one end and on the other a bank of galvanometers whose mirrors reflected the light back to the recording camera six feet away. The length of the light beam provided the amplification, as electronic amplifiers were not yet sufficiently stable. The electrical signals from the ECG, pressure transducers, and oximeters were fed directly to the galvanometers. At the end of a diagnostic procedure, the twelve-inch-wide role of film was removed from the camera and developed and the wiggly recorded lines analyzed by manual measurement.

At first, most of the cases were patients with congenital heart disease, since surgery for these lesions was new and many accumulated patients were potential candidates for treatment. In June of the second year, 1955, the hospital received a $220,000 grant from the Ford Foundation. The only constraint was that it had to be used for something other than direct hospital operating costs for patient services. Warner convinced Clarence Wonnacott that the grant should be used to set up a research foundation. The first $70,000 built a two-floor animal research facility on the roof, just above the little cath lab, with the animal quarters and Warner's office on top and two new research labs below. The remaining $150,000 represents the endowment for the Deseret Foundation, with the interest used to pay the diener who cared for the animal facilities.

The breakthrough that had attracted enough attention for the grant was a study of the way a pressure wave is distorted as it travels from the root of the aorta out to the periphery, a phenomenon Warner had encountered in his dissertation work. At the time (1955) Warner was taking a class in the mathematics department at the University, and the instructor presented the concept of harmonic or Fourier analysis in which a wave form can be represented as a series of sine waves, each a multiple or harmonic of the first or fundamental frequency. Warner decided to perform such an analysis on a pressure wave recorded from a catheter in the radial artery of a patient. It took most of a day to analyze a single heartbeat using a large slide rule and manual measurements from the pressure recording.

The next day in class the instructor talked about what happens to each of these harmonics as a wave form goes through some system, that is, the transfer function. For example, a radio has a tuner circuit with dials that permit one to adjust the properties of the circuit so that only certain frequencies will be amplified. All the other harmonics will be suppressed. That night Warner did a transfer function analysis of a single heartbeat, looking first at the harmonic content of the upstream pressure wave form, recorded through a catheter up in the root of the aorta, and then at the wave form recorded down at the radial artery. The harmonics of the two wave forms had different amplitudes. The plot looked very similar to the transfer function of the tuned circuit the instructor had used in his illustration.

Warner thought the artery might be distorting the pressure wave by amplifying certain frequencies and decided to build an electrical circuit that could be adjusted until it distorted an electrical wave form the same way the artery was distorting the pressure wave form.

With the help of Dietrich Gehmlich in the electrical engineering department, he built a tunable circuit with a resistor, a capacitor, and an inductor or coil, the properties of each component variable by turning knobs on the front panel. This was Warner's first analog computer. To test his idea, he waited for patients who needed catheters inserted for diagnostic studies. Once he had the catheters in the aorta and radial artery, Warner would leave the patient with his assistant while he ran upstairs to the research lab and quickly adjusted the knobs on the resonant circuit until it was distorting the electrical wave form in the same way the artery was distorting the pressure wave form (i.e., the two output wave forms were superimposed on the dual-beam oscilloscope). Then he could read off the resonant frequency and damping coefficient of the circuit and derive parameters of the artery, such as its elasticity, by analogy.

Warner and Dr. Alan Toronto studied a series of eighty patients using this technique and published the results. As one might expect, the resonant frequency of the aorta gets higher as the vessel begins to lose its elasticity with increasing age. This was the first time that kind of measurement had been made on living patients. Warner applied to the NIH and received funding to purchase the components for a general purpose analog computer for modeling or transfer function studies in other components of the circulatory system. In a few years the department had a whole roomful of these amplifiers that, with wires strung between them, could be used to build circuits to simulate very complex equations that couldn't possibly have been solved without a computer. For the first time, it was possible to describe various phenomena and relationships in a quantitative way.

Warner and his colleagues performed studies using a computer model of the sino-auricular node or pacemaker of the heart. Here, the input to the model was the frequency of nerve firings (action potentials) on the sympathetic and vagus nerves, and the output was the heart rate. Once they were satisfied that their model adequately described the relationship over a wide variety of input variations, they used it to explore the full range of input pattern combinations that might occur clinically.

When the University got its first digital computer, about 1960, Warner decided to study the way the concentration curve following a sudden dye injection is recorded at various points downstream. The transfer function of the upstream and downstream curves becomes a measure of the distribution of transit times of blood particles as they travel between recording sites. For example, transit time through the kidneys is very rapid, something less than ten seconds. However, for blood to flow through the legs and back to the heart may take as long as several minutes. Once again Warner and his coworkers had discovered a very powerful tool. It is useful to know the cardiac output and even more useful to know where the blood pumped by the heart goes.

The researchers were very excited about this work. Since the digital computer in the Merrill Engineering Building was available only after nine o'clock at night, a cot provided a place to rest while the computer ground out solutions to their simulations. Warner got acquainted with Professor Bob Stephenson, who directed the computer center and later became acting dean of the School of Engineering. Together they decided to try to model the diagnostic process using probability theory. Given a certain set of signs and symptoms and the frequency of each finding in patients with any one of a set of diseases, their program could calculate the likelihood that a patient had a particular disease.

To aid the patients coming through Warner's laboratory, they decided to make their model to diagnose thirty-five different forms of congenital heart disease. First, they collected data on how frequently each of fifty different findings, such as murmurs of different kinds and cyanosis, occurred in each disease and how common each disease was in the population of patients referred to the laboratory. After collecting several hundred such cases, a matrix showed the disease on one axis, the findings on the other. At each intersection of the symptom with the disease, a number represented the frequency of that finding in patients with that disease. This table formed the basis for diagnosing patients based on findings recorded by their referring physicians. A comparison of the computer diagnoses and those of the referring physicians showed the computer to be right more often than any of the physicians, based on diagnosis following heart catheterization. The average practitioner, who may see only two or three cases of congenital heart disease in a year, has little experience in diagnosis. These very exciting results were presented at the 1965 meeting of the American Heart Association and published in the *AMA Journal*.

Largely as a result of this groundbreaking study, Warner was successful in getting a grant from the NIH for a digital computer in his own LDS Hospital laboratory. In those days, machines were very expensive. The grant provided about $500,000 per year, and Warner felt a tremendous responsibility to use it productively. He stayed awake nights trying to think of new ways to use the computer to solve significant problems.

Over the next ten years, Warner and his colleagues developed many new computer applications with support from NIH and other sources. After the development phase of a given project (such as automated ECG interpretation) was complete, the hospital administration was asked to begin to charge patients for the service. If the medical staff thought a service was worthwhile, it was offered by the hospital, and in this way the HELP System grew.

The Beginnings of the HELP System

One of the first services Warner and his colleagues automated was the heart catheterization laboratory. They acquired an analog-to-digital converter, probably the first one ever used in a medical setting, and interfaced it to a digital computer. This permitted electrical signals from instruments such as pressure transducers to be fed directly to the computer in digital form. Programs were written which would recognize key features and then carry out whatever analysis was needed to interpret the data. In the cath lab this meant that by the time the physician had finished placing the catheter in the appropriate chambers of the heart and signaled the computer with a wand to make the measurements, he could ask for a display of the results on the oscilloscope, edit the data in any way he wished, and then call for a printout of the final report. This program cut the time for a catheterization and data analysis roughly in half.

Next, many of the group's cath lab programs were moved to the operating rooms. In the early days of open-heart surgery, it was apparent that patients undergoing extensive and prolonged surgery needed careful cardiovascular and respiratory status monitoring. Warner and his associates built programs that allowed the anesthesiologist to record other data, such as intravenous fluid intake, drug administration, and blood gas data, and generate a complete report as the patient left the operating room.

Most of these patients were moved immediately to an intensive care unit (ICU), so it was quite natural that the next phase of this research was designed to continue the monitoring there. The group developed a special console for the ten-bed post–open-heart-surgery unit. The console at the nursing station had a bank of lights — a red, a yellow, and a green light for each patient. The green light indicated that the computer was actively sampling data from a patient. At regular intervals the program would display the data being sampled—a pressure or an ECG waveform. The yellow light indicated that something had happened to that patient's data; that there was an abnormal trend in some variable. Maybe the pressure was dropping or the cardiac output was going down or the peripheral resistance was rising. The computer calculated each of these variables automatically from the shape of the aortic pressure waveform measured through a small arterial catheter introduced by a nurse the night before surgery. The red light indicated an emergency that required immediate action. The yellow and red lights were also interrupt buttons that would make the computer display a graph of the time course of the variable that was out-trending in the wrong direction.

One day Warner went down to visit the ICU and saw a nurse pumping up a blood pressure cuff on the left arm of a patient who had a pressure-monitoring catheter in the right arm. A yellow light showed on the panel. The nurse was embarrassed when she saw him watching her and explained that she didn't know what to do next. They sat down at the computer terminal and looked at all the data in both the computer and the chart. They called the resident and jointly decided that the patient probably was having a cardiac tamponade. The surgeon on call promptly took the patient back to the operating room.

This experience became another important turning point in Warner's approach to the application of computers to medicine. It was clear that just providing data and displaying it in a variety of ways might not be an adequate solution to the decision-making problem. This nurse clearly needed help in interpreting the data, and that interpretation required more data than just the hemodynamic measurements. It required data from other sources, such as the chemistry and hematology labs and x-ray interpretations, but most of all it required that the computer have some medical knowledge. They needed to build intelligence into the system.

Soon afterward, in 1970, Warner went to Europe to give papers at two meetings about ten days apart. In a little hotel overlooking Lake Geneva, he got the idea for computer-based knowledge representation which would provide the basis for the HELP hospital information system. He worked all night between meetings writing the first draft of that program, and by the time he came home, it was ready to try.

The next step was to put some flesh on the skeleton—to put medical knowledge into the shell program that the computer could execute. Two young physicians, Charles Olmstead and Barry Rutherford, were working with Warner, and together they developed a knowledge base of rules and relationships for management of patients in the ICU and for interpretation of measurements made in the cath lab. Their first paper on the HELP system was published in 1972 in *Computer and Biomedical Research*, a journal which Warner has edited for twenty-four years. It is the decision-making capability of the HELP System that distinguishes it from other hospital information systems.

Rutherford was a cardiologist who came to LDS from the Mayo Clinic and later moved to Iowa. Olmstead went on to become a radiation oncologist and moved to Missouri. The HELP System became the primary research effort of the Department of Medical Informatics at Utah, and Alan Pryor, Reed Gardner, and the whole group began working on building an integrated system that would support this kind of decision making. The first version was developed on a Control Data 3200 computer. After eighteen years the researchers could no longer buy parts for it and had to buy another used machine ("a junker for parts") to keep it going.

A newer machine was needed, but NIH was not interested in funding the second version of something. They finally took the problem to hospital administrator David Wirthlin, who made the decision to support the reprogramming effort and buy the new machine. LDS Hospital now owned the HELP programs. The reprogramming effort took several years because the original version had been written in assembly language for the 3200 machine. After the new system was up and running, the hospital worked out an arrangement with Control Data Corporation to market it. Income from the commercialization of the HELP system has provided a very important source of financial support for the department ever since. (Control Data sold the system to 3-M in 1987.)

Forming the Department at the University

When Warner first went to LDS Hospital in 1955, he sought out Horace Davenport and asked for a faculty appointment in the Department of Physiology at the University. As a result of his teaching activities there and his affiliations in the School of Engineering, by 1966 several graduate students were doing doctoral dissertation projects under his supervision at LDS. Henry Eyring, dean of the Graduate School, had invited Warner on several occasions to present his research to Eyring's graduate students in physical chemistry. After one such occasion, Eyring suggested that the University establish a new department so the students Warner was training could obtain a degree which reflected the nature of their training and experience.

Eyring contacted English professor Dr. Jack Adamson, who was then the academic vice president, and he in turn set up a meeting with Warner, Max Williams (dean of engineering), and Franklin Ebaugh (dean of the Medical School). Adamson asked both deans to explore with their faculties the idea of such a department. A few weeks later Ebaugh reported that the medical faculty felt the time was not right for such a move, but Dean Williams said the engineering faculty would welcome a bioengineering department since there were many areas of possible joint interest for both research and teaching. So the Department of Biophysics and Bioengineering was established, with laboratories at LDS Hospital and Merrill Engineering.

After about ten years, the department was divided. Bioengineering stayed in the engineering school, and a new Department of Medical Biophysics and Computing was established in the Medical School. Most of the faculty went with Warner into the Medical School, although the department's headquarters remained at LDS until 1985. The Department of Medical Informatics, with fifty-two students, is now the second largest graduate training program in the Medical School for the master's and PhD degrees.

The first graduate of the new program was Stanford Topham, an electrical engineer whose dissertation was a study of the control of cardiac output during exercise which significantly changed the way such clinical problems as the treatment of acute myocardial infarction are viewed today.

The Department Faculty

Alan Pryor came to the University in the mid-sixties with a background in mathematics and computer experience at NASA. For his doctoral dissertation he produced a program for the automated interpretation of the electrocardiogram that was used by the LDS Hospital until 1985, when it was replaced by a commercial system.

Getting automated ECG interpretation accepted by the cardiologists at the hospital was a real challenge. They could always find fault with it until Pryor got top electrocardiographer Alan Lindsay involved enough that Lindsay felt it was at least in part *his* program. Then Lindsay went to his colleagues in cardiology, showed them the facts, and convinced them that the program was doing a more consistent job of interpreting the electrocardiograms than they were. The department learned that to get this new technology accepted by users they must first convince someone respected in the field and then let that person sell it to his or her colleagues.

Pryor has been the architect of many of the underlying computer science aspects of the HELP System and has worked to achieve the goals originally set for the system and to make it a commercially viable product that can be used by other hospitals.

Reed Gardner's background was electrical engineering. He took responsibility for the hardware, and, in those early days of digital computers, expanded the ways for getting data in and out of the computer by designing systems for displaying information graphically and improving methods for interfacing analog equipment to digital computers for the operating room and ICU. He is prominent in the American Thoracic Society as the leader of the computer group.

Astrophysicist Paul Clayton was using television methods to observe and track the motion of the border of the sun that resembled very closely the methods Warner and his group were using to track the border of the left ventricle. Clayton had no initial background in physiology or medicine, but became knowledgeable in those fields by working closely with Dr. Hal Liddle, developing some special databases that allowed Liddle to track his patients closely. The fine papers produced from Clayton and Liddle's collaboration have had an impact on the direction the field of cardiology has taken. With Phil Frederick and the radiology department, Clayton developed the first automated radiology system. He is now head of the informatics unit at Columbia University and operates a multi-million-dollar IAIMS program there.

John Morgan, who had a degree in electrical engineering from BYU, developed a system for automatically coding diseases using the record room computer. He joined the faculty for a few years after graduation, then quit to develop a minicomputer-based version of the system he had created for LDS Hospital. In less than three years of selling his system to hospitals around the country from the back of a motor home, Morgan built a company which he sold to 3-M for $16 million. In appreciation, he gave the department a $100,000 grant which now supports the John Morgan Fellowship.

Justin Clark came to the department in the mid-sixties with a background in physics. After graduating, he joined the faculty and began working at Primary Children's Hospital on computer-based instrumentation for measuring physiological variables, particularly respiratory and cardiovascular parameters in newborns. Clark is a true

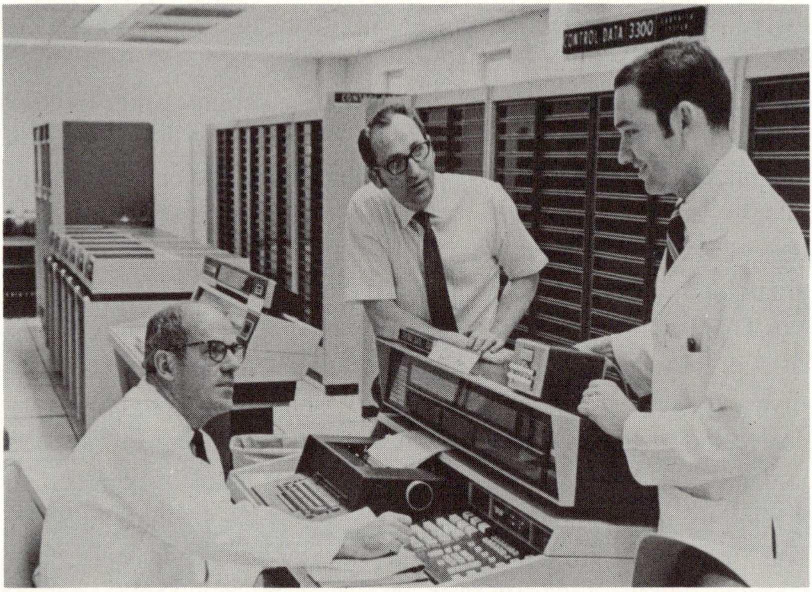

Drs. Homer R. Warner, Alan Pryor, and Reed Gardner with Control Data 3300 at LDS Hospital, about 1975.

inventor, and some of his patents are very remunerative for PCMC.

Mark Skolnick's arrival added a completely new dimension to the department's work. His computer applications in genetic epidemiology and genome mapping are discussed in his chapter elsewhere in this volume. The work of Skolnick and his group has brought the department international attention and has generated a new medical informatics subspecialty.

Peter Haug had received both his medical training and computer experience at the University of Wisconsin. After his residency at Utah, he stayed to become a member of the faculty. His areas of interest are natural language processing and decision support. Haug has worked with Warner on the decision-support algorithms for the Iliad project, and he is responsible for the latest version of the radiology component of the HELP System, replacing Paul Clayton.

Stan Huff, a Utah-trained pathologist, joined the medical informatics faculty in 1985. He has become a leader in the field of patient medical records and database design, and his concepts are being incorporated in the National Library of Medicine's massive Unified Medical Language project.

Dennis Parker, a medical informatics PhD, went to the radiology department of the University of California at San Francisco, where he developed one of the first high-speed CT devices for medical imaging of moving organs like the heart. He returned to the medical informatics faculty six years ago and has been pursuing his interest in spatial reconstruction of images and pattern recognition.

The Move to the University

In 1985 the University Hospital signed a contract for the HELP System with Control Data Corporation. Chase Peterson, vice president for health sciences, wrote Warner a letter, saying "We are installing your system. What are you going to do about it?" In a meeting it was decided that Warner rather than one of the younger faculty should move to the Medical School, since they perceived the task of getting HELP running at the University Hospital as integrally linked to the long-range future of the department and involving primarily political challenges. So Warner gave up his research career award and moved into space on the "A" level of the Medical School, across from the laundry.

The dean provided funds for a small TANDEM computer capable of running the HELP programs and intended for developing new applications tailored to the needs of the hospital and clinical staff. But Warner was not given access to the HELP System at the University because the "pure vanilla" version provided by Control Data was not allowed to be changed at all, and none of its clinical or decision–making features had been implemented as of this writing in mid-1991.

Frustrated by this situation, Warner responded to a need expressed by Dr. William Odell, chair of the Department of Medicine, for a program to supplement the learning experience of third-year medical students during their clerkship on the medical wards. Over the next few years, an expert system program was developed for the Macintosh computer with the help of experts from the Department of Internal Medicine representing nine different subspecialties. With support from a National Library of Medicine grant, a knowledge base was constructed representing more than 500 diseases which is currently being used by all medical students at Utah. The program, called Iliad, is marketed by Applied Informatics under contract from the University and is now used by more than thirty other medical schools.

Iliad has three modes of operation. It can act as a consultant on real cases by providing a differential diagnosis and suggestions and explanations at each stage of the work on a patient. In a second mode, Iliad can generate a simulated case of any disease in its knowledge base, allow a student to ask for findings (history, physical exam, laboratory, x-ray, etc.), and require the student to propose working hypotheses (diagnoses) based on what he or she knows at each stage of the workup. Students at Utah are required to work up simulations each week in both this learning mode and the test (Iliad's third) mode and are evaluated on their performance. It has been clearly demonstrated that students do improve their diagnostic proficiency by using Iliad, but that improvement is content specific.

It has been convincingly shown that one doesn't become a good generic problem solver: one becomes a good problem solver in a given area through experience in solving problems in that area. In other words, an expert cardiologist is not necessarily an expert hematologist. In the Iliad project, doctors have run the simulations to see how they do. They "muddle through" in areas where they are not experts, but in their own areas they focus quickly and get to the vital data in the most cost-efficient way. Iliad is designed to teach students in the same way. Rather than simply providing a list of findings to be memorized for a disease, Iliad organizes them into "clusters" or patho-physiological entities, and these entities are then formed into higher-level diagnostic entities. The students can take advantage of the patho-physiology Iliad has taught them to solve problems in clinical medicine.

The University is searching for Warner's successor as chair of medical informatics at Utah. The evolution of this new discipline over the last three decades has been exciting, with Utah playing a prominent role. Utah may lead the way in the next decade as well, since the necessary people, institutions, and attitudes are already well established.

CHAPTER FORTY

Pathology in the Salt Lake City Private Hospitals

JOHN H. CARLQUIST, MD • FRED MIYA, MD
CYRIL D. FULLMER, MD • SHELLEY SWIFT, MD
ASSEMBLED BY ERNST J. EICHWALD, MD

WHEN DR. JOHN H. (JACK) CARLQUIST arrived in Utah in the fall of 1939, only two pathologists, Drs. Lyman Daines and Orin Ogilvie, practiced in the city. The only other pathologists in the Intermountain West were in Cheyenne, Boise, and Reno. Dr. Daines was really a bacteriologist, and he was also part-time dean of the two-year Medical School. This all seems like an incredible load, especially in view of the seventy-nine pathologists now practicing in Utah. Even many of the smallest hospitals now have their own staff pathologists.

Pathologists had been involved primarily in anatomical pathology, and the early clinical pathology procedures were grafted onto the anatomical work, largely because no other physicians were interested in supervising laboratories.

LDS Hospital

The laboratory at LDS Hospital was typical of the period. Second-rate in both space and arrangement, it occupied about 600 square feet at the south end of the old east wing and housed five employees. A technologist covered hematology; others performed urinalyses and prepared tissue slides by frozen section technique; and a maid washed the glassware and helped in general. It was a far cry from the 168 people in all categories who worked in the laboratory and Blood Bank when Dr. Carlquist retired in 1976. In blood typing only the ABO system was known. Hematocrit determinations were not yet in use.

Basic Metabolic Rates (BMRs) were the only clue to thyroid disease. All procedures were manual, and quality control as it is practiced today was unknown. Pathologists limited themselves largely to tissue work, autopsies, and some supervision of laboratory procedures.

Dr. Carlquist performed his work at LDS on a part-time basis while teaching and assisting Dr. Ogilvie at his laboratory and the hospitals he serviced. Dr. Carlquist was called to active duty in the Army for a short time but was released at the request of the Medical School in order to continue teaching. Three things happened then: The four-year Medical School was established, Dr. Daines died in December 1941, and Dr. Ogilvie resigned his teaching position as a result of friction that developed during the reorganization of the school. Carlquist was now the only member of the Department of Pathology and Bacteriology.

The volume of work at LDS had picked up a little, and with all the classes in pathology and bacteriology, Carlquist carried a tremendous load. Dr. Louis P. Gebhardt came from Stanford in 1942 and the department was divided, with Gebhardt becoming head of bacteriology in 1943. Many efforts were made to recruit a full-time chair for the pathology department, and finally Dr. Francis D. Gunn was appointed in the summer of 1944. Shortly after his arrival early in 1945, Gunn developed active tuberculosis. He made a surprisingly good recovery, however, and was able to become active in teaching before the end of the year. Dr. Carlquist was then faced with four choices for full-time work: the Medical School, LDS Hospital, Holy Cross, or St. Mark's. He chose LDS Hospital, believing that it was "where the action would be." Dr. Crichton McNeil, Gunn's first resident, eventually took the job at Holy Cross, and Dr. Shelley Swift came later to St. Mark's.

LDS Hospital was an old H-shaped building. A low flight of stairs in front led to the second floor, which was the business and admitting area. The ground floor housed the kitchen on the east end, a radiology department as primitive as the laboratory, the autopsy room, and other utility areas.

The hospital faced numerous problems. The onset of tremendous evolutionary changes in medicine was not yet fully realized by either

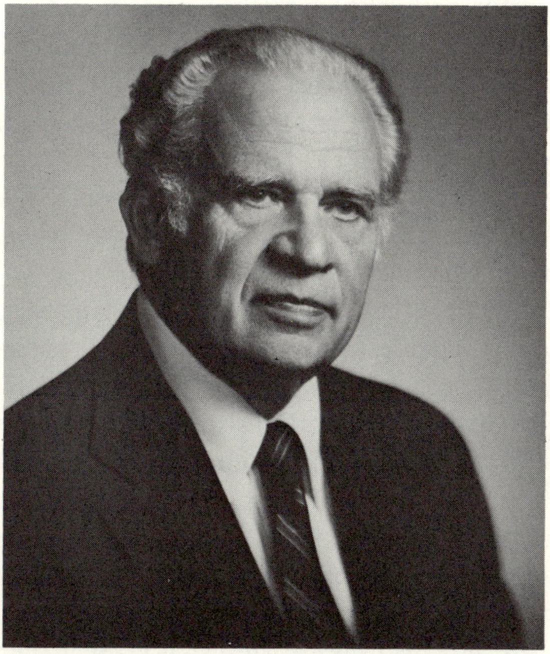

John H. Carlquist.

the medical staff or the early administrators. The laboratory did not work on a budget basis, and without such a guide, equipment and supplies had to be requested on a piecemeal basis. But a budget can be a powerful administrative tool, a great stimulus to future planning.

Dr. Carlquist's initial disappointment in the lack of progress gave way to hope with the arrival of new, well-trained specialists. Dr. Ray Rumel brought his skills in chest surgery. A year later Dr. Scott Smith arrived to be the first MD anesthetist, and this was another boost. In December 1947 Dr. Earl Crowder became the first full-time radiologist. He established a close relationship with the administrator, Clarence Wonnacott, and was able to build an outstanding department. The idea of "striving for excellence" was born.

Slowly but gradually the pathology department benefited from this philosophy. The first change in the laboratory was a new morgue. The basement autopsy room was dark, dingy, and dirty. It had only an embalming table without plumbing connection, not a true autopsy table. A pail was hung at one end to catch any washings from the body. A sink had one hose for water and another for suction. Since no "diener" or trained assistant was available in those days, the room got only a superficial cleaning after each post-mortem examination. At times the bucket at the end of the table would overflow, and the fluid would run out under the door and into the hallway, where it could be tracked into the adjacent kitchen and cafeteria.

The new morgue, large, clean, and well-equipped, served well. With increasing pressure, and the support of the Presiding Bishop of the LDS Church, a new laboratory replaced the original, long-outdated facility on the Sixth Floor East. Consisting of the entire seventh floor on the East Wing and a new addition of the eighth floor, the new laboratory was attractive and functional. For the first time, Carlquist had an office and a desk. However, it was not too long before space pressures began again. A newly constructed Central Wing included space on the south end for bacteriology and research. A former technology student provided the first research grant. A fair number of animals — Rhesus monkeys, rabbits, guinea pigs, and mice — were warehoused in the research area. Drs. Stanley Altman and Stanley Marcus participated in the research. Both tumor and bone marrow transplants were of interest to the staff. Fortunately, space on the first floor of the Central Wing originally planned for laundry storage became the Blood Bank. A small space near the business office was obtained for admitting laboratory staff to take routine blanket orders for lab work as patients entered the hospital.

One of Dr. Carlquist's most significant innovations was the placement of the surgical pathology suite adjacent to the operating room suites. This allowed the pathologist on duty to walk from the work area directly into an operating room to consult whenever the surgeon requested this service. In addition, this arrangement permitted nurses or other operating room personnel to bring surgical specimens to surgical pathology very quickly for frozen section examination or consultation. Not many large hospitals have this type of accommodation. In many instances the department of pathology is far removed from

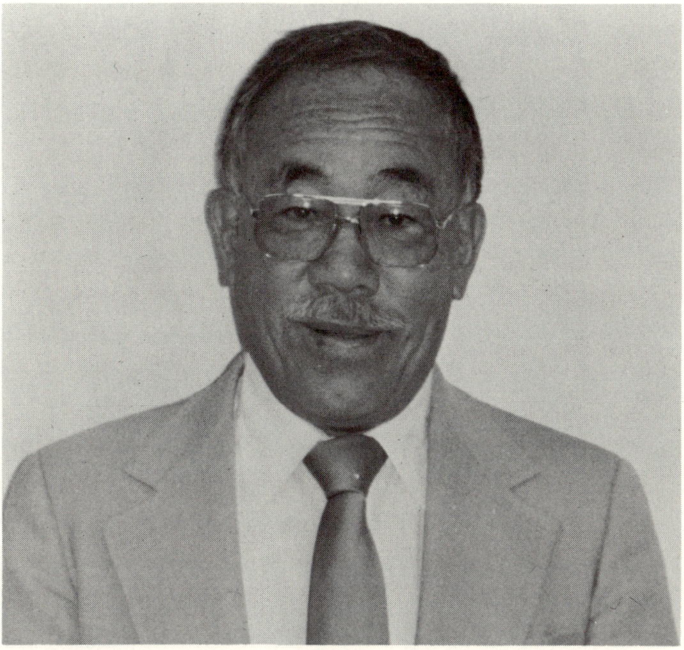

Fred Miya.

the operating rooms and communication must be by telephone, which creates the potential for dangerous communication failure.

When Dr. Carlquist joined the hospital staff, families were called in for typing for the occasional blood transfusion. Blood from the donor was drawn into an open flask which contained a citrate solution prepared by the hospital pharmacist. When the blood was given to the patient, it was poured into a glass cylinder with a sponge at the bottom to serve as a filter. World War II changed this. With the need for more transfusions on the battlefront, vacuum bottles were developed. As soon as they were available, in 1943, a Blood Bank was started, and the number of transfusions jumped from 60 in 1942 to 1,200 in 1943. The LDS Hospital Blood Bank was one of the first in the nation as well as the Intermountain West. The work volume increased explosively. One day during a busy heart surgery period, when more blood was used per case than is needed now, 26,000 pints were drawn,

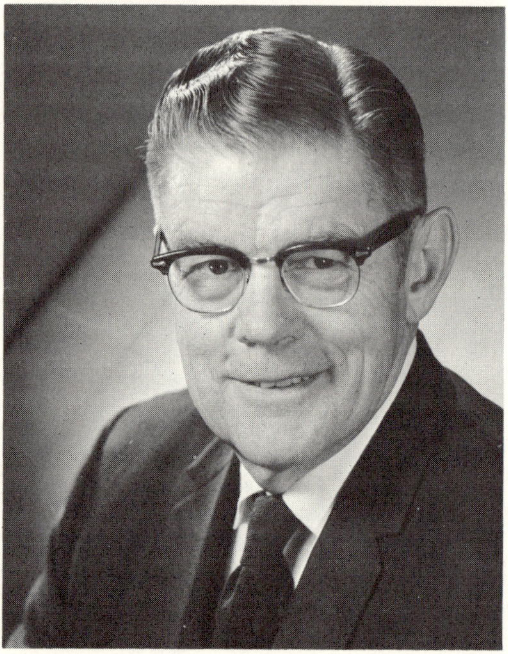

Cyril D. Fullmer.

indicating that it was the second largest in-hospital blood bank in the country after Johns Hopkins Hospital.

A major step forward was the installation of the laboratory computer. The brilliant Dr. DeWitt Hunter was assigned to work with the programmers. He left shortly thereafter, and Dr. Carlquist was obliged to assume his role. Automating the lab proved far more difficult and costly than the computer company, MedLab, had anticipated, and the company was taken over by Control Data Corporation. The system eventually developed was very flexible and paid for itself through charges previously lost and improved bookkeeping. The laboratory could never go back to the old paper slips and manual records.

Shortly before his retirement in 1976, Carlquist was asked to lecture to the pathology class on coronary artery disease and its effects on the heart. The class had grown from the old days and now numbered about 100 students. When he finished his lecture, he asked, as

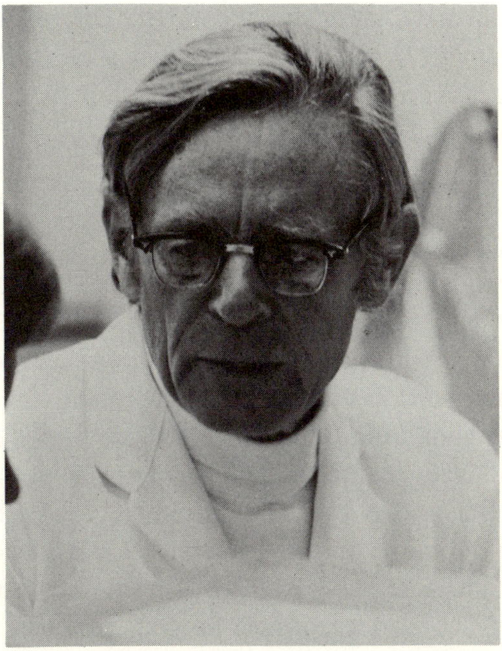

Ernst J. Eichwald.

always, "Ladies and Gentlemen, do you have any questions?" With this, the whole class rose to their feet and applauded — a very satisfactory way to finish a long teaching career.

Of Dr. Carlquist's many associates, Dr. William Weems distinguished himself for his interest in teaching and research. Appointed in 1971, he became the foremost expert on skin pathology, which led to his establishing a private dermatopathology laboratory in 1975.

Upon Dr. Carlquist's retirement in January 1976, Dr. Fred Miya became chair of the department. He had obtained a PhD in bacteriology at the University of Utah in 1959 and an MD in 1963 and had completed a pathology residency at the University and LDS. Dr. Miya was interested in immunology and had come to LDS in 1966 to take charge of the Blood Bank.

In July of 1976 he re-recruited Dr. Robert Flinner to chair the tissue pathology section. Flinner had trained and was an instructor at Tulane

Medical School and Charity Hospital in New Orleans and was on the LDS staff from 1971 to 1973. Dr. Flinner soon became the local consultant for many of the younger pathologists in the community, and Dr. Miya credits him for much of the present stability of the anatomic pathology services. With Dr. Elizabeth Hale Hammond, Flinner published a textbook on lesions of the Mediastinum. Both have taken an active part in teaching pathology to sophomore medical students.

Dr. Hammond was recruited from Massachusetts General Hospital in 1978 as an expert in electron microscopy and immunopathology. She became the first director of the Jack Carlquist Electron Microscopy (EM) Laboratory and has served on the University faculty for many years. On invitation from Dr. Henry Plenk, she joined the pathology section of the National Radiation Therapy Oncology Study Group (RTOG) and became its chair. Dr. Hammond has participated very actively in RTOG and has initiated several research projects, especially with Dr. William Sause. A key member of the heart transplant program, Dr. Hammond has been responsible for great advances in the field of immunopathology.

Dr. Miya reports as follows:

> In 1984 a $77 million replacement wing was constructed, and the Department of Pathology eventually occupied an area comprising more than 24,000 square feet. Thus, the department grew from its very modest beginnings in the 1920s into a superbly functional laboratory capable of providing most of the physician-requested laboratory tests and also providing skilled, highly service-oriented laboratory support for research and patient management for the clinical departments.
>
> Ironically, the Department of Pathology completed a circle, starting in a basement, rising to a wonderful height and view of the city, then moving back to the basement. "What goes around, comes around."

Holy Cross Hospital, Reported by Dr. Cyril D. Fullmer

With the completion of the transcontinental railroad in 1869, Utah's isolation ended; mines and smelters became profitable to develop and operate, and the growing activity created the necessity to provide places to care for injured workmen. In 1875 Sisters M. Holy Cross and M. Bartholomew came to Salt Lake City and arranged for the conversion of a two-story brick building into a hospital which could accommodate twelve to fourteen patients. In June 1883, a 125-bed hospital was opened on a ten-acre site between Tenth and Eleventh East on First South Street.

The few autopsies performed in those early years were, apparently, limited dissections authorized by verbal consent of relatives. Funeral homes provided the only facilities available for the procedure.

Laboratories with microscopes appeared at the University in 1906, when the first two-year School of Medicine was established, with Dr. Ralph Chamberlin as dean. In 1910 the Salt Lake City Health Department obtained a microscope and aniline dyes to stain and identify bacteria.

Laboratory facilities were extremely limited until the Sisters of the Holy Cross engaged Dr. Thomas A. Flood to take six months of pathology training in 1919 to become the first pathologist for a small laboratory in the hospital basement. The laboratory was equipped with a microscope, stains, reagents, and a sink for examination of surgical tissues.

In 1930 a small amphitheater was added to the basement morgue for teaching gross findings in disease. In the 1940s microscopic examination of tissues became a routine part of post-mortem study. The morgue sufficed until 1960, when a spacious new facility was constructed on the ground floor of the west wing, occupying 500 square feet, with a large morgue table, brilliant lighting, and a walk-in refrigerator to store bodies. A separate room was equipped with lockers and a shower for pathologists and the morgue diener.

On July 1, 1947, an expanded full-service laboratory was opened, and Dr. Crichton McNeil became the first full-time pathologist at Holy Cross Hospital. Dr. McNeil graduated from Buffalo Medical School in 1938, where he completed a residency in pathology in 1942. He served in the U.S. Army from 1942 to 1946, where he gained extensive experience in laboratory medicine, including blood banking using the new vacuum container. From 1946 to 1947 he was an instructor in pathology at the University of Utah. Dr. McNeil was a perfectionist dedicated to the advance of laboratory medicine with new tests and a tireless worker with an interest in research.

An expanded laboratory was designed, covering about 2,200 square feet. The work increased rapidly in the 1950s, and soon the lab overflowed into the attic, where spaces were developed for cytotechnologists to work with microscopes. A designated staining area actually existed in the attic stairwell. The entire hospital was reconstructed and modernized in 1958–59, opening to patients in 1960. The new laboratory in the west wing occupied about 12,000 square feet. The space was organized with state-of-the-art laboratory sections, a small research laboratory, pathologists' offices arranged in the center — adjacent to a library on the west — and cubicles for secretaries in an area immediately to the east.

In 1954 the first electrophoresis instrument was installed, as well as an autoanalyzer for chemistry and an automatic counting device for hematology. In 1964 a gas chromatography apparatus was supplied for steroid determinations. In 1966 protein-bound iodine determinations became automated, and a scanning device for radio isotopes was purchased.

Dr. McNeil resigned from Holy Cross Hospital in 1973 to complete a medical mission in Africa, where he had been on leave of absence twice before. He was followed by Dr. Cyril D. Fullmer, who obtained his medical degree at Utah in 1944. He interned at Cook County Hospital, Chicago, and served in the U.S. Army Medical Corps before returning to Salt Lake City.

On July 1, 1949, Dr. Fullmer had begun residency training in pathology under Dr. McNeil. He trained for two years and transferred to Salt Lake General Hospital July 1, 1951, where he attended two additional years under Dr. Francis Gunn. The relationship of work ethic and philosophy between Dr. McNeil and Fullmer was such that Dr. Fullmer was invited to return to Holy Cross Hospital on July 1, 1953.

In 1953 an autopsy on a patient who succumbed to cervical carcinoma caused a major change in the direction of Dr. Fullmer's activities. He had known the patient while he was a pathology resident. She was young, with four children, and she had sought medical assistance at the first sign of trouble. She had received state-of-the-art irradiation therapy and the best medical care available at that time.

Dr. Fullmer took a three-week course in cytology under Dr. Lauren Ackerman at Barnes Hospital in St. Louis. He reviewed numerous Papanicolaou slides from patients with cervical carcinoma before, during, and after radiation therapy, correlating his interpretations with the available opinions and the patients' history and follow-up. He returned to Holy Cross to establish a cytological diagnostic facility, new to the area.

A wall of public and professional skepticism existed, but a small corps of physician-believers at Holy Cross and a few nonstaff converts became active supporters of efforts to detect early cervical cancer. Drs. George Hinckley and Irving Ershler deserve special recognition.

In 1954 an unsuspected carcinoma was detected by cytological screening of an asymptomatic woman. A "cone" biopsy confirmed the cytological diagnosis. The "Pap smear" rapidly became the technique for control of cervical cancer, the second most common cause of death for women due to malignancy.

Dr. Fullmer developed cytological procedures in 1953-54, returning to the laboratory at night to screen cases until help from a screening cytotechnician became available in 1956. He established an accredited School of Cytotechnology in 1957. Cervical-vaginal specimens were mailed to the laboratory from physicians in surrounding states as well as local practitioners.

In 1968 Dr. Fullmer presented a scientific paper entitled "Pulmonary Cytology, a Diagnostic Method for Occult Carcinoma," in which ten early cases of lung cancer were detected and later proven surgically by Dr. Max Parrish. Multiple grants were then awarded to Holy Cross Hospital for support of cytological projects, the largest relating to study of smokers and bronchogenic carcinoma.

In 1970 Dr. Fullmer reported on 688 proven cervical carcinomas; 402 had *in-situ* disease. He worked on three major research grants funded from national sources until 1974. At one time, twenty research employees formed the successful study team. Expansion and research in a private hospital peaked and receded when Dr. Fullmer chose to return to full-time responsibilities for general pathology in 1974, after Dr. McNeil's departure added to the workload.

In 1958 Dr. Bruce A. Lloyd joined the pathology staff. He had trained at LDS Hospital and had spent one year with the Armed Forces Institute of Pathology, studying neuropathology and radioactive isotope procedures in Washington, D.C. He developed the isotope laboratory on the ground floor in the east wing in 1962 and started with blood volume determinations and simple isotope procedures. Several other excellent pathologists served Holy Cross Hospital between 1963 and 1979 for one to five years, moving on to greater opportunities. Dr. Fullmer resigned from active service July 1, 1985. Presently the laboratory at Holy Cross Hospital is being directed by four eminently qualified and experienced general pathologists: Dr. Joel R. Green, since 1977; Dr. Dennis L. Lombardi, since August 1977; Dr. Fred A. Hottes, since June 1979; and Dr. Eric Stark, since July 1990.

St. Mark's Hospital

Before 1949, the laboratory at St. Mark's Hospital was under contract with Dr. Orin Ogilvie, owner of the Wasatch Laboratory. Many of the tests and the processing of surgical tissues were done outside the hospital, and Dr. Ogilvie spent very little time at St. Mark's. The staff opted to terminate his contract and to search for a full-time pathologist; a general surgeon, Dr. Garner Meads, was appointed temporary laboratory director.

In November of 1949 Dr. Shelley A. Swift was asked to become director of the laboratory. A graduate of the two-year University of Utah Medical School, Swift had completed his medical studies at the University of Pennsylvania in 1940. In 1949 he had just completed an internship and residency at Philadelphia General Hospital, interrupted by four and a half years in the Army during World War II.

At that time, the laboratory was on the top floor, adjacent to the surgical suite. Although this was quite convenient for doing frozen sections, it was very inconvenient for servicing the emergency room and outpatients.

The laboratory occupied a single narrow room about 15 by 40 feet, with rows of counters along each side and at the ends. In this area all tests were done manually, and the equipment consisted of several microscopes, an incubator, centrifuges, water baths, and colorimeters. Almost all reagents were prepared by hand. Needles and glass syringes were autoclaved and the needles sharpened manually. (The risk of contracting hepatitis from this source was not yet appreciated.) At the north end of the laboratory was a small kitchen used occasionally by the adjacent ward. Pathology acquired this space and converted it to a bacteriology lab.

A glassed-in porch to the south of the laboratory, large enough to hold four donor beds with some work space, was acquired for the Blood Bank. The EKG and basal metabolism machines were housed here, since beds were required to perform these tests. All blood used in the hospital was drawn in-house. Typing and cross-matching were still done in the crowded main laboratory. An adequate amount of blood was maintained through a policy of requiring a two-for-one replacement for the first pint of blood used for each patient. In addition, donations were encouraged by groups so that their members could build up credit for future use. Companies such as Kennecott Copper and American Smelting and Refining, as well as LDS wards, were regular donors. A roster of unusual blood types, as well as 0-negatives, was built up. Blood from these donors was purchased for $25 a pint when needed.

During this period the staff consisted of about twelve full-time technicians. Several part-time persons, mostly students trained on the job, took night calls. For the first several years a surgical resident from the University of Utah rotated through histology for a six-month period. This practice continued until an adequate program was set up at the University.

An associate pathologist, Dr. Peter Crane, was recruited and held that position for several years until he became the director of the new Cottonwood Hospital laboratory. Several other temporary associate pathologists followed.

As the demand for services grew over the next several years, newly developed automated equipment was purchased. The already cramped quarters became totally impossible, with no space for expansion. Plans for a new south wing were under way, however. Pathology was assigned about half of the south portion of the second floor, just over the new cafeteria. In 1952 it seemed very adequate, but before long, space was again at a premium.

St. Mark's location on the northern outskirts of the city made it rather inconvenient for building up a large outpatient volume. Over the years a relationship with small hospitals in the region was developed, and specimens were received for histology and chemistry from about twenty hospitals and from doctors' offices in Utah, Idaho, Wyoming, Arizona, and Nevada. In some departments these specimens accounted for about a third of the workload.

St. Mark's was never in the forefront in purchasing the newer and more expensive equipment. The Technicon Company was a leader in automated chemical analyzers, and its 12/30 model had been out for years before the hospital administration finally agreed to purchase one. It was placed in the new wing, and shortly thereafter a similar machine was picked up, used. After about six months of research and development, the old machine was altered to allow for twelve additional tests, providing the capability for 24-channel chemistry surveys years before they were available at other hospitals. These two machines ran almost continuously, handling a large volume of the chemistry workload until they were replaced by the newer 12/60 machines at about the time of the move to the new hospital in 1973.

Dr. Swift retired upon reaching the age of sixty-five in April of 1982. Drs. John Croft and James Hathaway covered until St. Mark's contracted with the Department of Pathology at the University of Utah later that year. Dr. William Cathey and others filled in until Drs. Thomas Abbott in 1982 and David Head, from 1983 to 1988, committed most of their time at St. Mark's. Other temporary staff included Drs. Roger Arhelge, Ronald Weiss, Ed Egorshin, and James Avent — all of whom moved on to other positions or returned full-time to the University. Dr. Abbott became full-time chief in 1988, coincident with the sale of St. Mark's to the Hospital Corporation of America in January 1988, and Drs. David Knight and John M. Andrews are now also on full-time duty. The stable situation has improved the quality of work and the confidence of the staff. Residents in pathology also rotate through the service at St. Mark's.

The constantly increasing quality and sophistication of tissue pathology and laboratory procedures in the private hospitals have contributed greatly to the high standard of medicine practiced in the community. The history of the Department of Pathology at the University of Utah is covered in Part I of this volume, the history of the four-year Medical School.

CHAPTER FORTY-ONE

Physical Medicine and Rehabilitation

JAMES R. SWENSON, MD

PHYSICAL MEDICINE AND REHABILITATION (PM&R), one of the newest specialties, combines two distinct practice areas: physical medicine, the use of modalities, exercise, and other therapeutic techniques to treat various musculoskeletal problems; and rehabilitation, the comprehensive treatment of severe disability to lessen the patient's physical, psychological, social, and vocational impairments.

The roots of physical medicine have been traced to the ancients: The beneficial effects of heliotherapy and hydrotherapy have been understood since the time of the ancient Greek and Roman empires. In the eighteenth and nineteenth centuries, applications of electrical current were prescribed as a therapeutic modality. In France in 1890, D'Arsonval used high-frequency currents from a spark gap diathermy machine for both medical and surgical treatment.

During World War I, diathermy, electrical stimulation, heat, massage, and exercise were used increasingly as therapeutic tools in the United States. Physical and occupational therapy were utilized extensively in Army hospitals, and after the war Dr. John Coulter, an Army Medical Corps physician, continued to promote their medical use.

The modern-day concept of rehabilitation to assist in the recovery of injured and disabled military personnel was developed during World War II. Physical medicine and rehabilitation evolved as a specialty after the war because large numbers of physically disabled civilians needed restorative medical services. Dr. Howard Rusk, the

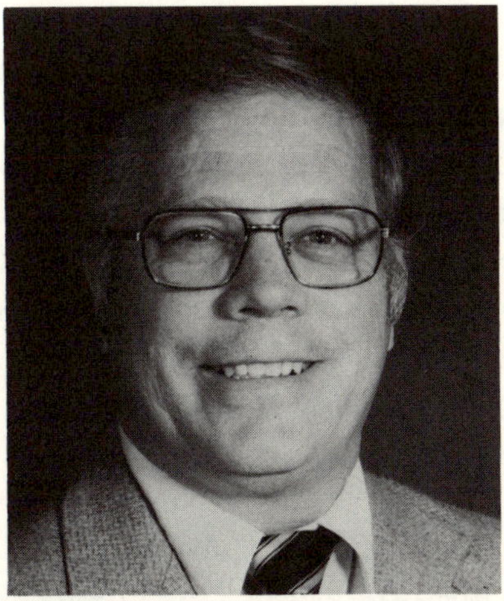

James R. Swenson.

father of rehabilitation medicine, established the first rehabilitation center at Bellevue Hospital in New York City in 1966.

In 1933 the American Physical Therapy Association was established. The American Academy of Physical Medicine and Rehabilitation had its official origin in 1938. Since 1947 Academy membership has been limited to physicians certified as diplomates of the American Board of Physical Medicine and Rehabilitation. The Board was founded in 1947 by Drs. Frank Krusen, John Coulter, and Walter Zeiter. The first exams were held that year, and ninety-one diplomates were certified. In June 1949 the body became the American Board of Physical Medicine and Rehabilitation, and from 1947 to 1990 a total of 3,454 diplomates have been certified.

University of Utah Rehabilitation Center

Chester Swinyard, MD, PhD, became interested in physical medicine and rehabilitation, so he divided his time between teaching neuroanatomy at the University of Utah School of Medicine and taking his own PM&R residency with Dr. Rusk at the Institute of Rehabilitation Medicine in New York City between 1951 and 1952. Swinyard developed a physical medicine and rehabilitation program at the Salt Lake General Hospital in 1952 and the Alcoholism Clinic at the University of Utah in 1953. In 1952, with the help of Clinton Vernon, the Attorney General, Reed Bullen, a legislator, and Louise Lake, a polio-paraplegic social worker, Dr. Swinyard made a very impressive presentation to the Utah State Legislature that resulted in the funding of the University of Utah Rehabilitation Center as part of the new University Medical Center, which opened in 1965. Dr. Swinyard left Utah in 1958 to join the faculty at New York University Institute of Rehabilitation Medicine.

Dr. Parley Madsen was an early Utah practitioner of PM&R. After residency training at New York University and the University of Colorado, he established a private practice in Salt Lake City from 1962 to 1965 and provided some patient care at the Weber County Convalescent Center in Roy, Utah. He describes those early years as a difficult time for him, as the community was just not ready for the rehabilitation specialty. He left the state to practice within the VA hospital system in Kansas and later in California.

Dr. James R. Swenson, a graduate of the University of Utah School of Medicine, completed a PM&R residency at New York University under the guidance of Drs. Rusk and Swinyard in July of 1965. He joined the University of Utah School of Medicine as the first chair of the Division of Physical Medicine and Rehabilitation, an autonomous division responsible to the dean.

In 1965 Swenson established a student training program and, in 1968, a residency program. When the new Medical Center was opened in 1965, only outpatient and consultative rehabilitation services were provided. An 8-bed dedicated inpatient center opened on January 1, 1966. By January 1967, 20 beds were available, and the unit was later expanded to 32 beds. This comprehensive rehabilitation program has provided local, state, and regional services for the past 25 years.

Dr. Howard Seeley joined the faculty from August 1968 to March 1970. He had received his PM&R residency training at the Long Beach VA Hospital and left the state to continue practicing in the VA hospital system.

Dr. Pedro Escobar completed his PM&R residency training at the University of Utah in 1972 and continued as a faculty member until 1984. He provided significant strength in teaching and patient care during those critical growth years. In 1984 he became chair at the University of Arizona.

Dr. Charles Sprague completed his PM&R residency at Utah in 1980 and served as a faculty member for one year before entering private practice in California.

After completing her residency at Utah in 1983, Dr. Jayne Clark was a member of the faculty until 1987, when she moved her practice to the Institute for Low Back Care in Salt Lake City. In 1989 Dr. Clark was appointed director of rehabilitation medicine of the Family Health Plan (FHP), a Utah health maintenance organization. She cares for a wide variety of outpatient musculoskeletal problems, performs electromyography, and supervises inpatients from the FHP program at the Holy Cross Rehabilitation Center.

Dr. Brian Buck completed a residency at the University of Utah in 1986 and was a faculty member until 1988. His interests included pediatric and neurologic rehabilitation and electromyography.

Dr. Judith L. Gooch completed her residency at the University of Michigan and joined the University of Utah in July 1986. She has been interested in amputee rehabilitation, sports medicine, electromyography, and pediatric rehabilitation. She currently provides pediatric rehabilitation services with Dr. Frances Tait, a pediatric neurologist, at the new Primary Children's Medical Center.

Dr. Janet Balbierz completed her PM&R residency at Sinai Hospital of Detroit in 1987, and after practicing there joined the faculty at the University of Utah in November 1988. She has been active teaching and consulting at the University Hospital, caring for inpatients with severe physical disabilities.

Dr. John Speed completed a PM&R residency at the University of Minnesota in 1987 and was appointed to the faculty there, doing clinical work in chronic pain rehabilitation through 1988. In January 1989 he joined the faculty of the University of Utah and is currently working in inpatient and chronic pain rehabilitation.

Since 1965 the University has had a teaching grant in PM&R from the federal government to assist in teaching 100 medical students each year. The grant has also supported two residents since 1975. The three-year program was established in 1966 and had grown to eight residents in 1990. Twenty-five physicians completed their training in physical medicine from 1968 to 1990. Since 1965 the faculty also has been teaching rehabilitation medicine to students of physical therapy, occupational therapy, speech therapy, social work, psychology, recreational therapy, rehabilitation nursing, and rehabilitation engineering and has been active in a wide variety of clinical research projects.

Salt Lake Veterans Administration Hospital

The first local physiatrist, Dr. Harold Rosenberg, took his residency in internal medicine at the University of Utah and received special training at the Universities of Colorado and Texas. He was employed by the Salt Lake Veterans Administration Hospital in PM&R in 1947. By virtue of his training in internal medicine, short-term training courses, and experience, he received Board certification number 237 in 1953. In 1952 he had moved to the new VA Hospital near the University as chief of the Department of Physical Medicine and Rehabilitation and begun to develop a comprehensive therapy program for both inpatient and outpatient veterans in the Intermountain area, although no Medical School teaching or inpatient rehabilitation bed service existed there during these years. Dr. Rosenberg practiced at the VA Hospital until his retirement in 1972. Dr. James Swenson was acting chief until 1975, when Dr. Ron Duerksen became chief.

Dr. Duerksen completed his residency training at the Portland Veterans Hospital in 1975. In 1981 he developed an inpatient service using eight beds loaned by the Department of Neurology. After working at the Salt Lake VA Hospital and Holy Cross, as well as three years (1985–88) at the Stewart Rehabilitation Center in Ogden, he opened an office in Provo and performs electromyography in Salt Lake City, Bountiful, Provo, Payson, St. George, Cedar City, and Price.

In 1981 Dr. Julian Ballesteros became director of rehabilitation medicine for one year. He completed PM&R residency training at the

University in 1977 and had four years' experience in the VA system. Dr. Robert Baer was chief from 1982 to 1985 and from 1988 to the present. He has had a special interest in electromyography and chronic pain rehabilitation, including the use of hypnosis and acupuncture as well as more standard Western therapeutic modalities. A 10-bed dedicated rehabilitation service was later expanded to 16 beds. Residents have been rotating through the VA Hospital since 1982 and have provided inpatient, outpatient, and outreach consultation services.

Dr. Jane Squires completed her PM&R residency at the Santa Clara Valley Medical Center in 1982 and a one-year fellowship in spinal cord injury at the Palo Alto VA Hospital. She joined the medical staff at the Salt Lake VA Hospital and the University of Utah from 1983 until 1985, when she became chief until October 1988. She then became associate medical director at the Western Rehabilitation Institute and program medical director in spinal cord injury.

In 1988 Dr. David Peifer joined the staff of the VA Medical Center. He completed a PM&R residency at the University of Utah in 1985 and then spent three years as director of the Brain Injury Unit of the Montebello Rehabilitation Hospital in Baltimore.

Private Rehabilitation Centers

In 1966 a third comprehensive rehabilitation center with six beds was established at Holy Cross Hospital by Dr. Wayman Spence, who continued as medical director until 1970, when he left the state to practice in Texas.

He was replaced as director by Dr. Robert Baer (1970–82 and 1985–88), who had been a resident at Ohio State University between 1960 and 1963 and then served on the faculty at the University of Missouri from 1963 to 1970. At Holy Cross Dr. Baer was joined by Dr. Dale Ream, trained at Stanford, who practiced from 1970 to his untimely death in 1980. In 1976 Drs. Ream and Baer expanded the Holy Cross Rehabilitation service to twelve beds. When Dr. Baer left in 1980, Dr. Richard Goka became medical director.

In 1986 the Holy Cross center was remodeled, expanded, and named the Quinney Rehabilitation Center. Dr. Max Root joined the staff from 1986 to 1988 and later worked at the LDS Hospital for a brief period before moving to Utah Valley Rehabilitation Center. In 1988 Dr. Goka left Holy Cross to practice in California. In 1989 Dr. Walter F. Haemmerle, a graduate of the Louisiana State Medical School PM&R residency, was appointed medical director. He was joined by Dr. J. Benjamin Griffin, who completed his residency at Utah in 1989. Drs. John Bender and Mark McGlothlin joined the Holy Cross medical staff in 1990 with an interest in outpatient and industrial rehabilitation therapy programs.

The fourth comprehensive rehabilitation center was established in 1974 at McKay-Dee Hospital under the direction of Dr. John M. Bender to serve patients from Ogden and the northern counties of Utah. As in the other comprehensive centers, a rehabilitation team of physical therapists, occupational therapists, speech pathologists, nurses, a social worker, recreational therapist, and psychologist was established. Within three years the unit was expanded to twenty beds, and Dr. Roger Davis, who received his PM&R residency training at the University of Utah, joined the medical staff.

In 1979 an annex to McKay-Dee was designated the Stewart Rehabilitation Center. When Dr. Davis left the community, Drs. Patrick Radecki and Robert Kukla, both of whom were trained in PM&R at Ohio State University, joined the medical staff, as did a rheumatologist, Dr. Jeffrey Booth. Dr. Milton Thomas completed a PM&R residency at Ohio State University and joined the practice in 1985, replacing Dr. Bender as medical director of the center in 1988. Stewart Rehabilitation Center has been active in the prevention of traumatic disabilities and created a multi-media production called *A Fine Line*.

Western Rehabilitation Institute, an eighty-bed free-standing, for-profit rehabilitation hospital in Sandy, Utah, became operational in March 1988 as the fifth comprehensive center, with Dr. John M. Bender as medical director. In 1990 the medical staff consists of Drs. Jane Squires, Warren Stadler, Richard Jackson, Michael Munhall, Richard Radecki, G. Lynn Rasmussen, and Sarah Jane Rasmussen.

Utah Valley Hospital established a comprehensive five-bed rehabilitation center in the acute hospital in 1988. Dr. Max Root, the center's first medical director, developed both inpatient and outpatient services. A new eighteen-bed unit opened in January of 1989.

LDS Hospital started to develop a comprehensive rehabilitation program in June of 1989. Dr. David K. Ryser headed the new nineteen-bed rehabilitation unit, opened in late December 1989.

Utah Society of PM&R

The Utah Society of Physical Medicine and Rehabilitation was organized on September 12, 1987. The founding members included Drs. Robert Baer, John M. Bender, Roger W. Davis, Pedro L. Escobar, Dale Ream, and James R. Swenson, with Dr. Bender serving as the first president. Dr. Janet Balbierz was elected president for 1990. The Society brings together on at least a quarterly basis all physician specialists in physical medicine and rehabilitation to discuss problems of mutual interest.

The amount of money spent for rehabilitation patients in Utah doubled from 1988 to 1989 because of the greater number of physicians and rehabilitation beds available. Many medical patients are now receiving skilled rehabilitation services in order to become more productive in society. The Utah State Medicaid program was not prepared for the financial demands involved, and a crisis has developed. A considerable conflict has arisen between the Medicaid payment program and the practitioners and the rehabilitation centers they represent. Instead of limiting services, a large number of services have been denied as a budget-saving maneuver. An ad hoc committee of physicians from the major rehabilitation centers and officials in the state Medicaid financial reimbursement section are trying to solve these difficulties to provide needed services for disabled Medicaid patients.

The Future

The future for the practice of physical medicine and rehabilitation in Utah remains bright. Many changes in practice locations, funding levels, and treatment procedures have occurred and will continue to occur. Over the past two years, rapid expansion of rehabilitation programs and the number of hospital beds has resulted in strong competition among the many rehabilitation centers. If the physiatrists of Utah will keep their focus on providing high-quality rehabilitation care for those in need and remain advocates for their disabled patients, this current period of competition and conflict will pass.

CHAPTER FORTY-TWO

Radiology

HENRY P. PLENK, MD, MS

THE FIRST X-RAY MACHINES made their appearance in Utah in several physicians' offices as early as 1902. The first hospital to require a unit was St. Mark's in 1907, with Dr. Warren Benjamin in charge of the department until 1919. At that time he was replaced by Dr. James P. Kerby, who was the state's first qualified radiologist, later to become a member of the American Board of Radiology. Kerby took over the Department of Radiology at Holy Cross Hospital, as well as St. Mark's, and added the Veterans Administration Hospital, the Veterans Outpatient Clinic, the Shriners' Unit, and the Utah State Hospital in Provo, continuing, nevertheless, to give most of his attention to his office in the Boston Building (343 South State Street).

By 1945 Dr. Kerby had developed squamous cell carcinoma of the ring finger from excessive radiation exposure due to fluoroscopy procedures and particularly the handling of radium sources without adequate protection. Hence Dr. Angus Wilson joined him from 1945 to 1952, later limiting his own activities to office practice until 1971.

Dr. Henry P. Plenk left the University to assume full-time responsibility for the Department of Radiology at St. Mark's Hospital in 1952. Dr. Kerby succumbed to his disease shortly thereafter.

Holy Cross Hospital

After Dr. Kerby had covered Holy Cross Hospital on a part-time basis from 1919 until 1948, Dr. Ralph R. Meyer became the first full-time radiologist, arriving in September of 1948 after completing a three-year residency in radiology at the University of Chicago followed by a year there as instructor. Dr. Meyer took an active part in medical student and resident teaching at the Salt Lake General Hospital (SLGH), as well as accepting junior students for externships in radiology. Meyer pioneered cerebral angiograms with Dr. Chester Powell. He established a residency program in radiology at Holy Cross Hospital in 1951 which he discontinued in favor of the other local programs in 1966.

Dr. Gerald Stevenson, who completed his residency at LDS Hospital, joined Dr. Meyer in 1957. Dr. Don Gowens, a resident at Holy Cross, joined the staff in 1962.

The department moved into well-designed quarters in a new wing in 1968. Dr. Robert Mitchell, a long-time University staff member, joined the group in 1970. Dr. Meyer resigned in 1978. The seventies saw the beginning of the development of special procedures requiring a new generation of radiologists who had training in ultrasound, interventional radiography, angioplasty, lithotripsy, etc. These procedures are largely carried out by Drs. Neel Bennett, George Baldwin, and Robert Brinton. A new CT scanner was installed in 1977.

Holy Cross pioneered in the use of mammography and has established a Breast Care Center in adjoining Moreau Hall. The Center also services a mobile mammography unit which travels far into outlying districts. Dr. Stevenson was the main force in developing mammography at Holy Cross, and Dr. Gowens has been chair of the group for many years.

LDS Hospital

The first x-ray unit at LDS Hospital was installed shortly after the arrival of Louis A. Thody, a British-trained electrician and recent convert to the LDS Church. The x-ray apparatus and the processing of films became his responsibility as well. He played a major role in upgrading the procedures, improving the quality of films, and for many years was also the only expert in the interpretation of radiographs. He took time off to visit prominent radiologists of the day at

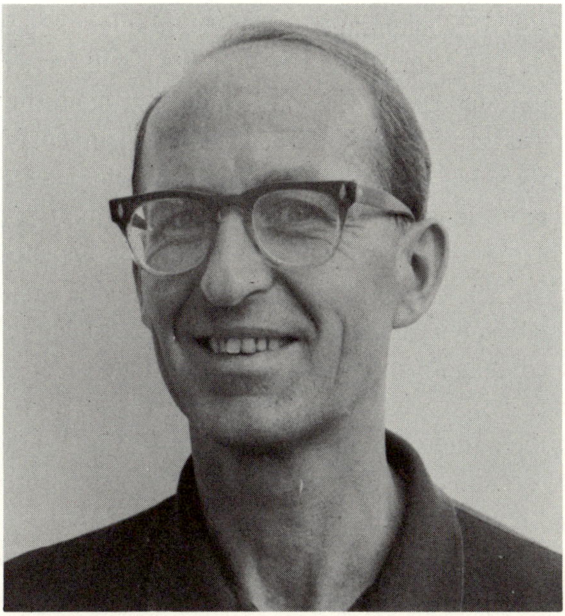

Henry P. Plenk.

the Mayo Clinic and in Philadelphia to increase his proficiency in interpretation. The demand for a physician trained in the field was satisfied by Dr. Q. B. Coray's return to Utah after he completed a residency in radiology at Washington University in St. Louis in 1926. Thody and Coray joined forces, and their firm continued to serve LDS Hospital on a part-time basis with an office in the Medical Arts Building. Mr. Thody was made an honorary member of the Utah State Medical Association in 1920; he retired in 1946.

Dr. Coray continued to serve as part-time radiologist at LDS until the arrival of Dr. Earl R. Crowder in 1948, who was recommended for the position by his friend Dean Richard Young of the University of Utah Medical School. Dr. Crowder was Dr. Plenk's mentor at Northwestern, where he had occupied the chair of the radiology department of Evanston Hospital since 1934.

When Crowder arrived in Salt Lake City on December 1, 1947, he found the x-ray department in deplorable condition. It consisted of two rooms — one containing a combined radiographic fluoroscopic unit, the other a combination office, file room, and x-ray reading area — and a small darkroom. An additional room housed a urographic unit which was unsafe for use and had to be condemned. For a 350-bed hospital, only about twelve to fifteen examinations were performed daily, and more myelograms and encephalograms were done than GI-series or barium enemas. The volume was low because many ambulatory patients were sent to clinics or private radiologists' offices, a practice widespread in all of the hospitals with part-time radiologic coverage. Crowder was able to double the x-ray department's space while waiting to build an excellent new department occupying the entire eighth floor of the new West Wing. When this space was occupied on January 1, 1950, it represented the most modern and luxurious department in the state of Utah.

Dr. Crowder established a radiology residency beginning with Dr. Phillip R. Frederick, a Northwestern graduate and intern at Evanston Hospital from 1947 to 1948. Crowder participated in the University's teaching program during the first year and held some physics seminars in the basement of his home. Frederick became the first additional staff member in the department after he returned from military service in the Korean War in 1953. Both doctors took courses at Oakridge Institute of Nuclear Studies in Tennessee to qualify for a radioactive isotope license from the Atomic Energy Commission. They opened the first nuclear medicine section of any department of radiology in the state.

The next resident, Dr. Jack Davis, became the first full-time radiologist at the Salt Lake Clinic in 1956. From 1948 to 1974, thirteen residents had all or part of their training in the program. Three graduates joined the department at LDS: Dr. J. Gordon Russell in 1957; Dr. Woodrow Copeland in 1961; and Dr. C. Richard Nixon in 1966.

Crowder, and particularly Frederick, were very innovative and inventive and did much pioneering work in nuclear medicine, cooperating with General Electric to promote improvements in the equipment. With the members of the Rumel Clinic, they pioneered angiocardiography. During 1965 and 1966 much of their time was absorbed by planning a new department to occupy the first three floors of another new wing. The availability of supervoltage equipment encouraged them to plan the first floor for the developing area of radiation oncology, the second floor for nuclear medicine and special procedures, and the third floor for a diagnostic department. The new facilities were ready for the diagnostic department in December 1968, and the Radiation Center was occupied on March 31, 1969.

The reading room of the x-ray department became a gathering place for house staff, and a great deal of informal teaching took place over a full coffee pot — the only coffee pot in the hospital. Crowder exerted a great deal of influence on the first post-war administrator, Clarence Wonnacott, who established the principle of excellence of service as a guide for expenditures.

Dr. Crowder retired on July 1, 1968, after suffering from a variety of physical ailments eventually requiring surgery with a very stormy postoperative course. He died of a stroke on September 14, 1970, at the age of seventy-one. A brief paragraph from Dr. Frederick's obituary for Dr. Crowder, published in *Radiology*, summarizes his life well:

> He will be long remembered especially for his gift of teaching. No matter how busy, he always made himself available to his students. Nothing brought him more satisfaction than watching his residents progress as they gained facility in study and learning through the radiology seminar program and the many informal teaching sessions that he held. A perennial student himself, Dr. Crowder had an excellent grasp of radiation physics and an unusual facility for explaining his concepts, thus making the subject an exciting adventure for his many students. His enthusiasm for learning never decreased during his retirement; he began to study biochemistry and did some informal tutoring in mathematics for his younger friends.

Dr. Phil Frederick was appointed head of the department and has provided outstanding leadership. The danger of in-breeding of the staff was recognized, and three additional radiologists were appointed between 1969 and 1971, none staying very long. Newer subspecialties such as neuroradiology, chest, nuclear medicine, ultrasound, CT, and magnetic resonance scanning revolutionized the whole field. An early-model CT scanner was installed in June 1976 and a second much better and faster GE 8800 in 1982; a second GE scanner was added in June 1983 and a magnetic resonance unit in May 1986. In 1976 Dr. Frederick began limiting himself to nuclear medicine and CT scanning and developed amazing competence in an entirely new field.

In July 1977 two outstanding new members with extensive experience in neuroradiology, angiography, and interventional procedures were recruited. Dr. A. Lee Bahr finished a fellowship in neuroradiology at Johns Hopkins from 1974 to 1976 and held a staff position as assistant professor from 1976 to 1977. Dr. Mark H. Miller followed Dr. Bahr by a few weeks. He had spent eight months in Lund, Sweden, for special training in angiography and invasive procedures and had served two years as neuroradiologist at M. D. Anderson and Hermann hospitals in Houston. Bahr and Miller introduced many invasive procedures that became an important part of the total volume of work, including percutaneous abscess drainage, percutaneous biliary drainage, assistance with percutaneous renal stone extraction, transarterial tumor embolization of the kidney or liver, and infusion or therapeutic embolization for hemorrhage control. With the development of LDS as a major trauma center, the frequency of emergencies — many of those at night relating to neurologic and vascular diagnoses as well as to CT scanning — produced a profound change in the practice of radiology.

William James Morrison joined the staff in July 1978 after a residency in diagnostic radiology at Johns Hopkins from 1972 to 1975, including neuroradiology, angiography, and CT scanning, followed by another year on the staff as an instructor. In the Army he became chief of diagnostic roentgenology at Fitzsimmons General Hospital in Denver. He has concentrated on general diagnostic radiology with some interest in ultrasound, nuclear medicine, and mammography.

Dr. Irena Tocino — a native of Spain, where she graduated from medical school in 1975 — completed her residency in radiology at Cincinnati General Hospital. She became a staff member at the University of Utah, concentrating on pulmonary radiology, and was appointed chair of the pulmonary section. She switched to LDS Hospital in 1982 because of the strength of the pulmonary department and the intensive care unit. Her research interests have been in trauma of the chest, especially the occurrence of pneumothorax in the ICU, and more recently mammography. She was the driving force behind the Utah division of the American Cancer Society's campaign on early breast cancer detection and was responsible for the formation of the Utah Breast Cancer Task Force, of which she is the chair. Dr. Tocino has become a national and international authority on chest diseases and has made regular lecture tours, particularly in Spain.

Ultrasonography at LDS Hospital received a tremendous boost with the appointment of Dr. Timothy G. Lee in 1985. He had completed a residency in radiology at Northwestern University and a fellowship in 1972-73 at the University of Oregon, where he became interested in ultrasound. He joined the faculty there, and over the next four years pioneered in the field of ultrasonography, rising to the rank of associate professor. In 1978 he came to the University of Utah, where he was promoted to professor in 1981. Dr. Lee has received numerous honors and has contributed greatly to the literature and textbooks on ultrasonography.

Under Frederick's leadership, with the influx of highly qualified new blood in various subspecialties, increase in the number of scientific presentations, published papers, guest lectureships, and teaching seminars demonstrates the dramatic change to a productive academic department during the last ten years.

St. Mark's Hospital

Between 1952 and 1960, Dr. Plenk operated in a very inadequate facility of two diagnostic examining rooms and a therapy room containing an orthovoltage unit. Dr. Richard Y. Card joined the staff on January 1, 1957, after one year of fellowship in nuclear medicine and radiation therapy at the University of Pennsylvania in Philadelphia and Memorial Hospital in New York City, where he gained experience in interstitial therapy with iridium seeds and intracavitary injection of radioactive isotopes. The move into a new department in

February 1960, with diagnosis on the ground floor and nuclear medicine and therapy on the lower floor, was an important milestone. The new CO^{60} machine, the first supervoltage unit between Denver and the Pacific Coast, inaugurated the era of supervoltage radiation in the Intermountain area.

Between 1961 and 1962, Dr. John Caffey, former Utahn and recently retired professor of pediatrics and radiology at Columbia University, New York City (author of *the* textbook on pediatric radiology), joined the staff on a one-third basis, spending his remaining time at Primary Children's and Salt Lake General hospitals. The next staff member to join was Dr. R. Newell Ford, after three years of radiology residency and two years on staff with Dr. Ben Felsen at the University of Cincinnati. Ford brought experience in cardiovascular procedures and took over lymphangiograms. Dr. Ken Orton trained and was on the radiology staff at Stanford for two years, in charge of angiography, special studies, and invasive procedures. His arrival in 1968 expanded the skills of the group greatly. Unfortunately Orton died suddenly of a heart attack in 1981, at the age of forty-eight.

After Ford's arrival in 1963, Dr. Plenk limited himself to radiation therapy, assisted by Card, who was also in charge of nuclear medicine. In February 1964 the second hyperbaric chamber in the United States was installed at St. Mark's. The use of oxygen under three atmospheres of pressure is based on the radiobiologists' observation that the sensitivity of tumor cells increased greatly with increased oxygen tension.

In 1968 Brent Goates, administrator of LDS Hospital, approached Dr. Plenk about the possibility of his taking over a new therapy facility then under construction, including a linear accelerator. After much discussion, the radiologists, administrators, and boards of St. Mark's and Holy Cross hospitals decided that it would be best for the community to develop a single strong radiation therapy center. The move to LDS took place on March 31, 1969, and included some equipment and all personnel and patient records.

St. Mark's moved into a brand-new, well-designed facility on Thirty-ninth South and Thirteenth East with an excellent physical plant for the radiology department. New staff members with the following expertise were: Drs. Richard Flynn, 1973, pediatrics and angiography; Larry Stevens, 1976, ultrasound; Dennis Y. Utani, 1980, neuroradiology and CT scanning; Ed Mineau, 1982, angiography and interventional radiography; George Boren, 1982–83, ultrasound and body CT; followed by Robert Bell, 1985; and Paul Weiss and Ron Ruff, 1986. Dr. Card retired in July 1984.

Primary Children's Medical Center

Utah's first active pediatric hospital started with the completion of a new building on Twelfth Avenue in 1952. The staff were all part-time practicing physicians with other hospital affiliations. Radiology was covered largely by the University staff.

In 1961–62 Dr. John Caffey spent one-third of his time as the first pediatric radiologist, trying to upgrade the service. Upon Caffey's return to Denver in August 1962, Dr. Virgil R. Condon became the first full-time pediatric radiologist after residency at the University–SLGH–VA Hospital and a year at Denver Children's Hospital under Drs. Allen and Caffey, followed by a year in radiation therapy at Ellis Fischel Hospital at the University of Missouri. Condon found a very inadequate physical plant performing only five to ten examinations per day. During the ensuing years many full-time specialists were attracted to the staff in pathology, surgery, pediatrics, neurology, cardiology, psychiatry, and later pediatric oncology, neurosurgery, and related subspecialties.

A new wing in 1970 provided a modern department occupying the entire third floor. In 1987 five radiologists were supervising more than 32,000 examinations a year compared with 2,000 in 1962. Additional staff members were Drs. William Nixon (1970), Richard Jaffey (1978), Barbara Reid (1983), and Richard Boyer (1986), each bringing special skills and interests. Milestones were the installation of a biplane cardiac catheterization lab, CT scanner, and ultrasound and participation in the Intermountain Health Corporation (IHC) magnetic resonance (MR) unit located at LDS Hospital. The rapid advances in radiology improved pediatric radiology with some added features, such as removal of foreign bodies from the trachea or esophagus.

Dr. Condon is the recipient of numerous honors and awards and has held many distinguished offices in state and national organizations.

Primary Children's crowning glory was the move in April 1990 into a new, much larger free-standing facility — with an anticipated full capacity of 200 beds — next to the University of Utah Medical Center, which promises to be one of the outstanding pediatric facilities in the country to provide tertiary care for infants and children.

University of Utah–SLGH, 1946 to 1952

Radiology at the University during this period is discussed in Part I of this volume, "Early History of the Four-Year Medical School at the University of Utah, 1942–1952."

University of Utah, 1952 to 1970

Dr. William R. Christensen received his MD at Harvard in 1942, then did research in biochemistry and served a medical internship at Massachusetts General Hospital in Boston. While serving in the U.S. Army from 1943 to 1946, he was assigned to the Climatic Research Lab in Lawrence, Massachusetts. He completed a residency in radiology at Peter Bent Brigham Hospital, Boston, in 1951, followed by a Fulbright Scholarship at Royal Marsden Hospital, London, to do work in radiobiology as well as in clinical oncology. Christensen took over as professor and chief radiologist at the Salt Lake General Hospital (SLGH) July 1, 1952, with Dr. Ru Kan Lin as his only staff member until 1954. Several residents stayed for one to two years after completion of their training until Dr. Blaine Brown returned in 1957 from a year's training in radiation therapy at the University of Chicago. He was placed in charge of therapy and nuclear medicine until his early death in 1969. Two other University of Utah residents completed the staff: Dr. Carlisle Smith from 1957 to 1970, and Dr. Robert Mitchell from 1966 to 1970.

In July 1965 the SLGH ceased to exist, and all patients and activities were transferred to the University Hospital at the north end of Fort Douglas. The new radiology facility was a great improvement, but the design (with only limited input by Christensen) left much to be desired. Dr. Christensen's major accomplishment was the training of forty-six residents who, upon graduation, staffed many hospitals of the Intermountain region and beyond. While he was not successful in attracting outside staff or grants to develop significant research projects on his own, cooperation with the radiobiology laboratory (Department of Anatomy) resulted in a number of publications. Blaine Brown's death precipitated a crisis of manpower and recruiting. Unable to obtain support from the dean, Christensen resigned in 1969, effective July 1, 1970, together with Drs. Smith, Mitchell, and Stowell.

The VA Hospital on Twelfth Avenue came under the direction of the Dean's Committee of the Medical School in 1946. The first full-time radiologist was Dr. Robert Crowder, 1949–52, followed by Paul Christensen, then Justin Wolfson, until William Stowell took over in 1957 and moved to the new VA Hospital on Fort Douglas when the two facilities were combined in 1962, and the VA became a general rather than a psychiatric and TB hospital. Stowell was the first to develop skills in catheterization techniques, which he taught to the residents. Christensen and Stowell resigned from the University in 1969 and became the radiologists for Valley West Hospital in 1970.

The year after Christensen's resignation was very difficult for everyone. Various radiologists were called upon to help out on a part-time or full-time basis. Dr. Ross Phillips from St. Benedict's Hospital in Ogden covered therapy almost full time after Dr. Brown's death. Earl Crowder, who recently had resigned his position at LDS, helped to read Medicare films in diagnosis and supervise residents. Drs. Mike Edson and Dale Bass stayed on as junior faculty after completing their residencies.

University of Utah, 1970 to Present

A search committee recommended Dr. David G. Bragg. Bragg was born in Oregon in 1933; he took his AB at Stanford in 1955 and his MD at the University of Oregon in 1959. After two years in the Army, he took a residency in radiology at Columbia Presbyterian

Hospital in New York City, 1962–65, and stayed on staff for one year, 1966–67. In 1967 he became chair of diagnosis at Sloan-Kettering-Memorial Hospital in New York City.

Bragg accepted the appointment as chair in April 1970, effective July 1; but neither he nor his two recruits, Drs. Ruben Koehler and David O. Davis from the staff of Mallinckrodt Institute of Radiology at Washington University in St. Louis, were available on a full-time basis until the end of August or mid-September. Bragg, Koehler, and Davis rotated coverage throughout the summer, two days at a time, commuting from New York and St. Louis, respectively. In mid–September Dr. Winston Mitchell, former staff radiologist at McKay-Dee Hospital in Ogden, who had spent time in Lund, Sweden, and at the University of California at San Francisco learning angiographic techniques, also joined the group.

During the decade from 1970 to 1980, the full-time radiology faculty at the University grew from four to fifteen, including four with the rank of full professor. The residency program was completely reorganized and increased to four slots per year, eventually increasing to four years in length. It is now one of the most sought-after programs in the United States.

In 1974 a diagnostic research pavilion was constructed, headed by Dr. James Nelson, who received an NIH Career Development award. Development of the Intermountain Radiopharmacy, installation of the first magnetic resonance unit (MR) in 1975, and of ultrasound imaging with the arrival of Dr. Tim Lee in 1977 added great sophistication. Total amounts of research grants grew from zero prior to 1970 to $2.7 million in 1980.

With the move into the new 450-bed University Hospital in September 1981, the physical plant was greatly enlarged and fully equipped with up-to-date machines, where required. Ingenious cooperation with several manufacturers enabled the staff to obtain equipment for reduced cost in return for their development and research contributions. Other firsts were the addition of an interventional neuroradiologist and interventional procedures such as lithotripsy, laser angioplasty, and a vascular ultrasound laboratory.

In 1983 the department was organized into three divisions: neuroradiology under Dr. Anne Osborne, abdominal imaging under Dr. Franklin J. Miller, and musculoskeletal-breast with Dr. B. J. Manaster as director. A new medical imaging research laboratory (MIRL) under the direction of Robert Kruger, PhD, was created in 1986. This section alone already boasts 153 publications. The scientific output of the entire department is most impressive, with about 200 publications a year, numerous books, and editorships of several yearbooks.

Many members of the faculty, but especially Dr. Bragg, have assumed positions of prominence in the National Institutes of Health as well as in major societies, both national and international. The department is one of the University's newly selected centers of research excellence. Of a total operating budget of $13 million, institutional support provides less than 2%; research grants in force have averaged $12 million since the 1980s.

The quality of radiologic practice in most hospitals of the Wasatch Front has improved greatly over the last twenty years, due largely to the recent recruitment of better-trained radiologists, many of whom have had additional years of faculty experience, especially at the University of Utah.

Two hospitals deserve particular mention for their pioneering efforts. Dr. Russell Nichols remained on the faculty of the University of Chicago from 1946 to 1951, after completing his residency. In 1951 he was recruited as the first full-time radiologist at the Dee (now McKay-Dee) Hospital in Ogden. He was joined by Dr. John Stucki in January 1955, but five months later Nichols accepted the position of professor and head of radiology at Jefferson Medical College in Philadelphia. After four years he returned to Ogden. He established a policy of mini-sabbaticals which allowed staff members to leave for one to four months to gain special skills not available in the department. Dr. Nichols and Dr. Mitchell, who joined in 1964, spent time in Lund, Sweden, to gain competence in cardiovascular procedures. Dr. Thorsten Lofgren from Sweden came on staff from 1966 to 1969.

Dr. Bruce McIff's arrival on January 15, 1973, at Utah Valley Hospital changed the character of the Department of Radiology there and the range of procedures utilized. A University of Utah graduate in medicine in 1968, McIff trained at Long Beach VA Hospital, the University of Southern California, and Children's Hospital in Los Angeles and brought state-of-the-art angiography and special procedures to the area. He also became very influential in hospital and IHC politics and was president of the Utah Medical Association in 1985–86. The state of Utah can be proud of the quality of radiology practiced throughout the area.

CHAPTER FORTY-THREE

Radiation Oncology

HENRY P. PLENK, MD, MS

WILLIAM KONRAD ROENTGEN, A GERMAN physicist, announced the discovery of "a new kind of ray" called x-ray on December 5, 1895. One month later a physician in Chicago applied these rays in the treatment of a patient with advanced breast cancer — undoubtedly the most rapid application of a scientific discovery to practical therapeutic use! As the field developed, radiologists were trained in this country first by the Army toward the end of World War I, and a specialty board was established in 1934. Most radiologists in the United States trained in and practiced both diagnostic and therapeutic radiology until the development of supervoltage machines (in excess of 1 M volts) in the fifties and early sixties. Because of the cost of the equipment and of the massive concrete walls required for protection against the high-energy rays, radiation therapy (later called radiation oncology) developed into a separate discipline.

In most European countries, under centralized systems of medical care delivery, therapy facilities were concentrated in selected university hospitals, and a number of centers stood in high regard for their facilities and for the professional skills and great volume of experience of their staffs. Stockholm, Paris, London, and Manchester had the most prominent schools. The few therapists in the U.S. prior to World War II all had their training abroad.

In Utah in 1947 most of the six practicing radiologists (four in Salt Lake City and two in Ogden), as well as most hospitals, treated patients with orthovoltage (100-400 KV) equipment, providing only a minimal number of patients per day for each facility.

Tumor Institute, St. Mark's Hospital, and Radiation Center, LDS Hospital

The installation of a 2,000 Curie CO^{60} unit (equivalent to 2 MeV photon beam) at St. Mark's Hospital in February 1960 and the creation of the Tumor Institute signaled the start of the modern era of radiation therapy. Efforts to recruit a certified radiation therapist were totally unsuccessful, since even in 1958 only fifty-four doctors in the U.S. limited their practice to therapy — a requirement for membership in the American Club of Therapeutic Radiologists.

Having an interest in therapy, Dr. Henry Plenk, head of the Department of Radiology, decided to learn what he could in several weeks' visit to three major supervoltage centers: Glockner-Penrose Cancer Hospital in Colorado Springs, Colorado (with Dr. Juan del Regato), Stanford University in Palo Alto, California (with Dr. Henry S. Kaplan), and M. D. Anderson Hospital in Houston, Texas (with Dr. Gilbert H. Fletcher). From the experience he gained, together with Dr. Richard Y. Card's exposure at Memorial Hospital in New York City, new techniques were established for use with supervoltage. Patient referral from the entire Intermountain area increased gradually to 428 patients per year in 1968, in spite of the installation of a comparable unit at the new University Hospital in 1965.

From January 1963 Dr. Plenk confined his activities to radiation therapy. Dr. Card spent almost half time on therapy and nuclear medicine after the arrival of Dr. Newell Ford, who limited himself to diagnosis.

Pioneering work in England, Australia, and Seattle, Washington, demonstrated the value of breathing 100% oxygen at 3 ATM of pressure, and in February 1964 a hyperbaric chamber, donated by Mr. Sidney Eliason, Sr., was installed — the second such unit in the United States. Over the next fifteen years, more than 600 patients were treated in this manner. Drs. Plenk and Card were asked to report their experience with their first 150 patients at the first International Hyperbaric Congress in San Francisco in 1966. This led to the invitation to St. Mark's Tumor Institute to become one of thirty members of the Radiation Therapy Oncology Group (RTOG), a national study group funded by the National Cancer Institute (NCI).

Unknown to anyone else, LDS Hospital was in the process of constructing a modern therapy facility when the administrator, Brent Goates, approached Dr. Plenk in 1968 about the possibility of his taking over the operation. After much soul-searching, Dr. Plenk and the radiologists, administrators, and boards of the three private hospitals — St Mark's, Holy Cross, and LDS — reached the conclusion that a single therapy center serving all three institutions would be best for the community from the standpoint of cost-effectiveness, staffing, and quality, because it could handle a larger volume than competing institutions could develop.

The new "Radiation Center" at LDS Hospital was ready for occupancy with an 8 MeV Linear Accelerator, a new CO^{60} unit, a 300 KV Orthovoltage unit purchased from Holy Cross Hospital, and a 50-100 KV Superficial unit from LDS Hospital. Harry Fry, a British radiation physicist, arrived in January 1969 to assist in preparations for the move. The hyperbaric chamber, a Cobalt Target, all patient therapy records and therapy personnel from St. Mark's moved between March 28 and 30, 1969, and the first patients were treated at LDS on March 31 without any interruption in service. The Siemens Mevatron 8 (linear accelerator) operated with an 8 MeV x-ray beam, and in October a 4, 7, and 11 MeV electron became operational.

A two-year technology training program was instituted in 1972 with the help of several Australian and British technologists and some cooperation from the University of Utah. By 1988 forty students had graduated from the LDS program, which contributed greatly to correcting the severe nationwide shortage of technologists. Since 1974 Carla Rich, an LDS graduate, has provided outstanding leadership in the operation of the Center as well as the training program. In 1976 Mr. Fry was replaced by David Matthes, MS, who has contributed greatly to improved treatment planning, teaching, quality control, and greater sophistication in the program's technical and physical aspects.

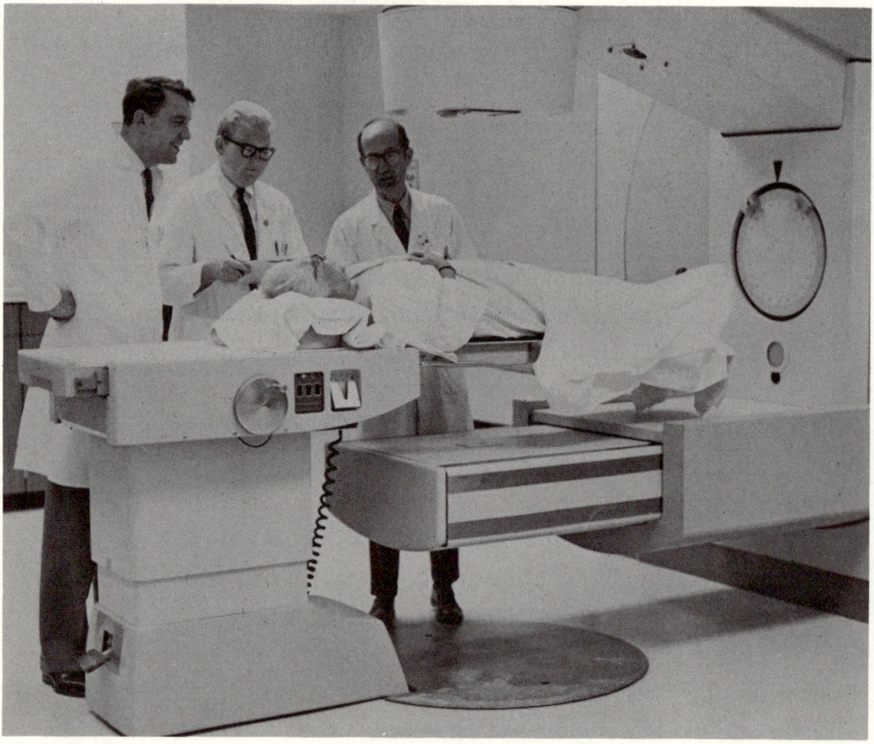

Harry Fry, physicist, Murray Schirmer, chief technologist, and Dr. Henry P. Plenk operate the first linear accelerator in Utah, an 8 MeV Siemens Mevatron, at the LDS Hospital Radiation Center, about 1970.

Rented radium sources were abandoned in 1971 in favor of a Cesium system; treatment plans were beginning to be computerized, and a dosimetrist was added in 1975.

An approved residency program was initiated in 1969, with one new resident per year (except for two who started in 1970). Between 1969 and 1989, most of the seventeen residents received almost all their training at the Radiation Center, with an additional three to twelve months of affiliated training at major cancer centers in the U.S., England, or the Continent and/or the University of Utah forming part of the program. Six of the best residents came on staff after completion of their training; three have since become chairs of academic departments of radiation oncology — Drs. Don Eisert at Vanderbilt, Len Gunderson at the Mayo Clinic, and Tom Roland at the University of Vermont.

Dr. Charles Votava, the first associate, joined the staff in February 1971 after a residency in radiology and an additional year as assistant in radiation therapy at the University of Iowa followed by a fellowship in radiation oncology at M. D. Anderson Hospital in Houston. Dr. Votava brought many new technical skills and a good clinical background of two years in medicine. He was an excellent teacher and was responsible for many innovations, especially in the treatment of gynecologic and "Head and Neck" problems. Dr. Votava left in November 1973 for a full-time academic position at the University of Tennessee.

The first two full-time residents, Drs. Richard C. Brown and Leonard L. Gunderson, arrived in 1970 and came on staff in 1973, after completing their training, initiating a very productive period for the Center. Drs. Gunderson and Votava became interested in the treatment of rectal carcinoma and wrote the chapter in Gilbert H. Fletcher's textbook *Radiotherapy*. Dr. Gunderson became the "sparkplug" for RTOG protocols on the subject.

Unfortunately for the Center, Dr. Gunderson accepted a full-time academic position at Massachusetts General Hospital and Harvard Medical School, with the opportunity to develop a gastrointestinal service on radiation medicine, and left Salt Lake City in March 1976. He later switched to the Mayo Clinic, where he became chair of the department in 1989. At almost the same time, in 1976, Dr. Brown left for a position at the University of Arizona and in 1981 returned to Utah to take over a new department at Utah Valley Medical Center. During the next three years, the Center experienced a period of instability, with rapid turnover of three new staff members until Dr. William Sause (1978) and Dr. John Thomson (1979), who had been residents at the Center, joined the staff. Sause became very active in RTOG and the Southwest Oncology Group (SWOG) and distinguished himself by his prolific scientific output, his teaching, and his ability to stimulate residents in their own research projects. Dr. Thomson took on pediatric oncology and the Children's Cancer Study

Group, participated in RTOG and SWOG activities, and played a leading role in research with hyperthermia.

Dr. Plenk relinquished his directorship of the Center in 1980 but continued in charge of the residency program and as principal investigator for RTOG. Dr. Sause took over as administrative chair at that time and assumed all functions upon Plenk's retirement in April 1986.

Dr. Jennifer Fischbach completed her residency in 1982 and had experience at St. Benedict's Hospital in Ogden before coming on staff in April 1986 as Dr. Plenk's replacement. She has actively participated in RTOG and has taken special interest and responsibility in the treatment of breast cancer.

The staff has participated actively in tumor conferences at St. Mark's, Holy Cross, and Cottonwood hospitals over many years and in October 1989 took charge of an elegant new satellite facility with a 6 MeV linear accelerator opened at Cottonwood Hospital to serve the south end of the Salt Lake Valley.

Under Dr. Sause's tenure as director, the physical plant was expanded by 1,000 square feet and a new higher energy linear accelerator (6-15 MeV photon and 3-20 MeV Electron beams) was installed. The department became one of the most active contributors to RTOG protocols, especially in intraoperative studies. Sause gained national and international recognition as chair of the lung committee and has been an invited panelist in the U.S. and in Europe on numerous occasions.

Between 1969 and 1986, the total grant support from various sources was almost $1.2 million. The Center's cumulative bibliography lists 135 papers. Major research areas over the years covered hyperbaric oxygen, cancer of cervix, cancer of rectum and anus, lung, brain and prostate tumors, hyperthermia, radiation sensitizers, multifractional daily treatment schedules, stereotactic localization of brain tumors, conservative treatment (lumpectomy and radiation therapy) of breast carcinoma, ovarian cancer, and intraoperative radiation.

University of Utah

Dr. Blaine Brown was a staff member from 1954 to 1956, when he became the first person to take an extra year of training in radiation therapy at the University of Chicago. He returned to Salt Lake General Hospital (SLGH) in 1957 to do therapy with orthovoltage equipment, moving to the new University Hospital in 1965, where a 2 MeV Van de Graaf unit was installed. Dr. Brown died of a heart attack in 1969. The next two years' therapy was supervised by several interval appointees until Dr. J. Robert Stewart arrived in July 1971. He was recruited by department chair Dr. David G. Bragg, who was also successful in getting a commitment for $250,000 to upgrade existing therapy facilities.

Stewart is a Provo native and University of Utah graduate with BS and MD degrees and two years of medicine at Boston City Hospital. After two years in the Army, he was a resident in radiation oncology at Stanford University (1963–66) and remained on the junior faculty there until 1971.

Dr. Karen Fu, also an ex-Stanford resident, joined Stewart for a year, after which she was replaced by Dr. James Eltringham, another former Stanford staff colleague. Dr. Eltringham became chief of the section of radiation therapy, played an active role in the residency and technology training program, and was the radiologic consultant for SWOG. He attained the rank of professor but left in 1986 to join the staff of the Tumor Institute of the Swedish Hospital in Seattle, Washington. In 1972 Stewart was able to attract Dr. Lyle A. Dethlefsen, DVM, PhD, to establish a very successful radiobiology laboratory.

The first resident, Dr. Joel Ohlson, started in July 1972 and joined the faculty from 1975 to 1978. Dr. R. Joseph Watson arrived in January 1973 to complete the last six months of a residency (begun in Wisconsin) and to assume a faculty position (1973–76). From 1972 to 1988, seventeen residents had completed all or part of their training at the University of Utah.

Dr. Frederic A. Gibbs, Jr., joined the faculty in 1977, after three years at Stanford and two years' research experience at NCI. He became chief of the section of radiation therapy in 1986 and has been the driving force in an active hyperthermia project, cooperating closely with the manufacturer BSD Corporation, located at the University Research Park.

Other junior faculty who stayed one to five years between 1978 and 1985 were Drs. Arthur Elman (1978–80), Lovered Peacock (1980–82), Michael Sapozink (1982–87), and Geraldine Jacobsen (1985–86). The present junior staff consists of John K. Hayes, a University graduate (1988), and Janalyn Prows, graduate of the Milwaukee County Medical Complex (1988).

The approximately 10,000-square-foot Radiation Therapy Pavilion in the newly constructed University Hospital was occupied in February 1982. The facility contains three Megavolt treatment rooms, housing 6 MeV, 4 MeV, and Varian 2100-C linear accelerators, and two "simulator" rooms containing one AECL simulator and a hyperthermia clinical research unit (BSD 1,000). Two physicists and two dosimetrists form the physics section staff.

Dr. Dethlefsen heads the section of experimental oncology with four other PhDs. Grants of $450,000 allowed complete renovation of 6,000 square feet of space and the purchase of very sophisticated equipment. Areas of major interest are basic molecular biology, *in vitro* cell biology, and hyperthermia as a radiation sensitizer.

Clinical research has been mainly in areas of cooperative studies: CCSG (Children's Cancer Study Group), SWOG, RTOG (as an LDS Hospital affiliate), innovative dosimetry, treatment aids, retrospective clinical studies, moving beam electron therapy, and hyperthermia.

Dr. Stewart became the principal investigator of a three-year, $900,000 cancer center support grant covering three universities, fifteen departments, and four hospitals. Among other support from NCI was a five-year program project grant in conjunction with LDS Radiation Center for "Preclinical and Clinical Cancer Research, Hyperthermia" in 1981. Numerous additional grants have supported the radiobiology lab. The University saw its largest patient volume, 869, in 1984. A satellite facility staffed by University radiation oncologists was opened at HCA–St. Mark's Hospital in May 1991.

St. Benedict's Hospital–Val A. Browning Cancer Treatment Center

While a member of the University staff, Dr. R. Joseph Watson was appointed director of the radiation oncology unit to be constructed as part of the new St. Benedict's Hospital. He was instrumental in decisions regarding layout of space and equipment, which consisted of a 6 MeV Siemens linear accelerator, a Cascade simulator, and a Copintech treatment planning computer. The center opened July 1977, when Watson resigned from the University and moved to Ogden.

Dr. Watson graduated from the University of West Virginia Medical School in 1965, and after a ten-month radiology residency switched to radiation oncology at the University of Wisconsin, where he learned M. D. Anderson and Stanford techniques under two chiefs. Sister Geanne of the Order of St. Benedict had a PhD in physics and became his physicist. Within a period of five years, the volume had increased to an average of 27 patients per day in 1982 and an annual average of about 400 patients in subsequent years.

In January 1983, Dr. Jennifer Fischbach, who had completed her training at LDS Hospital, joined Watson as an associate, but returned to LDS in April 1986. Dr. Watson was very active as an affiliate of LDS Hospital in RTOG and was a major contributor to prostatic and brain tumor protocols. In December 1985 a second linear accelerator (Varian 1800) with 6 and 18 MeV Photon and 6 and 20 MeV Electron beam capacity was installed, and an additional room was built. Unfortunately, Dr. Watson had to resign late in 1986 because of a severe illness which led to his death in March 1988.

Dr. Cleo E. Dymott succeeded Dr. Watson in July 1987. She had her training at the University of North Carolina and Joint Center at Harvard and was in practice in Olympia, Washington, before coming to Utah. Dr. Leslye Ingersoll, University of Utah graduate and Stanford trainee in radiation oncology, joined Dr. Dymott in 1989.

Utah Valley Regional Medical Center (UVRMC)

Dr. Richard C. Brown was appointed head of the Radiation Therapy Center at the Utah Valley Regional Medical Center and treated his first patient there on April 6, 1981. He obtained his MD at the University of Kansas, had a surgical internship at the University of Utah, and received his radiation oncology training at the Radiation Center at LDS Hospital. He has seven publications. The equipment in Provo consisted of a 6 MeV Varian 6100 Cascade simulator and superficial 100 KV unit. The volume continued to grow to an average of forty patients a day by the end of 1987. An associate, Dr. T. J. Blair, who trained at the Mayo Clinic, joined Dr. Brown in August of 1985.

A second 17 MeV linear accelerator was installed in Provo in 1981. The largest number of patients are treated for carcinoma of the prostate, either by external radiation or by transperineal implant with radioactive gold seeds. More than 100 prostate patients are seen in a year. The 380-bed UVRMC, one of Utah's largest hospitals, serves as a tertiary referral center for the central portion of the state. Two medical oncologists are now on the staff, making the oncology unit quite self-sufficient.

A satellite facility was opened at the Dixie Medical Center in St. George in May of 1986, and 150 patients were seen there during the first year. Drs. Brown and Blair originally alternated covering St. George for a period of two months, leaving Provo Thursday afternoon and returning Saturday morning. A medical oncologist assisted during the first part of the week, and a nurse practitioner was on location full time. Dr. Ray S. Richards, a University of Utah graduate, completed a residency in radiation oncology at Loma Linda University Hospital in 1989 and became the first full-time radiation oncologist in St. George. The radiation therapy needs of the central and southern parts of the state appear to be well met by these two centers.

CHAPTER FORTY-FOUR

Utah's Women Physicians Coming of Age

DENISE CALLISTER QUINN, MD

THE CHALLENGES AND CHANGES IN THE LIVES and practices of women in medicine in Utah in the last one hundred years are "mind–boggling." In 1990, sixty-eight or 17% of the students in the University of Utah College of Medicine were women. This may come as no surprise now, but few people know that during the last quarter of the nineteenth century, the number of women practicing medicine in Utah was unequaled anywhere else in the country.

From 1840 to 1850, emigrants surged westward for varied motives. The Mormons, led by Brigham Young, arrived in the Great Salt Lake Valley in 1847, and Utah became an official U.S. territory in 1850. In 1848 the first women's rights convention was held in New York, and newly formed women's suffrage organizations began their fight for the right to vote and hold office. While the number of women in industry and the professions already was increasing, the equal rights movement gave added support to those courageous pioneer women who chose to study medicine. Medical training still entailed great sacrifice on their part, however, because they had to leave husbands and children to study in eastern medical schools; and most of them had to work their way through school scrubbing floors and waiting tables. Why would they do this?

In 1850 only one state or territory topped Utah's death rate of one person in every forty-eight. Inadequate housing and food and infectious diseases took a heavy toll. As a result of plural marriages and

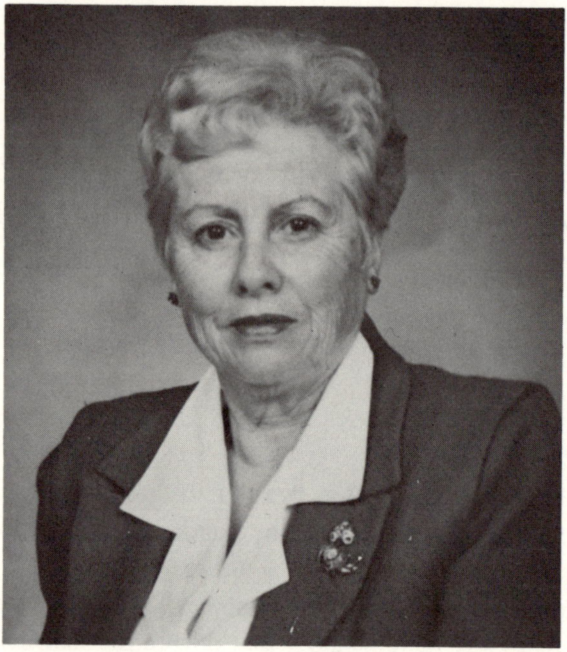

Denise Callister Quinn.

many new immigrants, childbirth and its complications added to the death rate. Doctors and well-trained midwives were scarce, and as rapid regional colonization moved families farther and farther from the Salt Lake Valley, babies often were delivered by midwives with no experience whatsoever. Brigham Young was acutely aware of the deplorable conditions and encouraged some of the "sisters" to study medicine. He wanted these women to practice medicine, but, in addition, to teach other women how to "serve competently and with scientific cleanliness in childbirth," and also to care properly for the many children who contracted diphtheria, cholera infantum, whooping cough, pneumonia, and other diseases.

Women were wanted as doctors for other reasons. In this era of Victorian prudery, most young women had a strong aversion to being assisted in childbirth by male physicians, a feeling shared by their husbands. Throughout the United States it was often proclaimed that attendance by men in obstetrical cases was offensive to modesty, and "once a mother's modesty was gone, chastity would soon follow."

So, in 1872, twenty-five years after the Mormons entered the Great Salt Lake Valley, Romania Bunnell Pratt set out to attend the Women's Medical College in Philadelphia. Dr. Pratt, a plural wife with children, gained an outstanding reputation in obstetrics as both teacher and practitioner. Later, after special training in the East in diseases of the eye and ear, she became the first ophthalmologist in Utah and was credited with performing the first cataract operation in the state. The first woman doctor actually to *practice* in Utah was probably Ellen B. Ferguson, who came to the Territory as a specialist in the diseases of women. She was also the first woman deputy sheriff in the U.S. and an enthusiastic suffragist as well.

Deseret Hospital was opened in 1882 as a maternity and emergency hospital and a women's health-care training center with Dr. Ferguson as the resident physician. The visiting staff included two male doctors plus three women physicians, Romania Pratt, Ellis R. Shipp, and Elvira S. Barney.

Dr. Shipp, often referred to as "the grand old lady of medicine in Utah," is credited with founding a school of obstetrics and nursing. An active practitioner and a prolific writer in many issues of *The Utah Sanitarian*, she was also a plural wife with ten children.

One of the most colorful personalities was Dr. Martha Hughes Paul Cannon, called Mattie, who obtained her MD at the University of Michigan in 1880. She too was a plural wife and mother, and she taught classes in nursing in addition to her practice. Eager to see a state board of health organized in Utah, and also to improve working conditions for women, she ran as a Democratic candidate for the state senate in 1896, defeating her own husband, who ran on the Republican ticket. It is said that he never forgave her for her boldness in not only running against but defeating him! She was the first elected woman state senator in the United States.

Among those receiving their MDs were Margaret Shipp Roberts, Mary Minor Green, Emma Atkins, Mary Emma Van Schoonhove, and later, Jane M. Skolfield (who practiced well into this century). Other early women physicians were Belle Anderson Gemmel and Justine Anderson McIntyre, whose father, Dr. W. F. Anderson, was an early Utah surgeon and a friend of Brigham Young.

These pioneer women physicians, though very different in personality from one another, shared the traits of intelligence, courage, persistence, and compassion. They were held in high regard as practitioners and teachers. They all took an active interest in women's suffrage, and another of them became a member of the state legislature. In spite of their stressful lives, several lived into their nineties and the majority into their late seventies.

The twentieth century, apparently bright with promise, became instead "an era of stagnation and regression" for women in medicine. Few were admitted to medical schools after the 1910 Flexner Report on the quality of U.S. medical education was acted upon, which resulted in few new women practitioners. Soon only *one* medical college for women (in Philadelphia) remained where previously several had existed. The admissions committees of most medical schools were convinced that women would not be as productive in their profession as their male colleagues. The women's rights movement had faded, and women applicants no longer had the support of their former crusaders. The medical profession was becoming oversupplied during the early years of the century, and greater economic competition prevailed. The rugged pioneer woman doctor was no longer a necessity, and the exclusion of women from the profession was justified by the traditional opinions voiced by *both* men and women that women "were less able to stand the strain of practice."

A crusade in the late 1840s had encouraged women to go into medicine to teach, but in the 1900s forgotten were Sylvester Graham's reforms in personal hygiene, which included dietary improvements, sex hygiene, dress reform, and physical exercise for women. It is interesting to note that as late as 1934 a woman physician advertised in the Salt Lake City telephone directory as a *dietitian* for fear she would not be accepted as a physician.

In the early years of the twentieth century, few hospitals accepted women regularly in internships and residencies. With the advent of

World War I and a marked decrease in the number of male interns, women were more readily accepted — but only while the war lasted.

By the end of the 1930s, the pessimism of women physicians stood in sharp contrast to the optimism with which they had welcomed the new century. The handful of women physicians in Utah were commonly called "the hen medics." Nationally, the percentage of women practicing medicine dropped from 6% in 1910 to 5.1% by 1940. The Utah scene was even worse.

With the entry of the United States into World War II in 1941, women doctors were once again a valuable national resource. President Roosevelt signed into law a bill enabling women doctors for the first time to hold commissions in the Army and Navy medical corps. The advent of the new four-year University of Utah College of Medicine, organized in 1942, gave women hope once again for equal opportunities. They represented 10% of that first four-year class, which graduated in September of 1944. In the early 1940s many women were accepted for internships in Utah hospitals as the supply of male interns dwindled rapidly. In fact, by January 1943 more than 2,300 intern slots in civilian hospitals across the nation remained unfilled. As the U.S. emerged from the war, women physicians hoped that their recent gains would be preserved and expanded. But, as it had a generation earlier, optimism faded in the face of reality. As one writer said, "Hospitals pitched women off their staffs as promptly as many shipyards told Rosie the Riveter to go home and peel potatoes."

The number of women medical students enrolled in the University of Utah College of Medicine peaked at 9.8% in 1945. From then on a downward trend in admissions continued until 1972, with *no* women admitted in some years.

From 1945 to 1950 the number of practicing women doctors listed in the Salt Lake City directory had doubled from four to eight, and by 1955 it had tripled to twelve (about 5% of the total doctors listed). About half were native daughters, the rest coming from elsewhere. None in this group had received their MDs in Utah, and the majority were engaged in general practice, obstetrics-gynecology, anesthesiology, or pediatrics. The women had developed a camaraderie and met at infrequent intervals in social gatherings to share much-needed emotional support. About three-fourths of the group were married; about half had children. Many were active on committees in their medical societies, and one, Dr. Esther Gross, was elected president of the Intermountain Pediatric Society in 1953.

In the 1960s, the number of women in private practice trained at the University of Utah increased again. They were bright, competent women and successful practitioners. They no longer seemed to have the need to "hang together" in order to have a professional identity, and most were active members of their local medical societies. Still, very few women physicians practiced outside metropolitan Salt Lake City and the surrounding areas.

With the 1970s came many national social and political changes which affected the future of women physicians in Utah directly. An increasing focus on women's rights and status had opened the way for women to enter male-dominated specialties. A dramatic increase in the number of women medical students throughout the nation kindled a rebirth of the optimism that had marked the late nineteenth century. Changes came from outside medicine — from federal laws and civil-liberties lawsuits. Changes also came from within medicine — from supportive doctors. In the previous twenty years, women admitted to the Utah College of Medicine averaged about 3% of the total. In 1972, 16.8% of the freshman class were women; in 1990 the percentage was almost identical at 17% or 68 women. The dropout rate had become similar for men and women; between 1970 and 1980, only *four* women were dropped or voluntarily withdrew from school in Utah.

By 1970, the Carnegie Commission reported that 91% of women physicians remained active in medical work. In 1975 Utah boasted 92 women doctors, 64 engaged in direct patient care; by 1988 the number had increased to 294. Most of those not in private practice were involved in medical administration, teaching, and research — 81 in 1988. In 1975 only 25% of the women physicians in the U.S. had earned their specialty board certification, compared with *33%* in Utah. By 1978, 47% in Utah had specialty board certification, compared with 38.4% nationally.

The seventies saw other significant changes as well. Most Utah women physicians now were married and had children. In 1975 the majority of residents were working in internal medicine, pediatrics, and psychiatry, and as yet there were no women in obstetrics and gynecology training. By 1978 the carefully guarded male domain of surgery had been invaded!

The number of women in private practice declined from the late 1970s to 1981. A few had retired, but the greatest shift was from single, private practices to medical group practice. Private practice made it more difficult to maintain the multiple roles of physician, wife, and mother, and about three-fourths of the women doctors now worked in family health plan groups, hospitals, and other agencies.

In the eighties most medical school programs were still relatively inflexible in meeting the unique individual needs of both male and female students. However, the residency programs (Utah's included) allowed for greater flexibility — an advantage for women with one or two children. In the "special arrangements program," for example, two residents could share one residency over a longer period of time.

In the eighties, almost as many female residents were in *training* as were women MDs in *practice* in direct patient care. More women were involved in medical research and education in academic medicine. Greater equity in salaries, promotions, and tenure had been achieved. No women physicians were departmental chairmen as yet, but one PhD held a chair. Among the eighteen women on the faculty, one was a full professor. Several were outstanding in their research, teaching, and publishing.

Utah's women physicians, now more than 10% of the total number of doctors (391 in 1991), are having a greater impact both individually and collectively on medical care, research, and education. As agents for change, women doctors have influenced many areas: winning more flexible training programs and reducing the old eighty-hour work week with its attendant "burnout" and poor quality of patient care. They have fostered greater recognition of the patient as a *person* and an *equal.* They have emphasized the *quality* rather than the quantity of services rendered patients, as well as the importance of *preventive* medicine.

Among many distinguished women physicians, the following have received awards and special recognition:

1965 Alma Nemir, MD (Public Health) — Woman of Distinction by University of Utah Faculty Women.

1966 Lenore Richards, MD (General Surgery) — Honorary President, Utah Medical Association (UMA).

UMA Presidential Awards:

1980 Joyce Johnson, MD (Internal Medicine).

1982 Elizabeth Boettcher, MD (Pathology).

1988 Kristen M. Ries, MD (Medicine, Infectious Diseases) — Special Award of Merit, Salt Lake County Medical Society, for pioneering work in the treatment of AIDS patients and AIDS education.

1989 Linda Leckman, MD (General Surgery).

1990–1991 Anne G. Osborne, MD (Neuroradiology) — Distinguished Scientist in Radiology, Armed Forces Institute of Pathology and American College of Radiology. Gold Medal and Memorial Lecture award, Chicago Radiological Society (1989).

1991 Elizabeth Hammond, MD (Electron-microscopy) — LDS Hospital, Hall of Honor.

All Utahns can be proud of their women physicians, past and present. They can look forward to their medical women becoming an even more productive and important human resource serving Utah.

Note: The author is indebted to Mrs. Elena F. Eyzaguirre and The Eccles Health Sciences Library for their assistance. Detailed bibliographical entries are available in the original manuscript of this volume, housed in the Special Collections of the Marriott Library, University of Utah.

CHAPTER FORTY-FIVE

Utah's Public Health

MELVIN M. OWENS, MBA • SUZANNE DANDOY, MD

MANY YEARS AGO, DR. M. J. ROSENAU, Professor of Public Health at Harvard University, defined public health as "the science and art of preventing disease, prolonging life and promoting physical and mental efficiency through organized community effort."

When Dr. G. D. Carlyle Thompson, director of the Utah Department of Health from 1961 to 1970, was asked for his definition, he responded that public health is whatever the Legislature wants it to be. Dr. Thompson's response reflects the state legislature's role in determining governing laws and funding for the Utah Department of Health — as well as the arduousness of the task of wresting that funding from the historically tight-fisted body.

In the Middle Ages, public health consisted of attempting to rid Europe of the plague. In more recent centuries, cholera, diphtheria, typhoid, and smallpox have flourished, often in epidemic proportions, but have been brought under control. To those raised in the 1930s, public health meant the visit of a public health nurse who provided what care and comfort she could, then placed a Measles, Mumps, Chicken Pox, or the dreaded Scarlet Fever sign in the front window of the home. Now the public health "plagues" of the industrialized nations are acquired immunodeficiency syndrome (AIDS) and present and potential contamination from hazardous wastes.

When Brigham Young led 143 pioneers into the Salt Lake Valley in 1847, sound scientific knowledge of sanitation and hygiene was

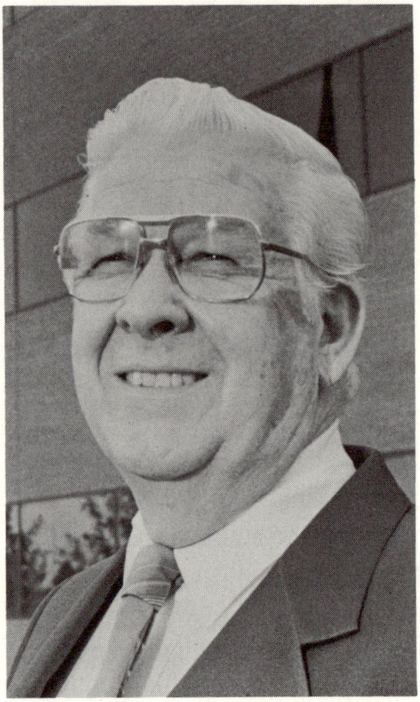

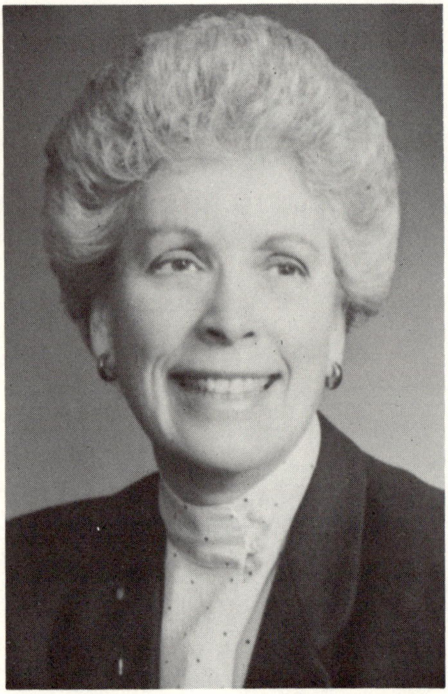

The late Melvin M. Owens, left; Suzanne Dandoy, right.

decades in the future. However, the famously practical leader was constantly advising as to the arrangement of barns, stables, and privies in their relationship to the pioneer homes and water supplies. He repeatedly told the people to "boil the water they drank," and a balanced diet and sufficient sleep were often subjects of discussion.

The Society of Health, "To give information to the masses of the people, to lessen their burdens, and to enable them to help themselves," was organized in the spring of 1849, twenty years before the first state Board of Health was founded in Massachusetts. Next a Council of Health was organized, which met weekly at the home of Mormon leader Willard Richards. Shocking death rates from endemic cholera, diphtheria, and typhoid were still a daily fact of life. Early recognition of the need to teach community health directly to the people created a priority for Utah's health practitioners.

As the nature of infectious diseases became better known, national and local campaigns for safer water systems and better sewage disposal had a major impact on general health. In 1889 and 1890 the *Deseret News* advocated construction of a downtown sewer system and city water pipelines to connect all residences. After Utah won statehood in 1896, Dr. Martha Hughes Paul Cannon, a physician who was the first woman in the nation elected a state senator, sponsored a successful bill to create a StateBoard of Health. Dr. Theodore Bruce Beatty was appointed health commissioner in 1898 by Governor Heber M. Wells at a salary of $1,000 per year, a part-time position until 1915. Dr. Beatty served as the state's health officer for thirty-six years, until 1934, and as an adviser and member of the Board of Health until 1947.

The Challenge: Public Health vs. Politics

A Utah legislator sang an ongoing refrain when he called Public Health "the bastard child of state government." It has never been an easy matter to secure sound public health legislation, as the interests of politicians have not always paralleled those of the public health officials. A case in point was Dr. Beatty's recommendation in 1900 that the State Board of Health adopt a compulsory smallpox vaccination ordinance. The Board acted, generating immediate statewide opposition led by the editorial writer of the *Deseret News* — despite the higher incidence of smallpox in Utah than in the surrounding states that had enacted compulsory vaccination laws, and despite support for the ordinance by the presidency of the LDS Church as well as the Utah State Medical Association. The compulsory vaccination ordinance was canceled by a bill passed by the state legislature and vetoed by Governor Wells, then passed again over the Governor's veto. It was many years before Utah rejoined the vaccination mainstream.

Other public health legislation was less controversial. In 1907 the teaching of sanitation and disease prevention in the public schools was authorized, and in 1911 it became possible to conduct physical examinations of preschool and school children, with discovered defects being called to their parents' attention. Health education for the prevention of venereal diseases also began that year, with laws enacted to require the reporting of all cases to the State Board of Health and the treatment of newborn infants' eyes to prevent gonorrhea. Still, Dr. Beatty's lot was never easy. He began advocating the construction of a state tuberculosis sanatorium in 1904, a facility which would not be built until 1940, in Ogden, where it was filled to capacity from its opening.

The Sheppard-Towner Act, passed by Congress in 1922, provided the first federal financial assistance for maternal and child health. Dr. Beatty turned to the Relief Society, the women's auxiliary of the LDS Church, as the most suitable organization through which to administer that law. The Relief Society soon had 194 clinics in operation throughout Utah, providing the quarters, necessary equipment, and volunteers to staff them. The federal money was used to pay the doctors. With the advent of the Social Security Law in the 1930s, federal funding made possible the implementation of a complete statewide educational program in preventive and public health.

The state legislature of 1937 adopted a law charging the State Board of Health with setting standards on testing before prophylactics (condoms and ointments) could be sold in Utah. After the prophylactics were tested at the State Health Laboratory, the Board issued a list of approved products.

A complete Utah Health Code was established in 1953, setting out the governing laws and the organization of the State Health Department. Chapters covered vital statistics, the control of communicable diseases, a state health laboratory, public health nursing, sanitation, hospital licensure, and maternal and child health. In the 1960s laws were enacted to control air pollution, to require testing of all newborns for phenylketonuria (PKU), and to establish a statewide Medical Examiner system.

The statutes were recodified in 1981, having been broadened in twenty-eight years to cover emergency medical services, solid and hazardous waste, radiation, health facility planning, and financial assistance for medical care. Protecting the health of the public was no longer restricted to the traditional areas of infectious diseases and the care of poor pregnant women and their children. It also included responsibilities for how health care was financed and how it was delivered.

Underfunding of the State Health Department began early, a fact that inspired severe criticism from the Utah State Medical Association in a report published in 1934 which declared that "the State Legislature has always been niggardly in its financial support of this Department, being more interested, apparently, in roads and cows than in the lives and health of human beings." Despite the lack of funds, Dr. Beatty maintained a high degree of efficiency, initiative, and loyalty among his staff, partly as a response to his own outstanding capabilities and tenaciousness. After he retired in 1934, the department was headed by Dr. J. L. Jones, followed by Dr. William M. McKay. After Dr. McKay's unexpected death in 1947, it was very difficult to find a qualified replacement at the salary offered. All salaries were very low, and key officers and employees in all divisions resigned. In 1949, at the urging of the Utah Public Health Association (which had been founded in 1916), Dr. Ira S. Hiscock, professor of public health at Yale, conducted a study which concluded that "The lack of satisfactory working conditions is alarming . . . . It is doubtful if there is a more acute or critical condition existing in any state."

These dismal conditions continued through the administration of Dr. George Spendlove, who became State Health Commissioner in 1950. In his Biennium Report of 1952–54, he reported 133 staff resignations out of a total of 175 employees. Even he left in 1955 for a higher salary and better support with the state of Washington. The turmoil didn't subside until 1961, when Dr. G. D. Carlyle Thompson was hired from the state of Montana with a gubernatorial promise of assistance in reorganizing the department and helping it regain and improve on the stature it had once enjoyed.

Public health was dealt another political blow in 1967, however, when the department's status was reduced in a government reorganization that made it a division in a new Department of Health and Welfare. The new department was predominantly a welfare organization, and Dr. Thompson retired in 1970 over philosophical differences with the executive director. Dr. Lyman Olsen served as director of the division during much of the agency's sojourn in the combined department — a difficult time politically for public health, since welfare services had a higher priority than their public health counterparts.

This period saw yet another political clash. Utah has consistently been among the states with the lowest percentage of the population served by fluoridated water supplies, a measure known to prevent tooth decay. Three attempts were made during the sixties to pass by popular vote a measure to fluoridate Salt Lake City's water; all failed. During 1976 the State Board of Health decided to try to remedy the situation by establishing a Board regulation requiring all public water supplies to be fluoridated. An aggressive campaign was launched to educate the citizens, and public hearings were held around the state. The regulation was actively opposed by the Libertarian Party and others who petitioned for a ballot initiative. Mandatory fluoridation was narrowly defeated amid complaints of voter fraud and ballot-box stuffing, and since then fluoridation decisions have been left to cities and require initiative votes. Only two small cities in Utah have chosen to fluoridate their water supplies.

By the 1980s the political wheel had turned sufficiently to allow Health to regain department status through legislation passed in 1981. At the same time, the State Board of Health was replaced with a Health Advisory Council, with the executive director of health reporting directly to and serving at the pleasure of the Governor. For cost–containment purposes, the state's Medicaid program was transferred from the Department of Social Services (the new name for the welfare agency) to the Department of Health. Replacing the State Board of Health with a Health Advisory Council was a departure from traditional state public health organization and tended, in the opinion of some, to politicize public health, since the executive director no longer enjoyed a political buffer by serving at the pleasure of the Board.

Beginning in 1979, Dr. James Mason became director and brought a new focus to public health, promoting wellness by urging people to change their lifestyles to eliminate the risk factors that cause poor health and disease. He left the department in 1983 to head the Centers for Disease Control (CDC) in Atlanta, Georgia, and in 1989 was appointed Assistant Secretary for Health in the Bush Administration. In 1985 Dr. Suzanne Dandoy was recruited from Arizona. A native of Los Angeles, Dr. Dandoy received her BS, MD, and MPH degrees from UCLA and took additional training in epidemiology and preventive medicine. She spent fourteen years in Arizona before coming to Utah, six as health director and four as professor of health administration. In 1991 the state legislature removed the environmental health function from the Department of Health and created a separate Department of Environmental Quality.

Public Health Programs

Dr. Beatty initially did laboratory exams for tuberculosis, typhoid fever, diphtheria, and glanders (a highly contagious disease of horses, mules, and asses transmittable to dogs, goats, sheep, and man) in his private medical office. In 1925 a public health laboratory was established at the State Capitol. With the development of vaccines, emphasis in the fifties and sixties was on mass immunization programs.

Poliomyelitis was rampant in Utah through the forties. In 1951 a major epidemic caused 577 cases, a rate of 84.39 per 100,000 population. Utah was the first state to have a statewide "Sabin on Sunday" program to distribute oral polio vaccine to the citizens. In the late sixties, a statewide TB eradication program combining health education and new TB drugs resulted in a dramatic reduction in TB cases and closure of the sanitorium a few years later. A "Muzzle the Measles" campaign in 1967 reached an estimated 96 percent of susceptible Utah children, and a "Rub Out Rubella" campaign was held in the seventies. While making great strides in eliminating these diseases, Utah had the highest 1965 rate for deaths from rheumatic fever and chronic rheumatic heart disease, 55 percent above the national average. In cooperation with the private medical community and the Utah Pharmaceutical Association, a major effort was launched to prevent this disease by treating all cases of streptococcal infection with low-cost penicillin. In the mid-eighties rheumatic fever resurfaced as a significant problem in the state, however, and AIDS also emerged as the new public health challenge.

Early programs in maternal and child health involved well-child conferences, dental clinics, and prenatal clinics. In the late 1930s, public health nurses demonstrated the value of prenatal and postnatal care and the proper preparation for home deliveries. At the same time, the Board of Health strengthened regulations for the twenty-two maternity homes in Utah. A special maternal and infant care program for enlisted men's wives and children was enacted by Congress and carried out in the forties through the use of federal funds. Identification of crippled children who needed surgery or other types of corrective care was begun in 1936; rheumatic heart disease was added to the program in 1952 and cerebral palsy and mental retardation in the 1960s. In the eighties the "Baby Your Baby" program was initiated to address an increasing infant mortality rate; the program became a model for the nation and was replicated in several other states.

As chronic diseases moved into the forefront in the seventies and eighties as causes of morbidity and mortality, public health efforts aimed at prevention and early detection were expanded. Cervical cancer and hypertension screening, education concerning the harmful effects of tobacco, identification of families at high risk for heart disease, and education of physicians regarding cholesterol in the diet were emphasized, with the support and cooperation of the private medical community.

One of the most significant areas of program growth has been environmental health. Early efforts were directed at proper sewage disposal, including the supervision of the construction of standardized pit privies throughout the state in the thirties. While in 1915 Salt Lake City became the first community in Utah to chlorinate its drinking water, the first state legislation authorizing regulation of water supplies and wastewater systems was not passed until 1953. What began as concern for sewage disposal and protection of drinking water grew after World War II to include programs involved with air pollution, industrial hygiene, radiological hazards, plumbing codes, food handling, control of pollution in all waters of the state, and disposal of solid wastes. Unique to Utah and the adjacent states was the necessity, beginning in the fifties, to monitor radiation from the Nevada Atomic Test Site. Because of contaminated hay and pasture lands, increased levels of radioactive iodine appeared in Utah milk in 1962, requiring extensive milk control efforts. All of these activities gave the State Health Department a much greater regulatory role than it had played in the past. The most recent addition to the environmental health arena has been the prevention and clean-up of pollution from hazardous substances such as toxic chemicals and uranium mill tailings.

As communities developed efforts to expand emergency medical services to their citizens, the state legislature authorized the department in the 1970s to organize these services into a statewide system and to train and certify those who delivered the services in the field. Utah developed one of the premier emergency medical services programs in the country.

In order to maintain Utah's past accomplishments in citizen health and to establish goals for the future, the department published "A Statement of Health Policy — A Prescription to Improve the Health Status of Utahns" in 1984. "A Prescription for Health Care Costs in Utah" emphasized competitive cost-control strategies. The department also published a document outlining social barriers to the health care system for ethnic minorities. Thus, public health began to focus on the operation of the health care system and citizens' access to health care.

Public Health Organizations

In the early part of this century, the LDS Church was involved with the delivery of public health services in the community. Later, local health departments were created to bring services to the people.

While the 1898 statutes provided for every county or district and every city to have a board of health and to appoint a local health officer, areas were slow to act. Salt Lake City appointed its first City Health Commissioner in 1903. Dr. Samuel G. Paul served on a part-time basis and was instrumental in developing well-baby clinics, milk stations, public health nursing, and a laboratory. The compensation for such appointees was roundly attacked by Dr. Beatty in 1912:

"Local authorities frequently employ as health officers men who are wholly unfit and incompetent, because more capable members of the community refuse to accept the miserable pittance doled out to them as compensation. It is only just to add that there are many competent and faithful health officers who do not consider the question of compensation. They know that lives may be saved by their efforts, and the consciousness of that fact is the reward for the performance of a responsible service which often engenders dislike and hostility of the very people whom they endeavor to protect."

The first fully organized local health department in Utah began in Davis County in 1937. During the next twenty years, local health services were organized in most of the major cities and larger counties. After a thirty-year effort, the Salt Lake City and County departments were merged in 1969. Still, public health services in the rural areas consisted primarily of a public health nurse and a sanitarian who were state employees serving a multi-county area, with local physicians often serving as part-time health officers.

In the 1970s the department made a concerted effort to develop multi-county health departments directed by full-time health officers for parts of the state where local health services had been only loosely organized. By the end of the decade, six local departments served single counties, and six more covered the rest of the state in multi-county combinations. These local health departments have undertaken a full slate of services for the communities they serve, including, for example, restaurant and water supply inspection, maternal and child health clinics, screening for chronic diseases, school health, control of sexually transmitted diseases, immunizations, and distribution of protective car seats for children.

The Utah Public Health Association was organized in 1916, with primary emphasis on tuberculosis control activities and responsibility for the Christmas Seal fund-raising campaign. Over time, the Association became involved in a wide range of public health services and education. In 1987 a coalition of volunteer organizations, working with the department, was successful in persuading the legislature to increase the cigarette tax, with the additional revenues directed in part to an expanded program of prenatal and maternal care. This effort would have been less successful if the department had launched it alone. Sometimes volunteer organizations are able to sponsor activities that government agencies are politically unable to manage.

Attention has been given here to the poor morale of state health department employees who felt that they had insufficient funding, low salaries, and inadequate working conditions during the forties and fifties. In June 1986 a new building was dedicated for the sole use of the department. The Martha Hughes Cannon Building was named in honor of this early physician and legislator who was such a strong advocate for public health. Innovative features such as a day-care center for employees' children and a physical fitness center were included as examples of the department's concern for its employees and their work environment. The Cannon Building was also the first government facility in Utah to be totally "smoke free," with no smoking permitted at any place inside. Some of the concerns expressed by Dr. Hiscock in his 1949 report have been addressed in this environment in which public health can receive the attention it deserves. In 1991 the most modern medical examiner facility in the nation was completed for that portion of Utah's public health work.

From comprehensive health data a gratifying improvement can be seen in the health status of Utah citizens over the years. Illness and death from diseases common to the early pioneers are now virtually nonexistent. Mortality rates are down, and further decline is expected as modern medical technology and increased attention to changes in lifestyle work together toward improving the health of Utah's citizens. These significant changes are the result of the combined efforts of the public health and private medical communities in Utah.

Note: The author is grateful to Drs. G. D. Carlyle Thompson and Lyman J. Olsen, who contributed information from their perspective as former state health officers in Utah. Dr. Thompson also provided his research on the terms and circumstances of tenure of the past state health officers. Regrettably, Melvin M. Owens died in 1987, soon after completing the first draft of the essay on which this chapter is based and never had the opportunity to see it in final form. S.D.

EPILOGUE

Reflections on the Relationship of Medicine and Society at Large

HENRY P. PLENK, MD, MS

HISTORIAN DANIEL J. BOORSTIN, in his recent book *Hidden History*, states that the historian's mission is to discover the uniqueness of people, places, and moments. It is hoped that the preceding essays have fulfilled at least some of these demands. How do events in the Beehive State over the last fifty years relate to the broader image of medicine in this country?

Professor Mark Siegler of the University of Chicago, pioneer of the new "Medical Ethics," divides the practice of medicine in the U.S. into three phases: (1) paternalism, lasting up to the sixties; (2) equality of doctor and patient (sixties and seventies); and (3) bureaucratic dictatorship for patients and doctors alike since the eighties.

Lewis Thomas, in *The Youngest Science; Notes of a Medicine Watcher*, describes medicine up to the thirties and forties as a period of "the laying on of hands." The number of conditions cured was very limited, some surgical conditions excepted. Pneumonia was a self-limiting disease with high mortality until the use of specific antisera and sulfa drugs in the thirties and antibiotics in the forties (the first penicillin became available to civilians only after World War II). Diabetic coma was treated with fluids and with insulin after its discovery in the twenties. Acute heart failure was treated with bleeding, digitalis, and oxygen; duodenal ulcers with Sippy powders and atropine; tuberculosis with rest, sunshine, and pneumothorax; syphilis with heavy metals — arsenicals, mercury, and bismuth.

In spite of the absence of the modern tools of scientific medicine, physicians and their opinions were held in high regard and were rarely questioned by their patients or the public at large. "The doctor knows best" was generally accepted. Popular magazines did not discuss diagnosis or treatment. Malpractice suits were rare until the fifties, and in many instances physicians were considered friends of the patients and of the family. Especially in the thirties, forties, and even fifties, doctors in general did not expect to get rich — though graduation from medical school was always an assured meal ticket, even in the depression years, when barter often replaced fees. Dr. Dorman's story of his days as a coal camp doctor (Chapter 2) is a wonderful reminder of this period.

Until Medicare was instituted in 1966, physicians treated charity patients (i.e., anybody who could not afford medical care) for free or for token payments. Men and women attracted to the field were motivated by the idea of rendering service to society and/or the excitement of being able to make a scientific contribution. The early recruits to the University of Utah Medical School certainly exemplify this group. They did not expect fortunes, mansions, or even assurance of support for their wisdom or endeavors. In many ways this was the golden age of medicine. The Roman poet Ovid, in his *Metamorphoses* (freely translated) describes the golden age this way: "The golden age was first without judges, soldiers, or laws [bureaucracies]. People were content, trusting, without fears." Yet some shortcomings of the period were discrimination against women and religious minorities and almost total exclusion of blacks by the majority of private schools.

The fifties represented the end of this era, with the beginnings of subspecialization, the knowledge revolution, and the increasing role — especially in the U.S. — of government support of science, research, and medical schools. By the mid-fifties the laying on of hands was changing to a loss of touch. The skills of physical diagnosis and history-taking were replaced by the reading of signals from machines. With the rapid subspecialization in the sixties and seventies, the role of the primary physician, whether general practitioner or general internist, diminished to the great detriment of the physician-patient relationship. House calls disappeared, charity became the responsibility of government, and malpractice suits became epidemic.

Dr. Siegler's second phase of emancipation of the patient from the doctor gave the patient a greater say regarding his care, occasionally creating an adversarial relationship between patient and physician. While the increased role and greater assertiveness of the patient in decision making was an important step forward, it sometimes brought with it a belief in unorthodox methods of treatment. Some patients refused the physicians' advice even if effective treatment was available. Quack cancer cures such as Krebiazin and Laetrile proliferated, causing many unnecessary deaths when used in lieu of accepted methods. Refusal to have children vaccinated because of religious beliefs and the use of prayer instead of early intervention in potentially curable but otherwise fatal diseases was detrimental if not disastrous.

We are now well into the third phase of bureaucratic dictatorship, where government regulations and insurance companies dictate in many cases not only the choice of physician, but also the length of hospital stay. The current situation deprives the physician of some control in decision making and the uninsured one-third of the population of access to the best care available. The enormous increase in the cost of medical care has brought about a national crisis, with many responsible voices calling for a complete change in the existing system.

Utah has been a part of all these changes — the revolutionary explosion of scientific discovery and knowledge on the one hand, some loss of the milk of human kindness and respect for the medical profession on the other.

Exit the Golden Age of Practice, Enter the Golden Age of Science

The golden age of the science of medicine, which started with the post–World War II involvement of government and private foundations in the support of research hospitals and medical schools, is still in full bloom. Dr. Maxwell Wintrobe's groundbreaking NIH grant of $100,000 in 1946 was the beginning trickle of the waterfall of hundreds of millions of dollars which allowed Utah to become one of the leading medical centers in the country. The total of awards to the

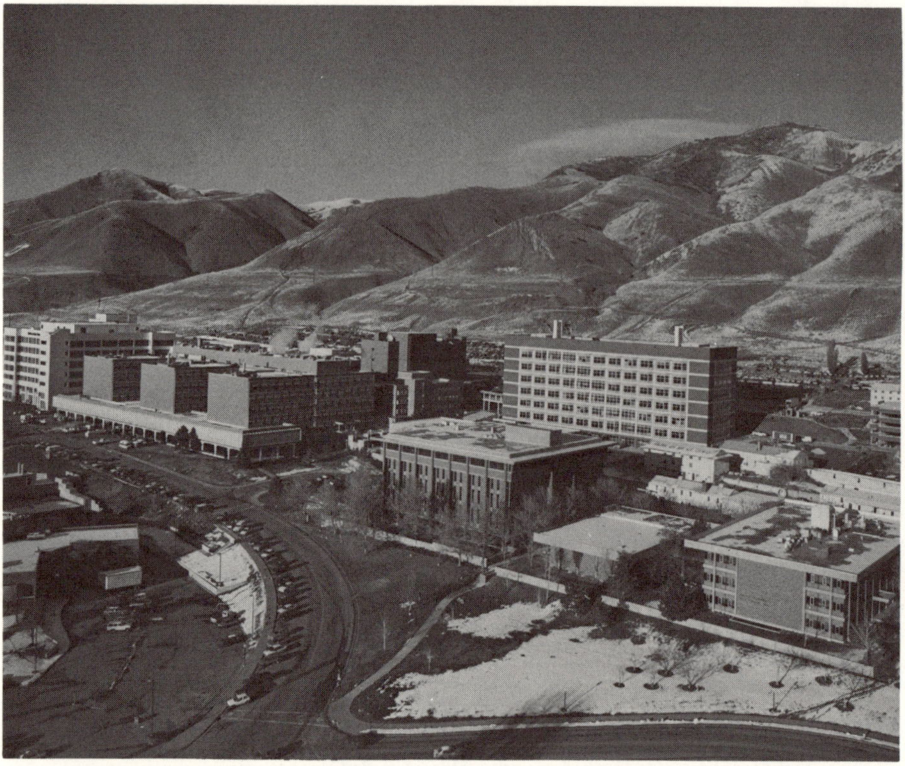

The Fort Douglas North Campus. Left to right: University Hospital, 1981, Medical School and Hospital, 1965, School of Nursing, School of Pharmacy. Behind Nursing stands the new eight-story Genetics Building, opened in 1991.

School of Medicine from 1968 to 1990 was $567,800,000. Of this, the University retains 48.5% as "overhead," an important sum for the maintenance of the School's operation.

An initial grant for a cancer research building (1948) was followed by construction of the original Medical School–University Hospital in 1965. The new University Hospital, built in 1981, and the latest addition of the splendid Primary Children's Medical Center form an impressive complex. Additional research facilities such as the Radiation Biology Laboratory, the Maxwell M. Wintrobe Research and Education Building, the Ezekial R. and Edna Wattis Dumke Building, and the George and Dolores Eccles Institute of

Human Genetics (1990), surrounded by the Schools of Pharmacy (in L. S. Skaggs Hall) and Nursing, and the Spencer S. Eccles Medical Library certainly provide the critical mass for outstanding research and medical care.

Many departments of the Medical School have distinguished themselves for their quality of service and outstanding research, and some have been named "centers of excellence":

— The Department of Radiology under Dr. David Bragg, for the center of diagnostic imaging research conducted by a multidisciplinary group, as well as leadership in obtaining a cancer center grant, Dr. J. Robert Stewart, director.

— The Laser Institute established in 1974 under the direction of Dr. John A. Dixon, for stimulating the development of early laser units suitable for medical use, for developing widespread clinical application of the tool, and for teaching the technique to scores of specialists in many fields of medicine.

— The Department of Ophthalmology, especially for its center of intraocular lens research by Dr. David Apple and corneal research by department chair Randall J. Olson.

— The Institute for Human Genetics, headed by Drs. Ray Gesteland and Ray White, and the section on population genetics directed by Dr. Mark Skolnick for demonstrating the role of genetics in many human diseases.

— The Division of Artificial Organs, under the leadership of Drs. Willem J. Kolff and Don D. Olsen, for imaginative contributions in providing artificial substitutes for failing hearts, ears, eyes, and missing limbs.

— Dr. William A. Gay, Jr., for initiating the combined University of Utah, Primary Children's Medical Center, VA, and LDS hospitals heart transplant program of 396 patients from March 1985 to July 1991, with some of the best results in the world (87.8% one-year survivals). (See Health Sciences Report, Special Edition of 1987, 1990.)

Major expansions have also taken place in the private hospitals in Salt Lake City, Ogden, and Provo during the past twenty years. A number of these institutions have made significant contributions to research and the training of residents.

Much innovation and research have originated at LDS Hospital, including the pioneering work in thoracic and vascular surgery of Drs. Ray Rumel, Russell Nelson, Hal Liddle, Kent W. Jones, Donald B. Doty, and others; the opening of the region's first intensive care and pulmonary intensive care units; and a very solid research program in pulmonary medicine under Drs. DuWayne Schmidt and Alan Morris and associates. A kidney transplant program came to fruition as a result of Dr. Larry Stevens' pioneering efforts, first started at the old Salt Lake General Hospital and leading to a combined LDS–University–PCMC organ transplant program, including heart, liver, and other organs. From 1983 to 1990, 546 kidney transplants were performed at LDS Hospital, with a five-year survival rate of 85% with "live related and 72% with cadaver donors." Since 1986, 42 pancreas/kidney transplants and 51 liver transplants have been performed. Of the 396 heart transplants by the combined program, 120 were performed at LDS.

A program in cardiology was established by Drs. Michael Vincent and Jeff Anderson and their colleagues. Dr. Clyde Ford originated a bone marrow transplant program in 1979; seventy transplants have been performed with results comparable to, but at one-third the cost of, many of the best-known centers in the country. Dr. Homer Warner started his career at LDS Hospital with cardiac catheterization and pioneered in the application of computers to medicine, the hospital serving as his workshop.

The staff of the Radiation Center at LDS Hospital initiated a number of original programs: The pioneering use of hyperbaric oxygen (HPO) during radiation therapy resulted in an invitation to join the Radiation Therapy Oncology Group. This allowed the Center to be at the forefront of research in radiation oncology and enabled Dr. William Sause to become one of the foremost authorities in lung cancer. The Center's donation of the hyperbaric chamber to the pulmonary service initiated the formation of an up-to-date hyperbaric medicine section with a full-time medical director and staff. Among other conditions, thirty-three patients were treated for carbon monoxide poisoning in 1990 alone, with striking reduction of loss of life. Treatment with hyperthermia plus radiation was used first at LDS, followed by a more comprehensive program at the University.

Dr. Leonard Gunderson, who moved to Harvard and the Mayo Clinic, got his start as the world expert in the study and treatment of colon cancer at the Radiation Center.

The study of cytology, especially in cervical and lung cancer, was initiated regionally by Dr. Cy Fullmer at Holy Cross Hospital. Holy Cross also pioneered in mammography and established the first "breast care center," while Dr. Irena Tocino at LDS Hospital deserves credit for improving the quality of mammography throughout the state and for initiating a breast cancer task force, which together with the Utah Cancer Society has done much to improve diagnosis and treatment of this most common tumor.

Holy Cross Hospital and McKay-Dee Hospital in Ogden have served as major training institutions for residents in the revitalized field of family practice.

The tremendous progress in the science of medicine requires the application of these gains to the population at large. We must re-examine our motivations and ethics and come to the conclusion that an affordable, excellent and comprehensive health care system is essential for the survival of our values and the health of the country as a whole.

INDEX OF NAMES

A

C

Q

R

Medicine in the Beehive State, 1940–1990,
was designed and produced for the publishers
by Howe Brothers of Salt Lake City.
The text of the book was prepared electronically, composed, and typeset
in Postscript Times Roman on Xerox Ventura Publisher.
Filmwork and imposition by Howe Brothers.
Printing by Publishers Press.